THE COMPLETE
BOOK OF
HERBS

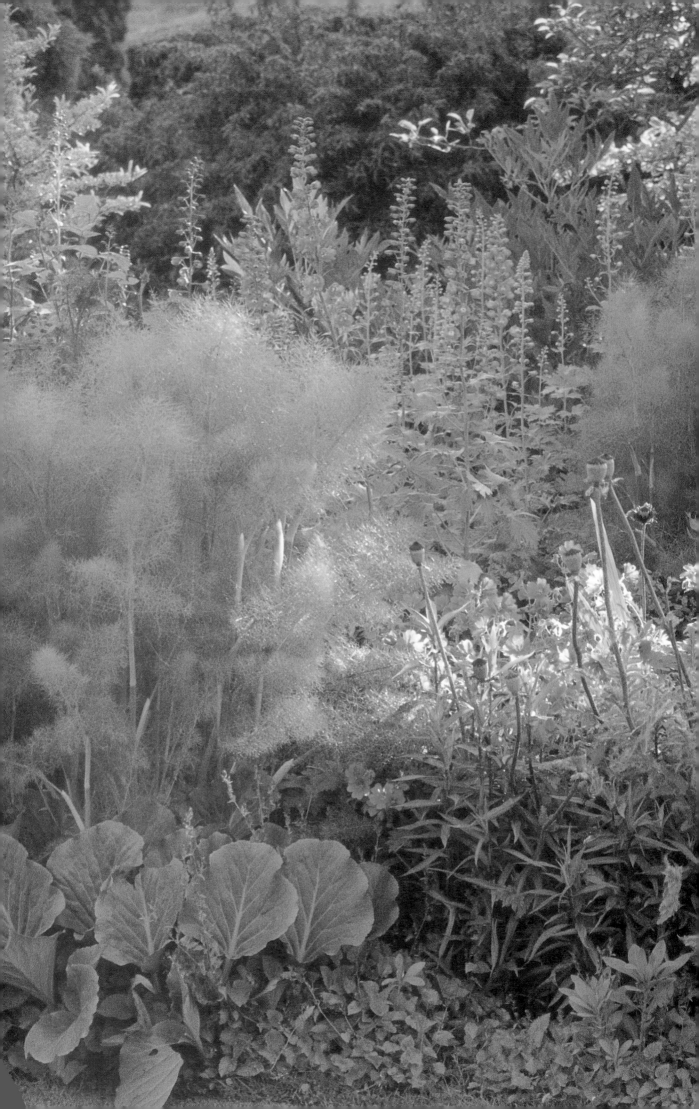

THE COMPLETE
BOOK OF
HERBS

LESLEY BREMNESS

PENGUIN
STUDIO

A DORLING KINDERSLEY BOOK

Project editor
Carolyn Ryden

Art editor
Tina Vaughan

Editor
Joanna Chisholm

Designers
Toni Rann & Nancy Chase

Managing editor
Daphne Razazan

Art director
Anne-Marie Bulat

Photography
Dave King

*To J. Roger Lowe for that rare combination of
inspiration and practical support*

PENGUIN STUDIO
Published by the Penguin Group
Penguin Books USA Inc., 375
Hudson Street, New York,
New York 10014, U.S.A.
Penguin Books Ltd.,
27 Wrights Lane,
London W8 5TZ, England
Penguin Books Australia Ltd, Ringwood, Victoria,
Australia
Penguin Books Canada Ltd, 10 Alcorn Avenue,
Toronto, Ontario, Canada M4V 3B2
Penguin Books (N.Z.) Ltd, 182-190 Wairau Road,
Auckland 10, New Zealand

Penguin Books Ltd, Registered Offices:
Harmondsworth, Middlesex, England

First published by Viking Penguin,
a division of Penguin Books USA Inc., 1988
Paperback edition published in 1994

10 9 8 7 6 5 4 3

Library of Congress Cataloging-in-Publication Data

Bremness, Lesley
   The complete book of herbs: a practical guide to
   growing and using herbs/by Lesley Bremness.
      p.   cm.
   Bibliography: p.
   Includes index.
   ISBN 0-670-81894-1 (hb)
   ISBN 0 14 02.3802 6 (pbk)
   1. Herb gardening – Handbooks, manuals, etc.
2. Herbs – Identification – Handbooks, manuals, etc.
3. Herbs – Utilization – Handbooks, manuals, etc.
I. Title.

SB351.H5B65B 1988 635'.7–dcl9   88-10197

Important notice
Herbs are very powerful healing tools. If they are misused, they can be harmful. This book is not a medical reference book. The advice it contains is general, not specific and neither the author nor the publishers can be held responsible for any adverse reactions to the recipes, formulas, recommendations or instructions contained herein. Before trying any herbal formula, sample a small quantity first in case you have any adverse or allergic reaction. Do not try self-diagnosis or attempt self-treatment for serious or long term problems without consulting a qualified medical herbalist. Do not take herbal remedies if you are undergoing any other course of medical treatment without seeking professional advice.

Typesetting
Southern Positives and Negatives (SPAN),
Lingfield, Surrey, Great Britain

Reproduction
Colourscan, Singapore

Printed and bound in the USA
by R R Donnelley & Sons

Contents

Foreword

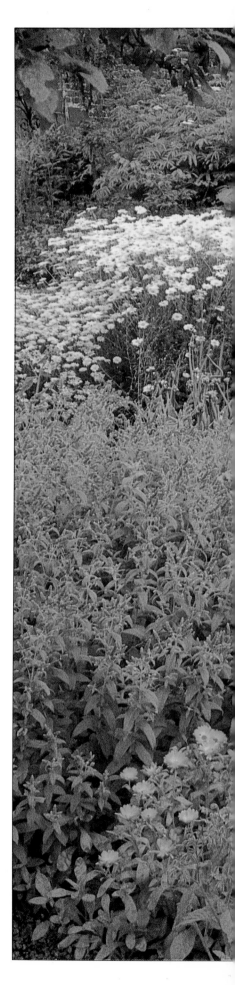

And where the marjoram once, and sage and rue,
And balm and mint, with curled-leaved parsley grew,
And double marigolds and silver thyme,
And pumpkins 'neath the window used to climb;
And where I often, when a child, for hours,
Tried through the pales to get the tempting flowers;
As lady's laces, everlasting peas,
True-love lies bleeding, with the hearts at ease;
And golden rods and tansy running high,
That o'er the pale top smiled on passer-by;
Flowers in my time which everyone would praise;
Though thrown like weeds from gardens nowadays.

John Clare (c. 1800)

> I would heartily advise all men of meanes,
> to be stirred up to bend their mindes, and spend
> a little more time and travell in these delights
> of herbes and flowers, than they have
> formerly done, which are not only harmlesse,
> but pleasurable in their turn,
> and profitable in their use.
>
> John Parkinson,
> *Theatrum Botanicum* (1640)

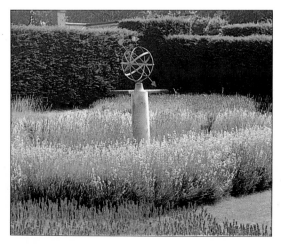

An ornamental sundial
(left) *surrounded by beds of
lavender in a traditional garden.*

**A colorful border of
flowering herbs** (opposite)
*including orange calendula, pink
marsh mallows and clusters of sky
blue borage flowers. They form part
of a highly attractive walled garden
which is planted with an enormous
variety of traditional medicinal and
culinary herbs.*

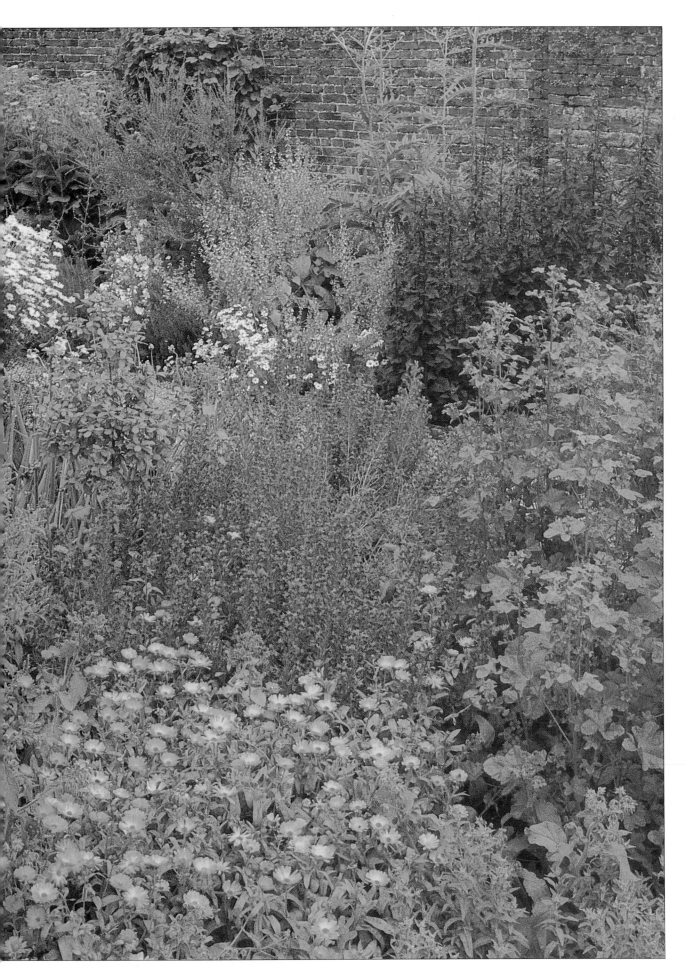

Introduction

Herbs are plants to serve and delight us, offering us an ever-increasing rapport with nature. Our changing understanding of the word "herb" reflects our changing relationship with the plant kingdom. There was a time when all plants were important to humankind; they were considered the children of the Earth Mother, each marked by divinity and worthy of respect. With industrialization, the rise of science and technology, our involvement with nature diminished. This change has led to a more limited concept of the term "herb," and even today, herbs are considered by many people to be only a dozen or so seasoning plants.

An early Western attempt to classify plants was made in the fourth century by the Greek philosopher Theophrastus, who divided the plant world into trees, shrubs and herbs, mainly by size; the herb category including a plant group similar to the large range now classified botanically as herbaceous. This broad concept of a herb was also reflected in the Book of Genesis, where God caused the earth "to bring forth grass, the herb yielding seed and the fruit tree yielding fruit." Such a large range of herbs included plants that were important to people on many levels – physical, mental and spiritual. Indeed, plants have often been used as symbols of spiritual progress, as with the "tree of knowledge" and the apple in the garden of Eden, and several cultures have a concept of paradise as a garden full of beautiful and useful plants capable of affecting all aspects of their lives.

Early writings
Early plant knowledge was passed on verbally. As both the body of knowledge and populations grew, it became more important to record accurately the accumulated information on herbs for the sake of safe identification and dosage. Many of the earliest writings are about herbs – the plants important to a community in ceremony, magic and medicine. Babylonian clay tablets from 3000 B.C. illustrate medical treatments; later they record herbal imports.

During the next 1,000 years, parallel cultures in China, Assyria, Egypt and India developed a written record, mainly of medicinal herbs. The Chinese *Canon of Herbs* is credited to a legendary emperor, Shen Nung, who died in 2698 B.C. (although the existing texts were compiled much later). This emperor, "the divine husbandman," tasted many plants on behalf of the Chinese people to discover which were poisonous. His canon includes 252 plant descriptions and notes on their effects on the human body, where they could be gathered, and how to preserve and administer them, thus setting the standard for future pharmacopeias.

From very early on, the Chinese tried to eliminate superstition and stressed the importance of practical knowledge. This is reflected in the more sophisticated *Nei Ching* or "Canon of Medicine" credited to another legendary emperor, Huang Ti (died 2598 B.C.), although the existing texts are also thought to have been compiled much later, probably around 600 B.C.

The Chinese have always held a wide view of plants. Herbs were not divided into compartments as they are in many Western minds today. To the Chinese the chrysanthemum is useful, beautiful and virtuous. Chrysanthemums were first grown for their medicinal properties and were a valued ingredient of the Taoist elixir. They were believed to be full of magic juices; perhaps that reason contributed to their beauty. One story tells of the people of Nanyang, in central China, who lived to be 100 years old because their drinking water came from a stream with many chrysanthemums growing beside it. The essence of the plants was thought to seep into the water and continually revitalize the inhabitants. Today in China, chrysanthemums are featured in spectacular flower displays and also used medicinally; one form is used in soups, salads and banquet dishes.

Early Western records of herbs describe a mixture of medicinal and magical uses of plants. Egyptian writings dating from 1550 B.C. contain medical prescriptions and notes on the aromatic and cosmetic uses of herbs, as these were important aspects of religious ceremonies. Around the same time, descriptions of herbs and magical charms were compiled in the sacred *Ayurvedas* of India.

The classical Greek and Roman writings made an attempt to remove superstition and eventually reached their peak in Dioscorides's *De Materia Medica* of 512 A.D. This describes 600 healing plants and is the earliest surviving herbal with illustrations. It became the basis of herbal knowledge until the seventeenth century.

Theophrastus also wrote a treatise on perfumes and cosmetics and described the effects of different herb and flower essences. A short time later another treatise on perfumes, by Apollonius, described where the best crops of herbs for perfume requirements could be found; the best marjoram essence came from the Aegean island of Cos, the best cypress from Egypt – and saffron reached high perfection on Rhodes.

Herbs and cookery
The use of herbs in cooking is a feature of the first-century cookbook written by the Roman epicure, Apicius. It uses fascinating and adventurous combinations of herb flavors. For example, artichokes were cooked in a mixture of

fresh fennel, coriander, mint and rue pounded together and added to pepper, lovage, honey, oil and liquamen (a strong, fish-based sauce that the Romans used in place of salt).

For centuries, herbs were a staple of daily life. In England in 1699, John Evelyn wrote *Acetaria: A Discourse of Sallets*, which listed 73 salad herbs, giving details of the part of each herb used, whether seed, flower, bud, leaf, stalk or root, and how it was best prepared – raw, chopped, steamed, blanched or pickled. This broad usage continued for centuries, demonstrated by the fact that even 200 years ago the word vegetable was not commonly used – we spoke of "pot herbs" (for bulk in the cooking pot), "salet" (salad) herbs, "sweet" herbs (flavorings) and "simples" (medicinal herbs from which "compounds" were made).

Herbs as garden plants

As communities became more secure and gardening developed for pleasure, books included the aesthetic appeal of herbs as garden plants. There was not the distinction between usefulness and aesthetic appeal that we apply now. *Herbys Necessary for a Gardyn* was compiled by Thomas Fromon around 1535 and included more than 30 species grown as much for pleasure as "for savour and beaute." Among them he included columbine, germander, stickadove (thought to be *Lavandula stoechas*) and wallflower.

In his essay *Of Gardens*, Francis Bacon includes many herbs in his sketch of an ideal garden. His famous opening is often quoted: "God Almighty first planted a garden. And indeed, it is the purest of human pleasures. It is the greatest refreshment

to the spirits of man." He goes on to describe possible fragrant delights month by month: "The breath of flowers is far sweeter in the air (where it comes and goes, like the warbling of music), than in the hand." He speaks of setting whole alleys of scented herbs; burnet, wild thyme and water mint "to have the pleasure when you walk or tread." He includes many garden elements of interest today: tall alleys or hedges for shade and shelter with openings to reveal distant views; a fountain or some watercourse in motion; knot gardens to be placed and planted so they can be viewed from a high window in the house; paths wide enough to walk comfortably on and a wild area with honeysuckle, sweetbrier, violets, strawberries and primroses.

The age of herbals

Herbals, books that provided plant descriptions and details of their medical uses, became increasingly popular in the sixteenth century. Although other botanic herbals had been written, it was fifteen centuries before any surpassed Dioscorides in botanic accuracy. In the sixteenth century, three famous herbals were printed in Germany; the third, Leonhart Fuch's *De Historia Stirpium* of 1542, has charming naturalistic illustrations of herbs drawn from direct observation, instead of being copied from old woodcuts as with most previous herbals. His text, however, was based mostly on the writings of Dioscorides. The tradition of botany and medicine continued in a number of publications, including

A seventeenth-century knot garden *features plants of the era, miniature box hedges and ornamental topiary.*

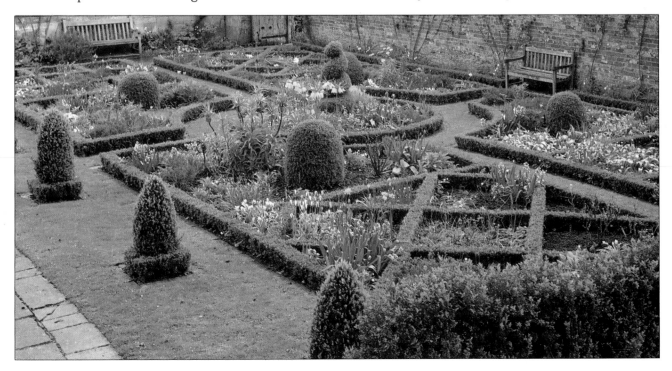

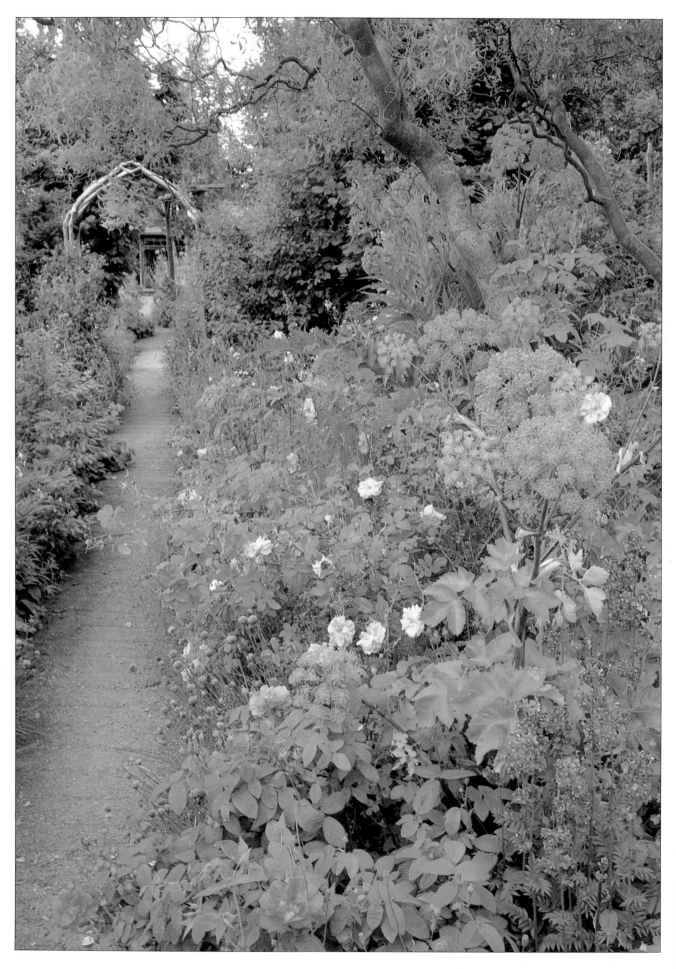

Gerard's Herbal (1597), by John Gerard, who grew over 1,000 species in his garden. In 1629, John Parkinson's herbal, Theatrum Botanicum, appeared, cataloguing over 3,000 species. This was followed in 1649 by the most famous of all herbals, *The English Physician* (also known as *The Complete Herbal*), by Nicholas Culpeper. Although this volume contained much useful medical knowledge, it was derided by many because Culpeper viewed the astrological aspects of plants as important. However, this had little effect on its popularity and it is still in print today.

Scholars made a valiant attempt to eliminate unscientific attitudes, but the common people held deep beliefs about the significance of plants: plants were deemed to serve humanity, each with a purpose for our benefit. The belief known as the Doctrine of Signatures, which emerged in the first century A.D., suggested that some aspect of a plant's appearance, usually its leaf shape or coloring, would give a clue to its medicinal properties. This notion remained popular for fifteen centuries, and appeared in several independent cultures at different times, from the Chinese to that of the North American Indians, although Culpeper was its last important champion.

Up to the seventeenth century, herbals had contained botany and medicine, but as science emerged, plants were classified, dissected and demystified, and botany and medicine went their separate ways. Great strides were made in herbal knowledge, using new technical skills to analyze a plant's components and to produce standardized tinctures and extracts. But in the face of science, with its skill in synthesizing drugs, and the rise in urban culture, herbalism declined and our involvement with nature seemed to diminish.

In 1931 an Englishwoman, Mrs. Maude Grieve, decided to change this situation and wrote *A Modern Herbal*, which drew together scientific and traditional information. Around this time a renewed interest in herbs began, partly spurred by the food and medical shortages of World War I. Old seasoning, salad and pot herbs were remembered, and, in the trenches, garlic, thyme and moss were rediscovered and used to play a lifesaving medical role.

The lure of herbs today

Recently, there has been a tremendous surge of interest in herbs. Research on their medicinal and cosmetic uses, and new ideas for their decorative and perfuming applications are continually adding to the large body of herbal knowledge and skills. The object of this book is again to combine traditional with scientific knowledge and present the many innovative ways in which herbs can be used to enhance life in the home and at work. This practical approach will, I hope, encourage you to further inventiveness by providing a glimpse of the inexhaustible potential of herbs.

The renewed interest in herbs has many branches. A revival of the culinary arts has prompted earnest efforts to grow and sell fresh herbs. A growing interest in the cuisine of other cultures has created a demand for unusual varieties of herbs. A desire for nutritious food, alternative medicines and a more balanced ecology has further extended the boundaries. A concern about the side effects of some modern chemicals has revived the use of herbal cosmetics, dyes and cleaning agents. Our growing sensitivity to scents has increased our desire for and appreciation of fresh herbal fragrances in all areas of our lives.

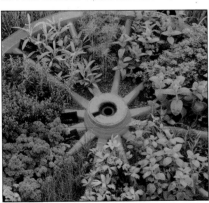

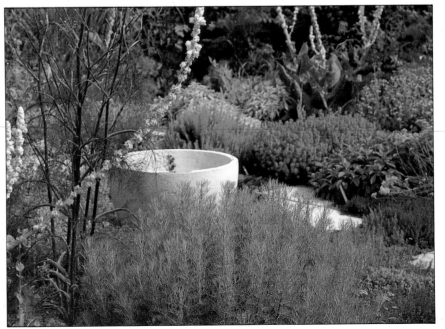

A bright red cartwheel (above) *makes an attractive and practical bed for planting a range of culinary herbs.*

Herbs and stone (right) *blend well together in this informal herb garden.*

A lush and colorful border (opposite) *with old roses and giant angelica flowers amid a range of traditional cottage garden plants.*

For many people, an interest in one aspect of herbs acts as a catalyst for other related subjects. Many begin with an interest in cooking, perhaps fueled by vacations abroad, and this may lead to the study of the nutritious and health-enhancing properties of herbs, and their medicinal qualities. Others may be interested in growing herbs and, having created a herb garden, may find unexpected further pleasure in the individual herbs, their fresh scents and many uses.

My own experience began with a great enthusiasm for organic gardening, but the prairie puritan in my background permitted me to devote my energies only to vegetables. When I discovered that herbs were useful and beautiful, I allowed a small door in my mind to open and found an enormous world of interesting plants waiting.

If pressed for the reason for my newfound enthusiasm, I would say how delicious herbs were, transforming an ordinary dish into a culinary delight; or that as the mother of a growing family I found them very handy for treating colds, coughs and other minor ailments; but in truth these were the extra benefits. The real pleasure for me was just being with the herbs. They are such pretty plants, with their soft and subtle colors; and they possess such an enthusiastic vitality, being mainly the same original wild species, left unhybridized. This makes them very easy to grow and generally trouble-free – indeed they often seem to promote the health of neighboring plants. They also give the whole garden and the gardener a pleasing sense of useful abundance.

Weeding became an unexpected delight; the fragrance, texture and shapes would lead my mind to thoughts of ancient rituals and ceremonies, the healing herb women of so many cultures, the exchange of secret messages through a cryptic posy of herbs; separate, colorful threads would emerge, linking the past with the present.

My range of herbs grew and I soon started to discover the many uses of these plants for myself. Herbal cosmetics were a real treasure – I could use the best-quality ingredients and make them for a fraction of the store-bought cost. Visitors would exchange stories about the craft use of herbs, about dye plants and herbal cleaning agents – the versatility and application of herbs seemed almost endless, and more and more areas of my existence seemed permeated by herbs.

As my original training was in art, I found myself considering how the aesthetics of herbs affected my life. They are certainly visually appealing, both in the garden and as fresh, simple decorations indoors. Through scent, I remembered the writers in history who have spoken of the ability of "sweet perfumes" to lift the spirits, an observation now confirmed by scientific research. And then there is their appeal to the sense of touch – the velvety leaves of marsh mallow must be among the most sensuous plants in existence – and taste. What could be more rewarding, when tidying a neglected corner of the herb garden, than to discover a wild strawberry waiting to be picked? Or to enhance a simple dish with a handful of fresh picked parsley and chives?

As my collection has grown into an herb garden, it has become an important retreat, a place that somehow has the ability to still the mind and encourage problem-solving. In a sense, I feel that the Earth Mother has returned to center stage. For me, these plants have regained their ancient significance as partners to be treated with reverence and gratitude; and the meaning of the word "herb" is expanding to its widest potential.

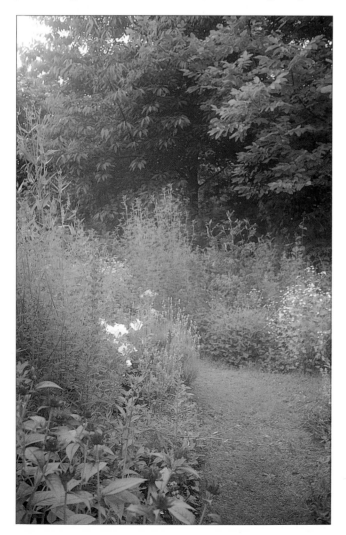

A tranquil corner of the author's garden (left) with colorful highlights provided by scarlet blooms of bergamot, white musk mallow and purple spires of viper's bugloss.

An overall view of the author's herb garden (opposite) shows a selection of medicinal, culinary and dye herbs planted in mixed beds.

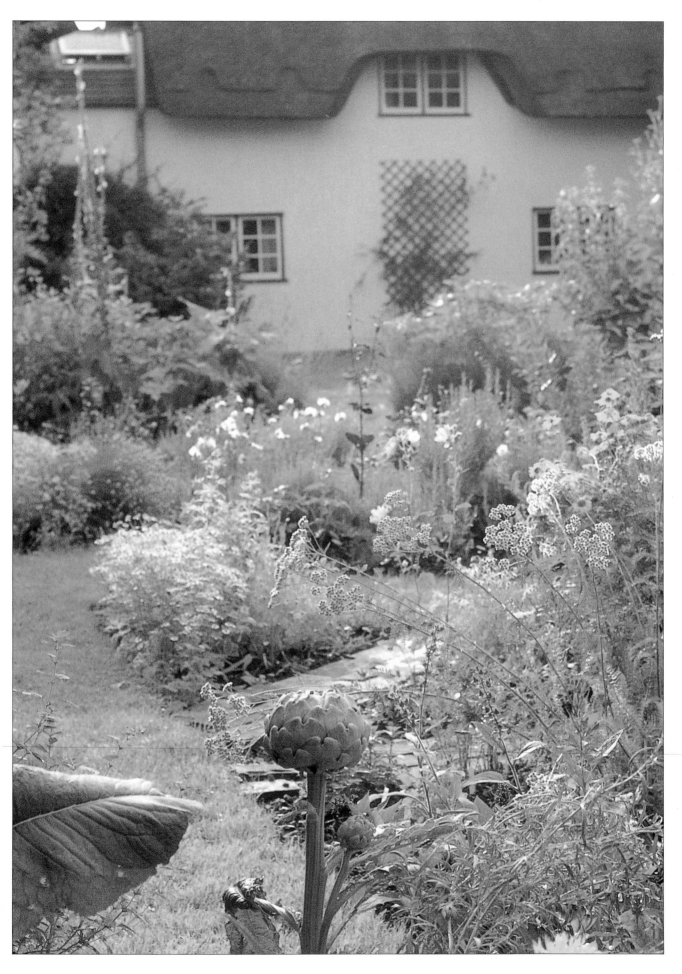

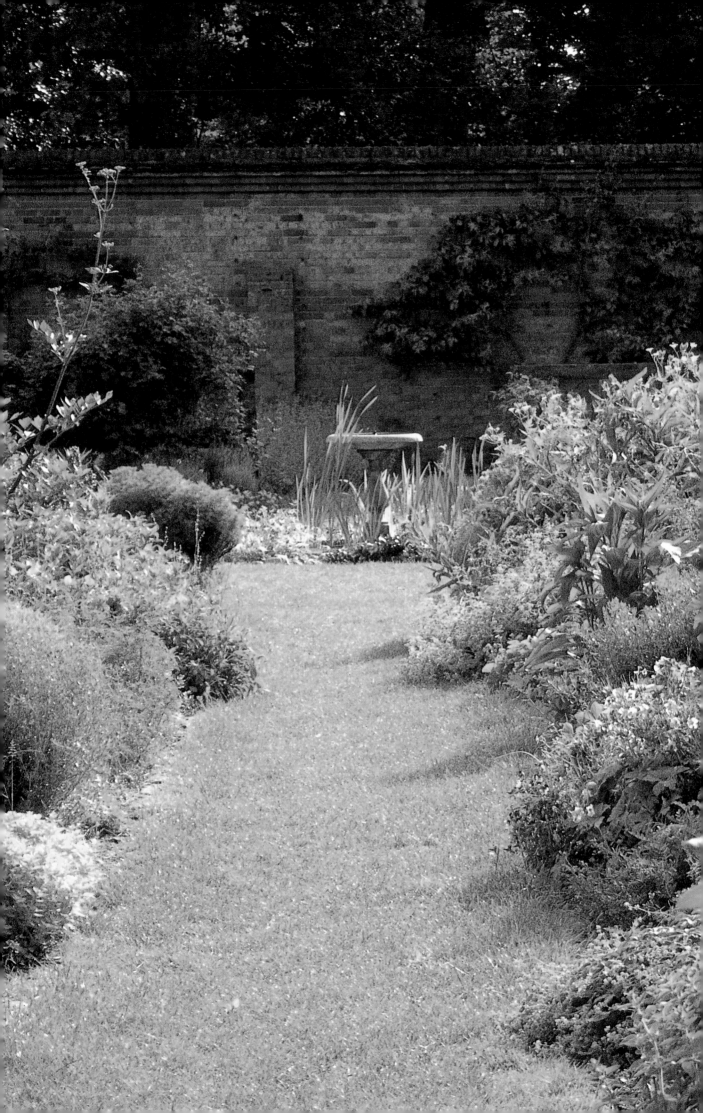

HERBS
IN THE
GARDEN

Herbs offer a rewarding combination of beauty and usefulness, and for those who have never felt the urge to grow plants, this benevolent and generous range is the perfect introduction to gardening. A small amount of effort is soon rewarded by aromatic silver and green foliage, scented decorative flowers, savory leaves and spicy seeds.

Herbs can be tucked into existing flower borders, vegetable beds or decorative pots. As adaptable plants, many will grow happily on a balcony or patio, or even indoors. When more space is available, a separate area set aside for herbs often becomes a special place for peace and enchantment. This may take the form of a traditional herb garden, neatly divided into beds and paths, or it may be more free-form and flowing. Herb garden styles and layouts are as varied as the people who cultivate and enjoy herbs. They can be as small or as large as space permits. The following pages describe how to set about designing an herb garden, and provide detailed plans for planting schemes in a variety of settings. There is also a wide range of inspiring ideas for theme herb gardens, designed to reflect personal interests.

A spacious path, flanked by well-stocked borders, leads to a stone sundial in this informal herb garden.

Planning an herb garden

Before embarking on your design, consider how much time and effort you are willing to put into your herb garden and how much maintenance any proposed scheme is likely to require. Don't be too ambitious or it will become a chore rather than a pleasure. If you are new to gardening, start with a small area or a few large containers and a limited number of herbs. As your enthusiasm grows, you can expand your herb garden and its contents.

SELECTING YOUR SITE

The ideal site is quiet and sunny with a protective surround. These conditions suit most herbs and will help to make a peaceful retreat. Such ready-made idyllic sites are few and far between but they are not difficult to create.

Aim for an area where at least three-quarters of the space is in the sun for most of the day. As many aromatic herbs are Mediterranean in origin, a slope that faces the sun for five to six hours each day is ideal as it will offer good drainage as well as extra solar energy. Spend time in the proposed site, noting the sun's passage over it, where shadows fall, which corners are sheltered from wind and the areas where water collects. If any part of the plot is waterlogged, it is worth making rubble-filled trenches, laying drainage pipes or making raised beds (see p. 261) before starting any further work, to avoid future frustration and loss of plants. Consider wind protection, particularly for evergreen herbs such as rosemary and sweet bay in the spring, and around a proposed seat or bench. A traditional hedge or wall (a frequent asset in small city gardens), or a screen supporting climbing plants, creates a feeling of seclusion, confines the perfumes of aromatic plants and reduces wind buffeting. It can also reduce outside noise and mask undesirable views.

Apart from considering the physical aspects of a site, think about its location in terms of how you plan to use it. Will herbs be close to your kitchen door for convenient picking? Will their scents drift indoors? Or do you want to create an herb garden retreat, removed from household activities?

DESIGNING YOUR GARDEN

Having selected your site, decide on the style of garden you want; whether it is to be a formal scheme following geometric patterns or an informal collection or grouping that dictates its own shape. The style of your home and neighborhood may give you a preference for formality or informality, or you may decide to try a combination of the two. Look at the pictures of other herb gardens in magazines and books and try to visit any in your area. Formal herb gardens are based on well-defined patterns and geometric shapes, with the beds and paths designed to give a sense of order and balance as well as access. Traditionally, the planting schemes were relatively sparse, with the emphasis on individual species. Today, many gardeners prefer to contrast the exuberant natural growth of herbs with the tidy formality of traditional designs.

In informal gardens, plants are massed together in a profusion of color and different species, with the herbs often intermingled with flowers and vegetables. The effect is natural and romantic. However, such seemingly disorganized growth requires planning so that neighboring plants complement rather than clash, and have sufficient sunlight. Paths must still provide access, so some structure is necessary to make the overall design work and to allow for maintenance.

DRAWING UP A PLAN

Once you have selected your site, measure its sides and prepare to draw up the area on squared grid paper, making each square on your grid represent a convenient measurement, such as 6 inches. Start the measurements from a baseline that is either parallel to your house or at right angles to it. Draw in the measured outline of your site in clear bold lines and mark in the main fixtures that will remain: fences, buildings, trees, etc. Be as accurate as possible and note any changes of level that may require steps or raised beds.

Now you are ready to try out some design schemes with tracing paper laid over the site plan. Establish the overall feel of a design before filling in any detail, and be prepared to discard page after page. Everyone has a natural sense of beauty and shape, often buried by looking too much at detail, but eventually you will know when a design feels right. Then you can start to mark in paths, beds and other details. If you wish to make a modern, free-flowing design, start with bold sweeping lines. People often have a tendency to draw small tight curves, but when translated into three dimensions, all lines are exaggerated. Hold up the design to a mirror to check its balance.

If you are designing a formal scheme, make a loose grid of lines on the plan based on the sur-roundings. Extend the lines of the house, doors, windows, garage, walls, and other boundaries so you have a selection of lines to choose your main pathways from. Each path should then line up with an existing structure, integrating your design.

Paths

For convenient access, herbs should never be more than 2 feet 6 inches from a path, so beds should measure no more than 4 or 5 feet across unless you insert stepping stones. Paths are also crucial to design for the color and patterns they can bring, as well as the way they can define shape (see below and pp. 260–1). In all garden plans, avoid putting a path straight through the space. It suggests rushing ahead, whereas an herb garden should be a place where you linger. Have a path change direction, or break its flow by altering the pattern of its fabric or adding a piece of sculpture or a tall herb.

FILLING IN THE DETAILS

Your design should now be an interesting pattern of lines. This is the time to extend your conception into three dimensions. Imagine you are sculpting paths and layers through a large cube of greenery. Consider adding different levels and further interest to the design. Three parallel lines on a plan need not necessarily mean a path and a border, they could represent three steps, a change of pattern in the path, or an edging herb.

Decide what form of enclosure to have (see pp. 255–9), bearing in mind any views you may wish either to hide or to emphasize. Place a chair where you propose to have a seat and stick canes into the ground at different heights to consider the effect various enclosures may have.

GARDEN DESIGNS

The illustrations below show some of the ways in which a rectangular or square space can be divided to make a formal arrangement of beds and linking paths. Other traditional designs are a simple ladder shape with square beds between narrow brick paths or wooden planks, and stepping stones arranged in a checkerboard pattern.

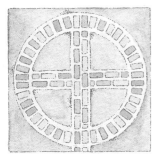

Brick circle
Bricks arranged in a circular path enclose two intersecting paths which cross at the center.

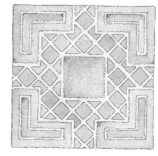

Brick diamond
Bricks arranged in a herringbone pattern add extra interest and flow to this design.

Square within a square
Tiles arranged as diamonds and laid in concrete give a simple design an ornate effect.

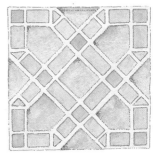

Diagonal paths
A mixture of paving materials emphasizing lines to create a knot garden effect.

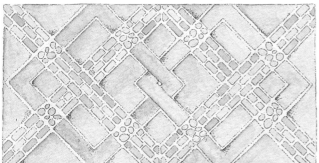

Interlocking diamonds
A diamond ribbon of santolina entwines with one of dwarf box. Where a hedge meets a brick path, the pattern is continued with a line of pebbles.

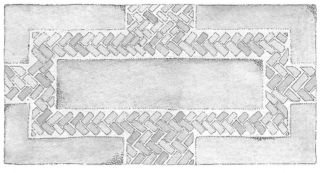

Oblongs and right angles
A long central bed is enclosed by bricks that have been laid out in a herringbone pattern to add extra interest to the design.

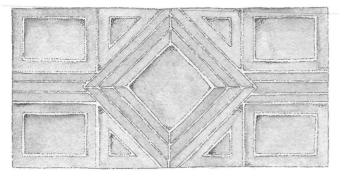

Diamonds and squares
A brick path divides square beds and creates a central diamond shape. The beds are edged with curry plants and box to emphasize their shape.

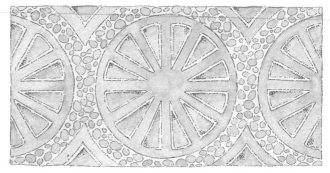

Wheel beds
Cartwheels are a practical and effective way to divide beds into separate planting areas. Here, a gravel path surrounds and links each wheel.

WORKING OUT A PLANTING SCHEME

Once you have planned the garden's physical layout, plot out where you might position the plants you want to grow in terms of their requirements and usage: culinary plants by the kitchen door, aromatic plants under the windows, further beds of dye, historical or medicinal plants, depending on your interests. Check the respective requirements of individual plants, and plot out their positions, bearing in mind aspects like contrasting leaf size and color, complementary plant shapes and heights. As a guide, one plant per square foot or ten per square yard allows plenty of space for perennials to grow.

Position annuals so you don't have to disturb perennials when planting or removing them. Use tall plants as focal points in central beds or as screens. Where you have the space, group several plants of the same species together to increase their effect. Use grid paper to plot out their eventual ground size as well as their colors and height. Often plants are drawn as tiny circles when in fact they are exuberant growers. Close planting may look effective but soon leads to overcrowding. Fortunately, most herbs are easy to transplant.

MARKING OUT THE SITE

Once the soil has been prepared for planting as described on p. 251, transfer your design to the ground. Mark out the boundaries of the plot with stakes, then start to mark out the beds and paths. You can use a large cardboard box as a set square to help indicate right angles in the soil for geometric designs. As a guide for angles of 45°, mark the two diagonals on the square end of a box with colored tape. To draw out circles, make a compass using a cane as a central stake and a marker that reaches the ground on a taut piece of string. To mark out small repeated shapes, use a card template and trace around it. Delineate areas with string and pegs or a sprinkling of lime.

The author's herb garden is a mixture of formal and informal styles. It has paved areas, lawn, knot garden beds, species beds and informal, cottage-style borders. Its design is flexible so it can expand as new interests demand.

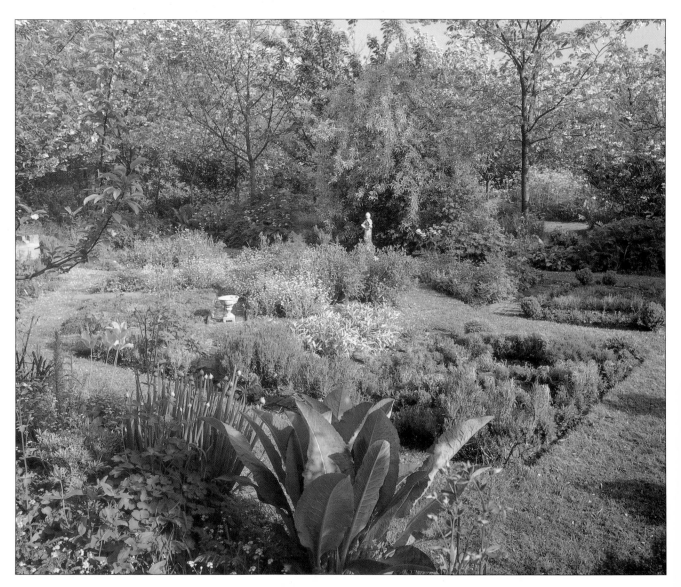

A small all-purpose herb garden

As most herbs require very little space, you can grow a surprising variety in a relatively small area. Many herbs have more than one use so you can satisfy a wide range of interests with comparatively few plants. Of those shown in this garden, fennel, rosemary, sage and thyme are culinary, medicinal, cosmetic and aromatic; lavender, bergamot and balm can be used to make scented gifts and comforting teas; tansy can be used to keep away flies, and marsh mallow makes a soothing ingredient for skin creams. In addition to offering many uses, these herbs are delightful flowering plants that will attract butterflies, bees and birds to your garden.

This design makes the most of a small space with its sweeping, curved path around the bed of low-growing culinary herbs, the backdrop of majestic plants such as angelica, sweet Joe Pye and marsh mallows, the ornamental bowl of water to attract birds, and the wooden bench surrounded by sweet-scented plants. Even in such a confined space, it is worth making room for a seat so you can relax in your garden.

Plant key

1 Honeysuckle *Lonicera periclymenum* Fragrant pale yellow flowers
2 Angelica *Angelica archangelica* Provides stature
3 Tansy *Tanacetum vulgare* Adds height and pungent foliage
4 Marsh mallow *Althaea officinalis* Adds height, velvet foliage and pale pink flowers
5 Sweet Joe Pye *Eupatorium purpureum* Majestic with large pink flower heads
6 Bronze fennel *Foeniculum vulgare* Highly decorative
7 Lungwort *Pulmonaria officinalis* Provides attractive green spotted leaves
8 Purple sage *Salvia officinalis* 'Purpurascens' Attractive purple leaves have strong flavor
9 Foxgloves *Digitalis purpurea* Statuesque and colorful
10 Variegated lemon balm *Melissa officinalis* 'Variegata' Fresh citrus scent
11 Chives *Allium schoenoprasum* Edible and attractive
12 Calendula *Calendula officinalis* Cheery orange flowers
13 Lavender *Lavandula angustifolia* 'Hidcote' Dwarf

form with silver leaves and dark purple flowers
14 Bergamot *Monarda didyma* Striking, decorative flowers and scented leaves
15 Lawn chamomile *Chamaemelum nobile* Makes a thick, sweet-smelling path border when clipped
16 Parsley *Petroselinum crispum* An essential culinary herb with dense green foliage
17 Salad burnet *Poterium sanguisorba* Add young leaves to salads and drinks
18 Golden marjoram *Origanum vulgare* 'Aureum' Aromatic golden leaves
19 Rosemary *Rosmarinus officinalis* Blue flowers appear in early spring
20 Thyme *Thymus praecox* 'Coccineus' Creeping thyme
21 Sweet woodruff *Galium odoratum* Plant under tall herbs

Features
Terra-cotta container of water to reflect the sky and attract small birds
Gravel path with larger pebbles along the inside curve to accentuate its shape
Wooden bench surrounded by aromatic plants

GARDEN PLAN

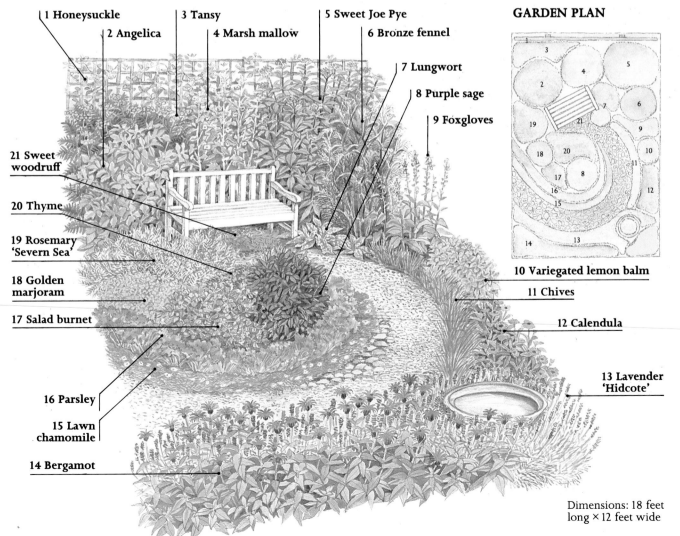

1 Honeysuckle
2 Angelica
3 Tansy
4 Marsh mallow
5 Sweet Joe Pye
6 Bronze fennel
7 Lungwort
8 Purple sage
9 Foxgloves
21 Sweet woodruff
20 Thyme
19 Rosemary 'Severn Sea'
18 Golden marjoram
17 Salad burnet
16 Parsley
15 Lawn chamomile
14 Bergamot
10 Variegated lemon balm
11 Chives
12 Calendula
13 Lavender 'Hidcote'

Dimensions: 18 feet long × 12 feet wide

A large all-purpose herb garden

Having a generous-sized plot in which to make an herb garden offers enormous scope for the creative gardener. With such space, you can have separate areas that reflect your various interests and can expand with them. Corners or beds may be planted along different themes; for example, Shakespearean herbs in one corner (see p. 35) and Anglo-Saxon amulet herbs (betony, vervain, peony, plantain, yarrow and rose) in another.

Space for a wide range of plants provides the opportunity to grow collections of species: a whole bed of thymes, one of sages, one of rosemary and another of marjorams. A large garden also gives scope for growing herbal trees.

This design is based on our family herb garden with its informal border containing dye herbs, cosmetic herbs and tall culinary herbs on either side of the entrance, a scented arbor, ceramic sinks planted with collections of alpine varieties, and many decorative, flowering herbs.

The beds are divided into groupings of medicinal herbs, salad plants, species collections (which form a patchwork of color in summer), aromatic shrubs and miniature knot beds, each planted with different colored santolinas in interweaving patterns. The layout of the lawn and brick paths allows access to all plants and defines the overall shape of the garden.

GARDEN PLAN

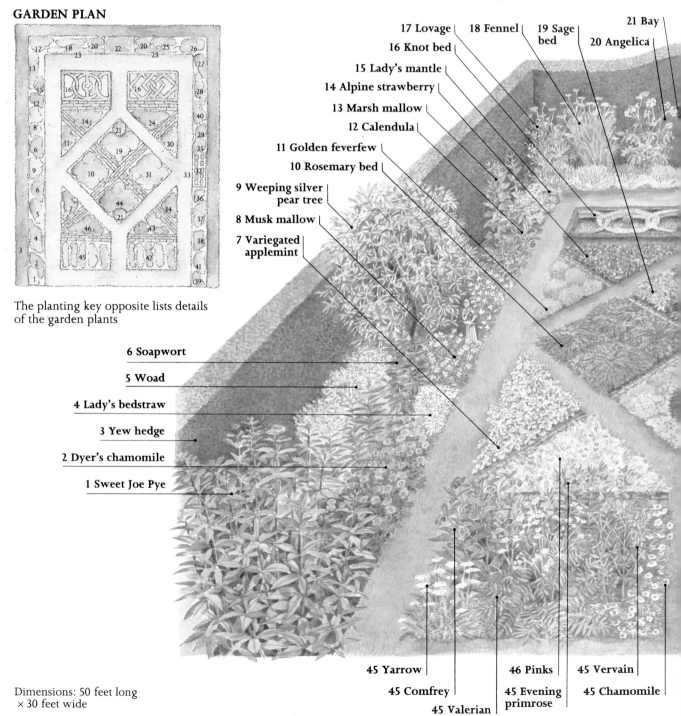

The planting key opposite lists details of the garden plants

17 Lovage
16 Knot bed
15 Lady's mantle
14 Alpine strawberry
13 Marsh mallow
12 Calendula
11 Golden feverfew
10 Rosemary bed
9 Weeping silver pear tree
8 Musk mallow
7 Variegated applemint

18 Fennel
19 Sage bed
21 Bay
20 Angelica

6 Soapwort
5 Woad
4 Lady's bedstraw
3 Yew hedge
2 Dyer's chamomile
1 Sweet Joe Pye

45 Yarrow
45 Comfrey
45 Valerian
46 Pinks
45 Evening primrose
45 Vervain
45 Chamomile

Dimensions: 50 feet long × 30 feet wide

Plant key

1 Sweet Joe Pye *Eupatorium purpureum* Majestic plant with pink-tinged flowers and sturdy purple stems
2 Dyer's chamomile *Anthemis tinctoria* Yields a yellow dye
3 Yew hedge *Taxus baccata* Provides shelter and an evergreen backdrop
4 Lady's bedstraw *Galium verum* Produces masses of tiny yellow flowers
5 Woad *Isatis tinctoria* Yields a rich blue dye
6 Soapwort *Saponaria officinalis* For cleansing fragile fabrics

7 Variegated applemint *Mentha suaveolens* 'Variegata' Attractive leaves and scent
8 Musk mallow *Malva moschata* Produces white or pale pink flowers; faintly scented
9 Weeping silver pear tree *Pyrus salicifolia* 'Pendula' Attractive, silver-leaved pendulous branches
10 Rosemary *Rosmarinus officinalis* Collection of species and varieties
11 Golden feverfew *Tanacetum parthenium* 'Aureum' Aromatic with daisy flowers
12 Calendula *Calendula officinalis* Bright orange flowers that

have cosmetic and culinary uses
13 Marsh mallow *Althaea officinalis* Skin-softening herb
14 Alpine strawberry *Fragaria vesca* Provides edible fruits
15 Lady's mantle *Alchemilla vulgaris* Large round leaves for cosmetic use
16 Knot beds with overlapping lines of **santolinas** (see No. 43) surrounded by a **box hedge** *Buxus sempervirens* 'Suffruticosa'
17 Lovage *Levisticum officinale* A decorative plant with strong savory flavor
18 Fennel *Foeniculum vulgare* A handsome, feathery plant

19 Sage *Salvia* Species bed
20 Angelica *Angelica archangelica* Grows to monumental height
21 Bay *Laurus nobilis* Trained to form a ball of foliage
22 Lawn chamomile *Chamaemelum nobile* 'Treneague' A sweet-scented welcome mat
23 Lavenders *Lavandula* species Select for color and height
24 Curry plant *Helichrysum angustifolium* Spicy, silver foliage
25 Bronze fennel *Foeniculum vulgare* Rich, bronze leaves
26 Elecampane *Inula helenium* Statuesque, with yellow flowers and enormous leaves
27 Sorrel *Rumex acetosa* Lush foliage and spires of flowers
28 Welsh onion *Allium fistulosum* Provides winter leaves for flavoring
29 Bugle *Ajuga reptans* Pretty blue flowers
30 Orris *Iris florentina* Striking plant with scented root
31 Thymes *Thymus* species A bed of colorful thymes
32 Akebia *Akebia quinata* Scented climber trained to form an arbor
33 Sweet woodruff *Galium odoratum* Plant where its sweet scent can be appreciated
34 Bergamot *Monarda didyma* Aromatic and attractive
35 Madonna lily *Lilium candidum* Exotic blooms
36 Sweet cicely *Myrrhis odorata* Edible fresh seeds
37 Lemon balm *Melissa officinalis* Strong lemon scent
38 Foxgloves *Digitalis purpurea* Spires of flowers add color to the back of the border
39 Medicinal rhubarb *Rheum officinale* Large, ornate leaves
40 Alpine herbs in sink
41 Catmint *Nepeta mussinii* Decorative purple flowers
42 Salad herbs Bed with **purple basil** *Ocimum basilicum* 'Dark Opal,' **coriander** *Coriandrum sativum*, **parsley** *Petroselinum crispum*, **chives** *Allium schoenoprasum*, **purslane** *Portulaca oleracea*
43 Green and silver-leafed santolinas *Santolina virens, S. chamaecyparissus* and *S.c.* 'Lemon Queen'
44 Marjorams *Origanum* species Marjoram collection
45 Medicinal herbs: chamomile *Matricaria recutita*, **vervain** *Verbena officinalis*, **evening primrose** *Oenothera biennis*, **valerian** *Valeriana officinalis*, **comfrey** *Symphytum officinale*, **yarrow** *Achillea millefolium*
46 Pinks *Dianthus* cultivars

Features
Garden bench sheltered by the planted arbor
Brick paths and **lawn paths** crisscross the garden
A stone statue of Pan

22 Lawn chamomile
23 Lavenders
24 Curry plant
25 Bronze fennel
26 Elecampane
27 Sorrel
28 Welsh onion
29 Bugle
30 Orris
31 Thyme bed
32 Akebia
33 Sweet woodruff
34 Bergamot
35 Madonna lily
36 Sweet cicely
37 Lemon balm
38 Foxgloves

42 Coriander
42 Purple basil
44 Marjoram bed
43 Santolinas
42 Chives
42 Parsley
42 Purslane
41 Catmint
40 Sink of Alpine herbs
39 Medicinal rhubarb

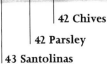

Patios and balconies

As cities continue to grow, space becomes more limited and, increasingly, people live in high-rise dwellings far removed from the earth and its soothing greenery. Those with a balcony or patio have the opportunity to create a private outdoor space in which to daydream and cultivate a selection of aromatic herbs.

To make the best use of such limited space, it is important to plant in all three dimensions, as shown in the scheme below. Use troughs, barrels, sinks and pots on the floor; tiers of pots or shelves up the walls; hanging baskets, and trellis or some other form of screening with plants trained over to add height, shade and shelter. Make the most of the space you have by planting creeping thymes

between bricks and pavers, or in cracks in walls, and by arranging containers in groups that complement each other. Over large areas of wall, fix interlocking clay pots so you can plant a vertical garden. This type of scheme is useful and attractive when filled with small culinary and trailing herbs, particularly if you include some bright, flowering varieties such as the wild strawberries, nasturtiums and chives featured here.

In sheltered areas that get sun only some of the day, take advantage of those herbs that thrive in part shade: angelica, bergamot, bugle, chervil, comfrey, feverfew, foxglove, lungwort, mints, parsley, sweet cicely and sweet violets. Try bay, bistort, clary sage, lady's mantle, lovage, marsh

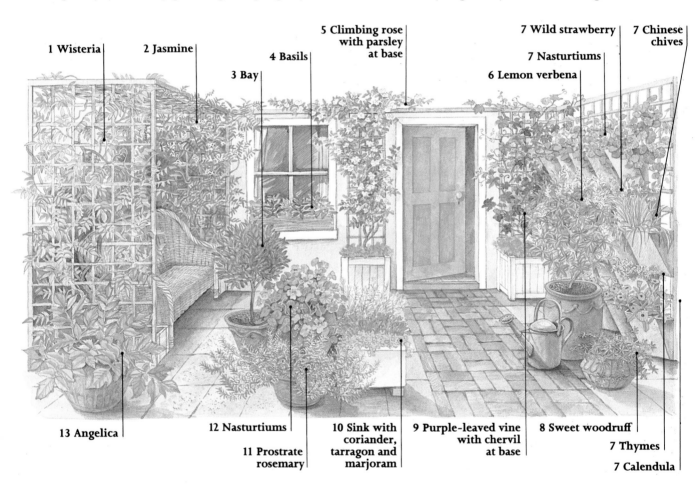

1 Wisteria
2 Jasmine
3 Bay
4 Basils
5 Climbing rose with parsley at base
6 Lemon verbena
7 Wild strawberry
7 Nasturtiums
7 Chinese chives
13 Angelica
12 Nasturtiums
11 Prostrate rosemary
10 Sink with coriander, tarragon and marjoram
9 Purple-leaved vine with chervil at base
8 Sweet woodruff
7 Thymes
7 Calendula

Plant key

1 Wisteria *Wisteria sinensis* Fragrant lilac flowers appear in spring
2 Jasmine *Jasminum x stephanense* Vigorous climber with fragrant pink flowers
3 Bay *Laurus nobilis* trimmed to form a neat tree
4 Basil *Ocimum basilicum* A selection of basils including dark opal and the smaller-leaved bush basil. These are grown in pots on the window sill for easy access and to make their transition indoors easier

5 Versailles box planted with climbing **rose** *Rosa* 'Mme Alfred Carrière' with **parsley** *Petroselinum crispum* at the base
6 A tall pot of fragrant **lemon verbena** *Aloysia triphylla*
7 Wall of ceramic pot units planted with (top row) **nasturtiums** *Tropaeolum majus*; (2nd row) **wild strawberry** *Fragaria vesca*; (3rd row) **Chinese chives** *Allium tuberosum*, salad herbs such as **orach** *Atriplex hortensis*, and **purslane** *Portulaca oleracea*; (4th row) **thymes** *Thymus* species; (bottom row)

Calendula *Calendula officinalis* and **mints** *Mentha* species
8 A pot of fragrant **sweet woodruff** *Galium odoratum*
9 Versailles box planted with flavorsome **chervil** *Anthriscus cerefolium* and a purple-leaved **vine** *Vitis vinifera* 'Purpurea' which may produce grapes on a sheltered, sunny patio
10 Culinary herbs Old porcelain sink positioned conveniently near the door and planted with favorite culinary herbs: **coriander** *Coriandrum sativum*, **tarragon**

Artemisia dracunculus and **marjoram** *Origanum onites*
11 Prostrate rosemary *Rosmarinus officinalis* 'Prostratus' An attractive, trailing form to grow in pots
12 Nasturtium *Tropaeolum majus* Attractive, bright and edible flowers and leaves spill over container's edges
13 Angelica *Angelica archangelica* Potentially tall plant anchored in a large pot which its roots can spread in

mallow, rue, salad burnet, sorrel, tansy and yarrow as well. To help them along, white tiles or white walls will intensify the available light.

If you have a roof garden or high-level balcony, consider structural safety and shelter. If it is windy, some form of screening should come high on your list of planning considerations. Everything will need careful anchoring, including the soil, which should be topped with gravel chippings to prevent it blowing away. Soft-leaved herbs such as lemon balm or angelica will become tattered in high winds, whereas narrow-leaved evergreens such as rosemary and lavender are more suited to such a location, although their appearance may become irregular and gnarled if winds are strong.

Careful placing of plant-filled pots can soften the harsh angles of walled yards and balconies. Rearrange containers frequently either to vary the aesthetic effect or simply so that you maximize the amount of sunlight they enjoy.

For container-grown herbs, life is often a cycle of feast and famine. They experience thorough wetness when watered, but in hot sun, when the soil dries out, their roots have nowhere to extend to in their search for extra moisture. The sun may blaze down for several hours, then disappear behind a building, bringing a sharp drop in temperature. Bear all these factors in mind (see p. 264) when selecting herbs and positioning containers on your patio or balcony.

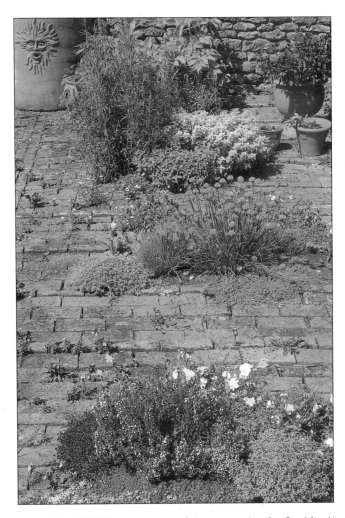

Clusters of tiny, creeping herbs (above) add color and softness to a brick-paved area.

A stately stone urn (left) planted with lemon-scented pelargoniums makes a showpiece in this patio garden.

An attractive collection of patio pots (below) filled with parsley, nasturtiums, sage, rosemary, flowering and scented pelargoniums and thyme, indicate an orderly gardener with civilized priorities.

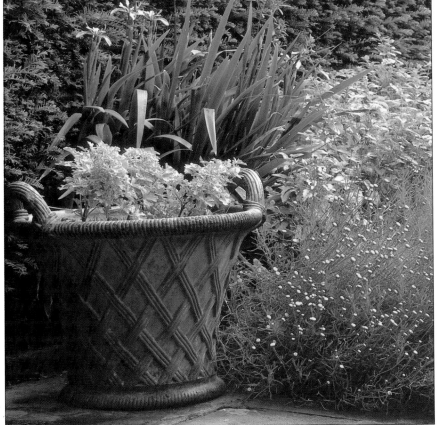

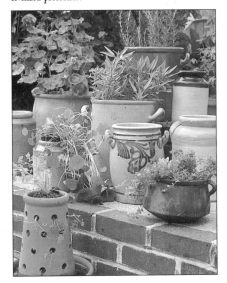

An indoor herb garden

Herbs grown indoors add a fresh fragrance to interiors, and because they're near to hand, encourage you to make maximum use of their leaves. For their part, the herbs gain a longer growing season and protection from severe weather conditions.

"Green fingers" are a result of interested observation and being sensitive to your plants' needs. Basically, herbs require a sunny or light area, water and air humidity, and freedom from draughts and extremes of temperature. Most herbs fare better and look more attractive in groups. Watering is easier and the plants respond well to the micro-climate that grouping creates.

A window sill is the most convenient location, especially if you can make full use of the light,

incorporating shelves or pots on the surrounding walls. The indoor garden illustrated below is designed all around the light source with a hanging basket at the top, climbing herbs and potted herbs on shelves at the sides and a trough full of potted herbs at the base.

Consider growing herbs to enhance different rooms: a clipped bay or sweet myrtle in a sunny entrance hall; peppermint in the moist air of a bathroom; healing aloe vera next to the medicine chest; scented geraniums, pineapple sage and lemon verbena to scent a living room; soothing lavender in the bedroom; hanging baskets planted with prostrate sage and trailing catmint in a stair-well and a grid system on which to bracket pots of culinary herbs on a sunny kitchen wall.

A window garden
Herbs grouped together around a window enjoy maximum light and improved humidity. Turn pots when necessary to prevent uneven growth.

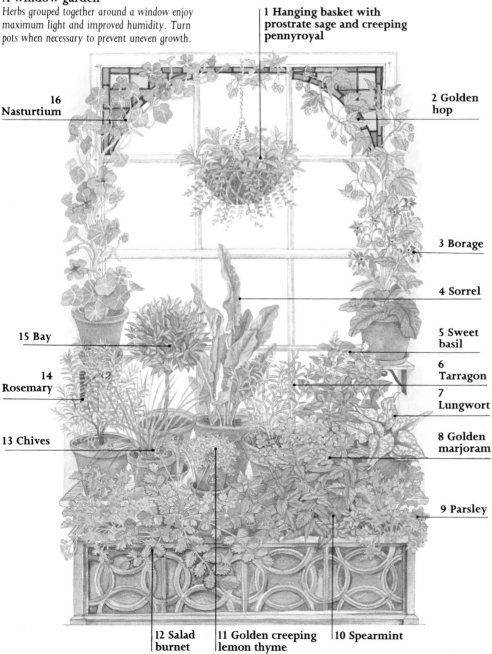

1 Hanging basket with prostrate sage and creeping pennyroyal

16 Nasturtium

2 Golden hop

3 Borage

4 Sorrel

15 Bay

5 Sweet basil

14 Rosemary

6 Tarragon

7 Lungwort

13 Chives

8 Golden marjoram

9 Parsley

12 Salad burnet

11 Golden creeping lemon thyme

10 Spearmint

Plant key

1 Hanging basket with **prostrate sage** *Salvia officinalis* 'Prostratus' which has blue flowers in early summer, and **creeping pennyroyal** *Mentha pulegium*, which has lilac flowers in midsummer
2 **Golden hop** *Humulus lupulus* 'Aureus' trained to grow around the window frame. Female plants produce flowers in late summer
3 **Borage** *Borago officinalis* Use its flowers to garnish food and drinks
4 **Sorrel** *Rumex acetosa* Lush leaves can be used as spinach
5 **Sweet basil** *Ocimum basilicum* An excellent indoor plant. Pinch off flowers to encourage leaf production
6 **Tarragon** *Artemisia dracunculus* Aromatic leaves
7 **Lungwort** *Pulmonaria officinalis* Pink/blue flowers in spring
8 **Golden marjoram** *Origanum vulgare* 'Aureum' Attractive leaves with good flavor
9 **Parsley** *Petroselinum crispum* Grow two plants so you always have a good supply
10 **Spearmint** *Mentha spicata* Refreshing flavor for teas and garnishes. Pinch off flowers for better leaf production
11 **Golden creeping lemon thyme** *Thymus x citriodorus* 'Aureus' Aromatic and colorful foliage
12 **Salad burnet** *Poterium sanguisorba* Use in salads
13 **Chives** *Allium schoenoprasum* Cut off the attractive flowers for better leaf production
14 **Rosemary** *Rosmarinus officinalis* Blue flowers appear in late spring
15 **Bay** *Laurus nobilis* Trimmed into a ball
16 **Nasturtium** *Tropaeolum majus* Trained on a wire around the window

Theme gardens

Much of the allure of herbs is in their many practical and historical associations. Stories, myths and legends featuring herbs abound. The more you find out about herbs, the more you are encouraged to investigate further. This increase in knowledge enhances the pleasure of planning and having an herb garden, and can be used as the basis for making a thematic herb garden.

To plan a theme garden, select plants according to your interests. You may wish to grow solely culinary herbs, or cosmetic, dye or medicinal herbs. If you enjoy discovering how people lived in other ages, you could plant a Roman cook's garden (see p. 34) or a Tudor "My lady's garden" featuring cosmetic and aromatic herbs laid out in a formal scheme.

As the following pages show, you can plant a bed or a whole garden of herbs according to their usage, or you can create a garden based on another culture's style and interests, such as the Chinese and Persian designs shown later in this chapter.

Herbs are excellent plants to grow in community gardens but are often overlooked in favor of more ornamental plants. A school garden could be planned around a period of local history; a church garden could feature herbs mentioned in the Bible or particularly associated with the Virgin Mary. In such gardens, clear labeling is important and paths should be wide, comfortable and safe. Some ideas are illustrated on the following pages.

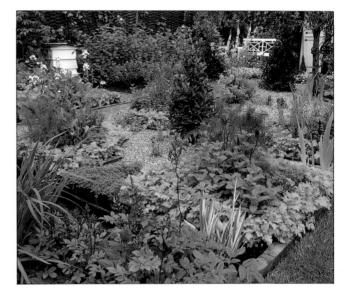

A country kitchen garden (above) planted with herbs and vegetables that are both attractive and useful.

A garden of Chinese medicinal herbs (below) with a statue of Li Shizhen, a Chinese doctor who wrote a practical compendium of medical plants in 1578 after 27 years of traveling through China collecting and testing remedies. His work lists 1,173 plants and 11,000 recipes and has been translated into Japanese, English, Latin, French and German.

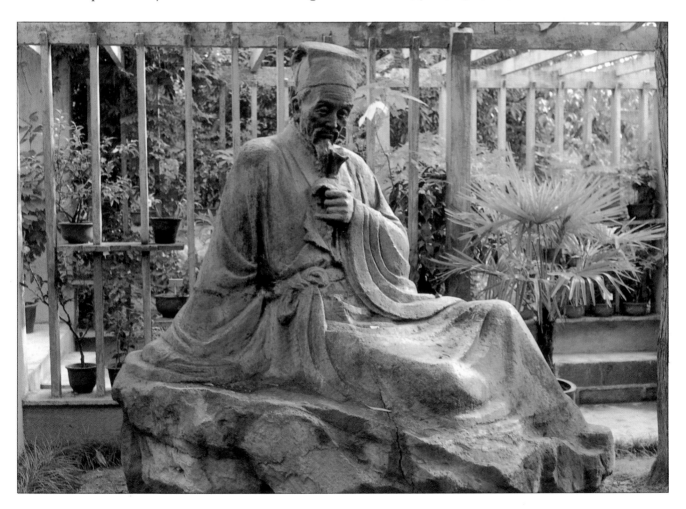

An aromatic herb garden

A garden specially created for its qualities of scent is a continuing delight, both for the gardener and for those who visit it. The aromatic herb garden is a place for perfumed plants of all kinds and sizes – from roses and scented climbers with herbal properties to tiny creeping herbs. Softly scented herbaceous plants can be planted beside some of the more fragrant varieties of culinary favorites, such as sages, rosemarys, mints and thymes, listed in the key below.

A fragrant corner can be created in almost any garden, including a balcony, provided you consider three main elements. First, plan for herbs on several levels: at your feet, at hand and nose height and above your head (use trellises, arbors and hanging baskets). Second, consider some form of enclosure to still the wind, confine the perfume and create a feeling of pleasurable seclusion. Third,

have a garden seat on which you can linger and enjoy this special place while watching the many bees, butterflies and birds that will visit it.

The design opposite has all of these ingredients: aromatic plants at different levels, from underfoot to overhead, an enclosure created by the sweetbrier hedge and trellis, and a relaxing garden bench designed with its armrests and seat as planting areas for creeping thymes, chamomile, sweet myrtle and lemon verbena. As you approach the seat, your feet will release aromas from the creeping herbs planted in the path.

The plan is based on a series of semicircles, most of which are planted symmetrically, with the same herbs appearing on either side. The formal, circular shape of the overall scheme marks out the area and increases the feeling of stepping into a peaceful, private garden.

GARDEN PLAN

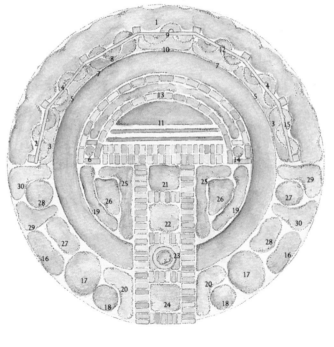

Plant key

1 Sweetbrier rose *Rosa eglanteria* A climbing rose with sweet pink blooms and apple-scented leaves
2 Climbing rose *Rosa* 'Mme Alfred Carrière' Beautiful, scented blush-pink blooms
3 Parsley *Petroselinum crispum* Offers fresh green leaves for nibbling. Benefits from shade of taller plants
4 Early Dutch honeysuckle *Lonicera periclymenum* 'Belgica' Early flowering and sweetly scented, especially in the evenings
5 Sweet woodruff *Galium odoratum* White, starlike flowers and aromatic leaves when dried
6 Lemon verbena *Aloysia triphylla* Lemon-scented foliage and pink flowers
7 Eau de cologne mint *Mentha x piperita* 'Citrata' Attractive and aromatic

8 Akebia *Akebia quinata* Semi-evergreen with fragrant red-purple flowers
9 White jasmine *Jasminum officinale* Sweet-scented flowers
10 Sweet violet *Viola odorata* Early spring flowers
11 Lawn chamomile *Chamaemelum nobile* 'Treneague' Bright green leaves with a delicious apple scent
12 Golden hop *Humulus lupulus* 'Aureus' Attractive gold foliage
13 Green, gold and silver creeping thymes *Thymus praecox* 'Coccineus,' *T.p.* 'Doone Valley,' *T.p.* 'Silver Lemon Queen' All have attractive leaf-colorings and flowers

14 Sweet myrtle *Myrtus communis* 'Tarentina' Spicy orange scent
15 Climbing rose *Rosa* 'New Dawn' Continuous, scented blooms
16 Madonna lily *Lilium candidum* Honey-scented, waxy white flowers
17 Clary sage *Salvia sclarea* Pungent large leaves
18 Rosemary *Rosmarinus officinalis* 'Miss Jessup's Upright' Pale blue flowers appear in spring
19 Clove pink *Dianthus plumarius* Sweet-scented, pretty flowers and silver-blue leaves

20 Catmint *Nepeta mussinii* Pungent leaves and pretty mauve flowers
21 Corsican mint *Mentha requienii* Tiny peppermint-scented leaves form a refreshing square mat to walk on
22 Pine-scented thyme *Thymus caespititius* (*T. azoricus*) Fresh scent and tiny pink flowers planted as a fragrant square mat
23 Creeping lemon thyme *Thymus praecox* 'Citriodorus' Lemon-scented; pink flowering mat to walk on
24 Caraway-scented thyme *Thymus herba-barona* Deep rose-purple flowers

25 Lavender *Lavandula angustifolia* 'Hidcote' Deep purple flowers, strong scent and attractive silver leaves
26 Bergamot *Monarda didyma* Rich red flowers and eau de cologne scent
27 Musk mallow *Malva moschata* Faintly musk-scented with small pink and white flowers
28 Variegated lemon balm *Melissa officinalis* 'Variegata' Gold-splashed, lemon-scented leaves
29 Sweet rocket *Hesperis matronalis* Sweet scented, purple and white flowers. Their fragrance becomes much stronger in the evening, once the sun has gone down
30 Soapwort *Saponaria officinalis* Soft pink summer flowers scent the air with a raspberry fragrance

Features
Wooden slatted seat set on a brick base (see p. 262). This is backed by a semicircular cavity wall, which forms a planter for a collection of thymes. The seat is planted with chamomile and beside it are herbs that need handling to coax out their scent
Brick path constructed with old floor bricks or pavers (see p. 261). The path is designed with planting areas for creeping aromatic herbs
Trellis planted with sweet-scented climbing plants to form a fragrant windbreak
Ornamental urn filled with water for floating scented flower heads

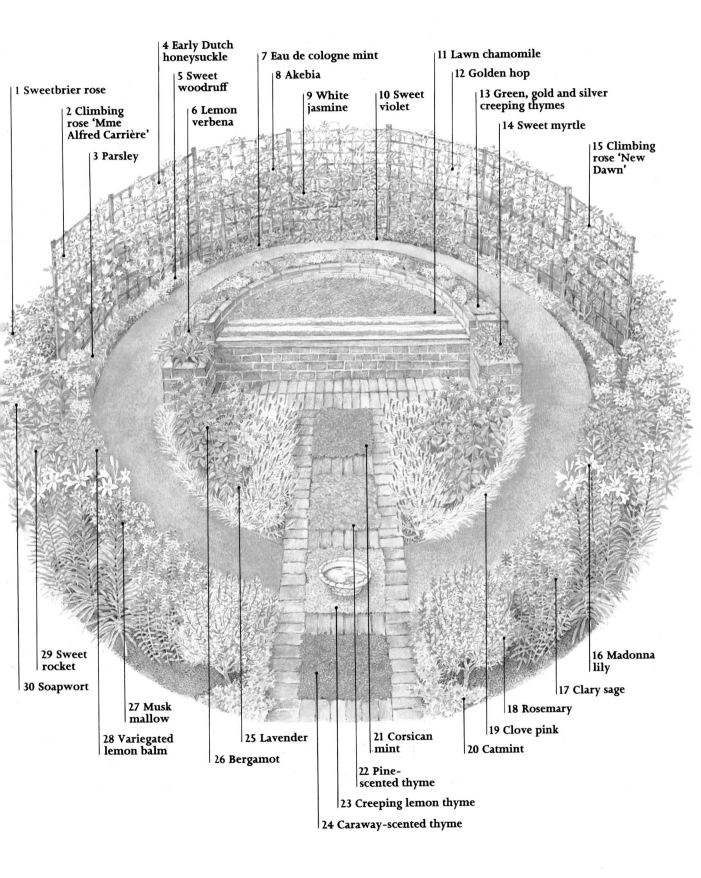

1 Sweetbrier rose

2 Climbing rose 'Mme Alfred Carrière'

3 Parsley

4 Early Dutch honeysuckle

5 Sweet woodruff

6 Lemon verbena

7 Eau de cologne mint

8 Akebia

9 White jasmine

10 Sweet violet

11 Lawn chamomile

12 Golden hop

13 Green, gold and silver creeping thymes

14 Sweet myrtle

15 Climbing rose 'New Dawn'

16 Madonna lily

17 Clary sage

18 Rosemary

19 Clove pink

20 Catmint

21 Corsican mint

22 Pine-scented thyme

23 Creeping lemon thyme

24 Caraway-scented thyme

25 Lavender

26 Bergamot

27 Musk mallow

28 Variegated lemon balm

29 Sweet rocket

30 Soapwort

Overall diameter 24 feet

A children's herb garden

Growing herbs is both a learning experience and a great deal of fun. There is the excitement of planting seeds and seeing if they sprout; the appearance of leaves, flowers and visiting insects; and finally the harvesting and using of different plant parts. All these aspects offer children the opportunity to see how useful plants can be.

As most herbs are easy to grow, select plants that children can enjoy in different ways. For preschool children, prepare a small, sunny plot and help them to sow mustard and cress seed. They will have the fun of watching them germinate and then be able to pick and eat the leaves.

The garden below contains plants with highly aromatic leaves to crush and smell; plants with edible leaves and seeds; flowers that will attract bees and butterflies, and plants with striking seed heads that are fun to play with. As children become older they will want to extend the range to suit their own interests.

Sensible advice for planning a children's garden is to keep it simple, but when I consulted my offspring, all four wanted a maze. We arrived at the compromise below, which is ideal for chasing games, with its linked, curved paths radiating out from a central point.

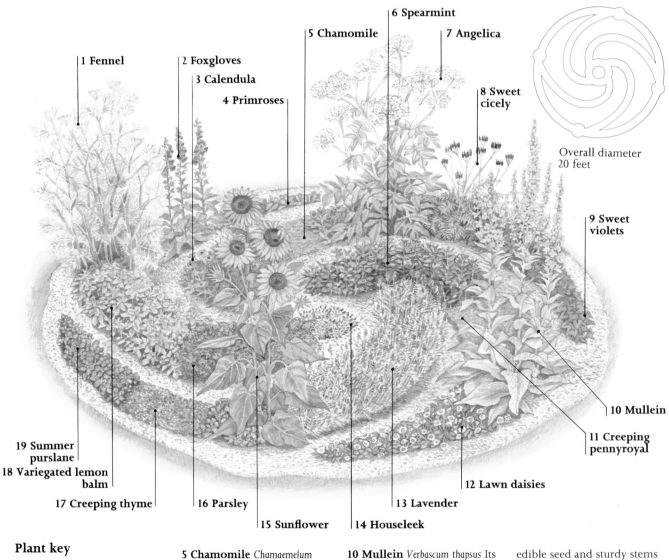

KEYLINE

Overall diameter 20 feet

1 Fennel
2 Foxgloves
3 Calendula
4 Primroses
5 Chamomile
6 Spearmint
7 Angelica
8 Sweet cicely
9 Sweet violets
10 Mullein
11 Creeping pennyroyal
12 Lawn daisies
13 Lavender
14 Houseleek
15 Sunflower
16 Parsley
17 Creeping thyme
18 Variegated lemon balm
19 Summer purslane

Plant key

1 Fennel *Foeniculum vulgare* Edible leaves and seeds
2 Foxglove *Digitalis purpurea* Interesting flowers that attract bees. Ensure your child is responsible enough not to eat any of the plant
3 Calendula *Calendula officinalis* Colorful flowers with edible petals for budding cooks
4 Primroses *Primula vulgaris* Produces early flowers

5 Chamomile *Chamaemelum nobile* Carpeting herb with flowers for a soothing bedtime drink
6 Spearmint *Mentha spicata* Minty leaves to nibble
7 Angelica *Angelica archangelica* Offers soothing leaves for car journeys
8 Sweet cicely *Myrrhis odorata* Edible green seeds
9 Sweet violets *Viola odorata* Scented flowers for candying

10 Mullein *Verbascum thapsus* Its stalks make good rods
11 Creeping pennyroyal *Mentha pulegium* Mint-flavored leaves; can be walked on
12 Lawn daisy *Bellis perennis* Flowers for daisy chains
13 Lavender *Lavandula angustifolia* Offers fragrant flowers
14 Houseleek *Sempervivum tectorum* Soothes cuts and stings
15 Sunflower *Helianthus annuus* A delight to watch growing;

edible seed and sturdy stems for building sticks
16 Parsley *Petroselinum crispum* Edible leaves and currency for bribing the cook
17 Creeping thyme *Thymus praecox* Sweet-scented and able to withstand children's straying footsteps
18 Lemon balm *Melissa officinalis* 'Variegata' Refreshing leaves
19 Summer purslane *Portulaca oleracea* Instant snack food

A moonlight garden

As a rule, gardens are planned for their appeal in daylight hours. However, many plants take on a quite magical appearance when viewed by the light of the moon.

Our eyes see differently by moonlight; most colors vanish, blue becomes white, and white and light gray appear almost fluorescent. A garden or border planted for viewing by moonlight should contain plants of these colors. For further impact, add white stones, statues and other garden features that will reflect the moon's light.

The photograph below was taken in my garden by the light of a full moon in May. Traditionally, this is considered a special night during the season of growth and renewal. I went out to sit on the wooden bench in my herb garden and waited for my eyes to adjust to the dark. At first the moon was hidden by clouds; then it slowly appeared and the garden was transformed. I recognized a froth of white dots as forget-me-nots, a silver curved line as a hedge of curry plant, the luminous fronds of a weeping silver pear tree, and an iridescent canopy of cherry blossom. Artemisias, lavenders, silver thymes and lamiums stood out with their silver leaves, as did the white flowers of daisies, sweet cicely, chervil, caraway, comfrey and sage.

All the silvery tones were intensified by the moon's light. The scent of unseen wild wall-flowers and narcissus drifted across the garden to complete the enchanted moment.

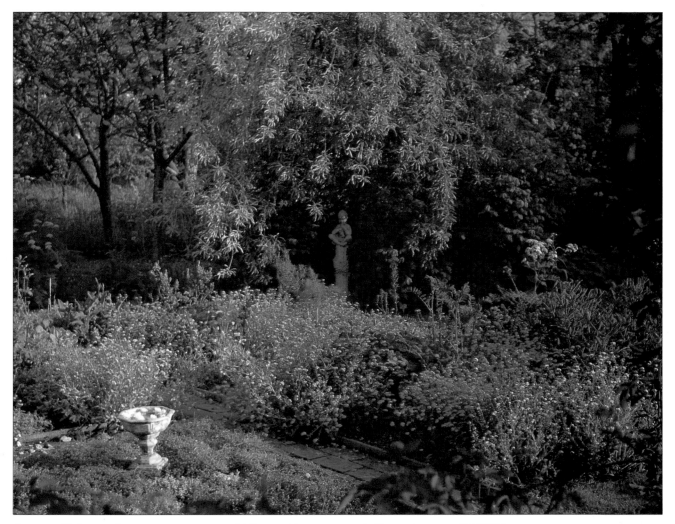

A moonlight garden
Viewed by the light of a full moon, a garden full of herbs takes on a magical quality.

Plant key

1 Cherry tree *Prunus avium* Covered in fragrant, pale pink blossom
2 Weeping silver pear tree *Pyrus salicifolia* Graceful hanging silvery branches
3 Sweet rocket *Hesperis matronalis* Sweetly scented white flowers
4 Forget-me-nots *Myosotis sylvatica* A mass of pale blue and white flowers
5 Thymes *Thymus* species Different thymes planted in a bed to fill it with color
6 Sweet cicely *Myrrhis odorata* Masses of flat white flower heads
7 Rosemary *Rosmarinus officinalis* A bush with pale blue flowers glowing in the moonlight
8 Evening primrose *Oenothera biennis* Tall stem outlined by the light

Feature
A stone urn containing water and floating cherry blossom
A stone statue of Pan

KEYLINE

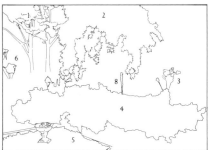

Culinary herb gardens

Although some herbs can be bought dried with their aroma intact (bay, sage, rosemary and thyme) and more shops now sell fresh-cut herbs in season, growing your own is the only sure way to taste the tangy first flavors of chervil, basil, lovage and other less common culinary herbs that are being rediscovered.

A pot of the two most useful garnishing herbs – parsley and chives – will serve you well near to the kitchen door, but immediate access is not so necessary for most culinary herbs. A walk into the herb garden adds to the pleasure of cooking and the sight of other fresh herbs can inspire you to try new combinations.

Most of the culinary herbs are sun lovers and appreciate good drainage plus wind protection. Two other considerations are a hard-surfaced, all-weather path from which you can conveniently reach the plants, and some form of exterior light or a flashlight kept near the door for late forages.

When deciding which herbs to grow, consider how much you are likely to use them. One plant of each of the evergreen herbs and the large perennials is enough for most households. If you are interested in salad herbs and vegetables, you will need more than one of each plant and should allow a patch at least 1 foot square or a row about 4 feet long.

An orderly garden layout makes for convenient picking. The cartwheel and star designs shown here are both attractive and practical. The scheme for a potager (right) is more ambitious.

TWO SIMPLE PLANS
Both these designs allow for expansion as interests develop. Bricks separate the beds to provide access and delineate blocks of herbs.

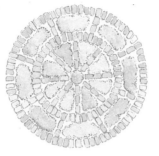

Cartwheel *Start by planting the inner wheel, adding on outer circles as needed.*

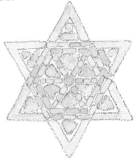

Star *A hexagon forms the inner core and is transformed into a star by the six outer points.*

A potager
This plan adapts the traditional French idea of a potager, where herbs, vegetables and fruit are grown together to make a space-saving and decorative garden. It includes a choice selection of vegetables, salad plants and herbs, and fruit trees trained around arches to form a walkway. Separate beds make crop rotation possible and each bed is edged in traditional dwarf box.

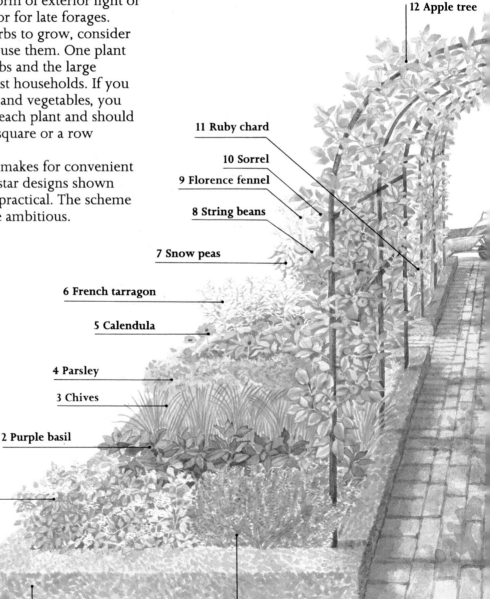

12 Apple tree

11 Ruby chard

10 Sorrel

9 Florence fennel

8 String beans

7 Snow peas

6 French tarragon

5 Calendula

4 Parsley

3 Chives

2 Purple basil

1 Compact marjoram

25 Dwarf box

24 Shrubby thymes

Dimensions: 15 feet square

Plant key

1 Compact marjoram
Origanum vulgare 'Compactum'
Dwarf variety with well-flavored leaves
2 Purple basil *Ocimum basilicum*
'Dark Opal' Deep purple leaves
and a slightly spicier flavor
than the standard sweet basil
3 Chives *Allium schoenoprasum*
Flavorsome leaves and pretty
purple flowers, also edible
4 Parsley *Petroselinum crispum*
Bright green leaves, essential
for any kitchen garden
5 Calendula *Calendula officinalis*
Add color to any garden and
attractive as a garnish
6 French tarragon *Artemisia dracunculus* For delicate and
distinctive flavor

7 Snow peas *Pisum sativum var. macrocarpon* Produce delicately
flavored pods for eating whole
8 String beans *Phaseolus vulgaris*
Provide bright orange flowers
as well as edible pods
9 Florence fennel *Foeniculum vulgare dulce* Cultivate for the
sweet swollen stems
10 Sorrel *Rumex acetosa* Lush
leaves and red-green flowers
11 Ruby chard *Beta vulgaris*
'Rhubarb beet' Bright red
stalks and leaves
12 Two pear trees *Pyrus communis* and two **apple trees**
Malus pumila Trained
(espaliered) over a system of
arches to make a covered
walkway

13 Artichokes *Cynara scolymus*
Magnificent thistle-like
flowers and delicious
vegetable heads
14 Red cabbage *Brassica oleracea*
'Ruby Red' Quick-growing
and attractive, edible leaves
15 Leeks *Allium porrum* Easy to
grow, valuable winter
vegetable
16 Chinese leaves *Brassica rapa*
'Pekinensis' Good in salads
and as a vegetable
17 Sage *Salvia officinalis* Attracts
bees and has many uses in and
out of the kitchen
18 Dill *Anethum graveolens* Good
for flavoring
19 Coriander *Coriandrum sativum* Grow for its leaves
and seeds

20 Chervil *Anthriscus cerefolium*
Delicious culinary herb
21 Arugula *Eruca vesicaria* Spicy
leaves to add to salads
22 Lettuce *Lactuca sativa* 'Lollo'
Attractive red-tipped leaves
23 Purple chicory *Cichorium intybus* Attractive red leaves
24 Thymes *Thymus vulgaris, T. x citriodorus, T. herba-barona* A
selection of shrubby thymes
grown for their different
flavors
25 Dwarf box *Buxus sempervirens*
'Suffruticosa' A 6 inch hedge
surrounds each bed

Feature
Brick path constructed with
weatherproofed pavers
provides access to all the beds

GARDEN PLAN

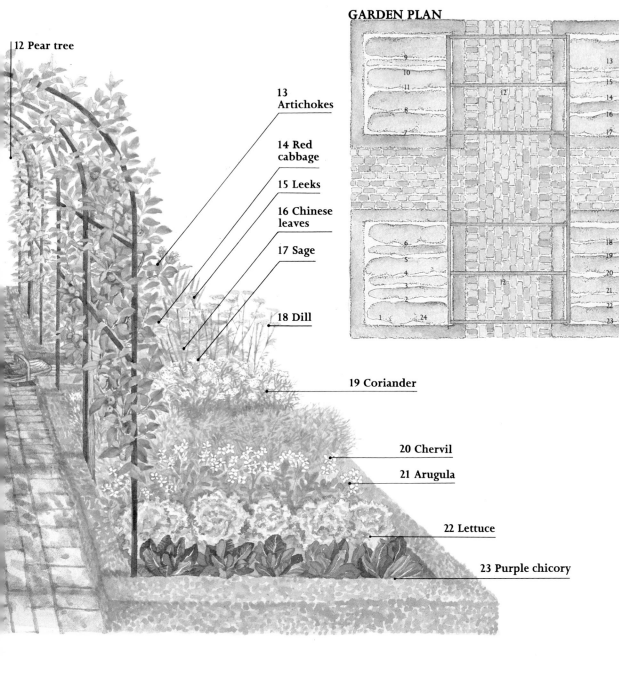

12 Pear tree

13 Artichokes

14 Red cabbage

15 Leeks

16 Chinese leaves

17 Sage

18 Dill

19 Coriander

20 Chervil

21 Arugula

22 Lettuce

23 Purple chicory

A Chinese herb garden

The Chinese have long been experts in the art of gardening in small courtyards. They create privacy, serenity and an air of mystery by dividing their space into still smaller areas with bamboo screens, moon gates (circular entrances in walls) and skilled use of texture, light and shade.

Although the concept of a domestic herb garden does not exist in China, medicinal herbs have been highly valued for over 4,000 years and are grown in botanic gardens. In Kunming, the city of eternal spring, botanists make regular trips to the Yunnan mountains to collect herbs for display in a national garden with rocks, water and shady pergolas.

The garden below is based on a small courtyard near the theater pavilion of the Summer Palace,

Beijing. Planting is kept very simple, with each bed devoted to showing only one species, yet it is planned so there is something of interest in each season. Here we have bamboo, known as one of the "three friends of winter," peonies for spring blooms, roses and poppies for summer and chrysanthemums for autumn. All have medicinal properties. I have made a small concession to Western ideas by underplanting with delicious Chinese culinary herbs.

The curved top to the surrounding wall gives extra lightness and the white surface provides a backdrop for the graceful shadows of the bamboo. The moon gate frames the view and provides a distinct entrance.

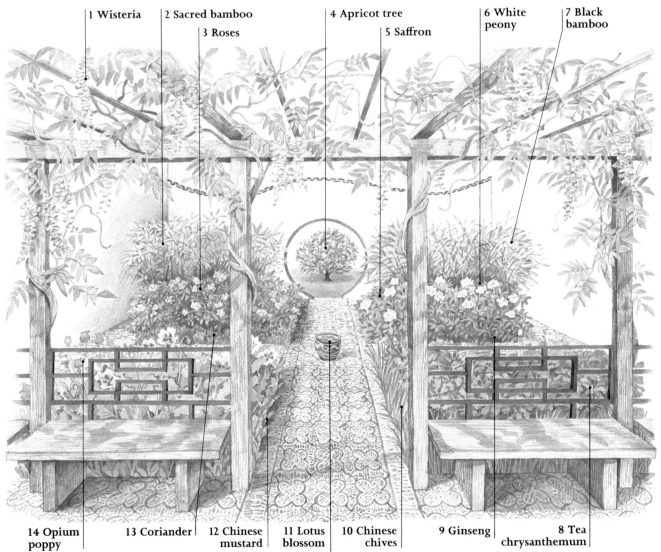

1 Wisteria 2 Sacred bamboo 3 Roses 4 Apricot tree 5 Saffron 6 White peony 7 Black bamboo

14 Opium poppy 13 Coriander 12 Chinese mustard 11 Lotus blossom 10 Chinese chives 9 Ginseng 8 Tea chrysanthemum

Plant key

1 Wisteria Wisteria floribunda Fragrant flowers in early summer; galls used medicinally
2 Sacred bamboo Nandina domestica Used medicinally
3 Roses Rosa 'Old Blush' Continuous clusters of pale pink roses; hips used as a digestive tonic

4 Apricot tree Prunus armeniaca Blossom appears in spring; seeds used in longevity pills
5 Saffron Crocus sativus Rich purple flowers in autumn
6 Peony Paeonia lactiflora Magnificent white blooms; roots used medicinally
7 Black bamboo Phyllostachys nigra Roots used medicinally

8 Tea chrysanthemum Chrysanthemum morifolium White, yellow or pink flowers used medicinally
9 Ginseng Panax pseudoginseng Takes 3–7 years to mature. Pink flowers late summer. Root used as a tonic and elixir
10 Chinese chives Allium tuberosum Mild garlic flavor

11 Lotus blossom Nelumbo nucifera Floating in a glazed pot; beautiful aroma and flowers
12 Chinese mustard Brassica rapa 'Chinensis' Flavorsome leaves
13 Coriander Coriandrum sativum Aromatic seeds
14 Opium poppy Papaver somniferum Luscious blooms from midsummer

A paradise garden

An enclosed pleasure garden, a paradise garden contains axial water channels, aromatic trees, fruits, fragrant herbs and colorful flowers. Developed in Egypt 4,000 years ago as a formal oasis, it reached its perfection under the Persians and the Moghuls in India. The style of geometric paths and rectangular beds was repeated in the monastic gardens of Europe.

This design follows the Persian tradition, with shallow pools lined with deep blue tiles, and decorative paving tiles. The central feature is an open pavilion, lavishly decorated with mosaic tiles in the traditional style, to give the effect of a sparkling jeweled retreat. Bright, flowering herbs add to this tapestry of color.

Although the season for flowers is short in very hot climates, the aromatic evergreen trees and herbs, perpetual flowering roses, ornamental tiles and blue water channels provide color, shade and pleasure all year round.

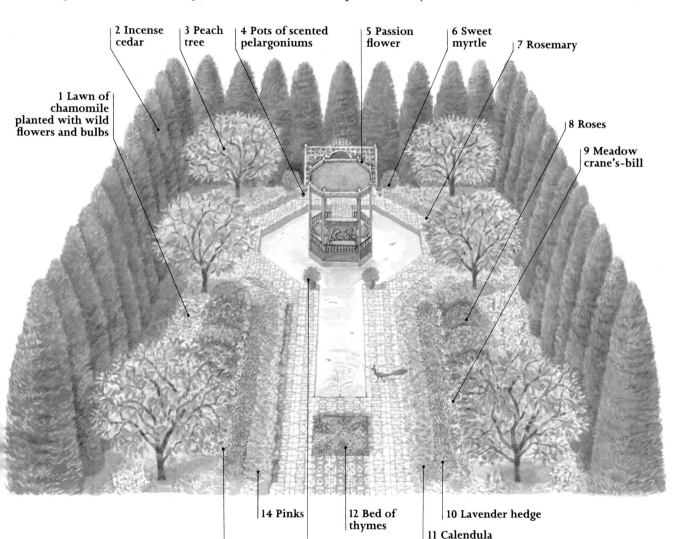

1 Lawn of chamomile planted with wild flowers and bulbs
2 Incense cedar
3 Peach tree
4 Pots of scented pelargoniums
5 Passion flower
6 Sweet myrtle
7 Rosemary
8 Roses
9 Meadow crane's-bill
10 Lavender hedge
11 Calendula
12 Bed of thymes
13 Pots of lemon verbena
14 Pinks
15 Golden-rayed lilies

Plant key

1 Lawn of chamomile *Chamaemelum nobile* An apple-scented lawn planted meadow fashion with colorful flowers and bulbs
2 Incense cedar *Calocedrus decurrens* A hedge of tall trees provides shelter and creates welcome shade
3 Peach trees *Prunus persica* Provide blossom and refreshing fruit
4 Pots of scented pelargoniums *Pelargonium graveolens* and other species interplanted with lemon grass. Pots positioned so plants release their aroma when brushed against
5 Passion flower *Passiflora caerulea* Striking flowers
6 Sweet myrtle *Myrtus communis* 'Tarentina' A low fragrant bush
7 Rosemary *Rosamarinus officinalis* 'Prostratus' A border of low-growing rosemary
8 Roses *Rosa foetida* with bright red flowers and *Rosa damascena* with deep pink flowers, planted in alternating colors

9 Meadow cranesbill *Geranium pratens* Planted by the roses to enhance their color
10 Lavender hedge *Lavandula dentata* Clipped to form a low hedge of fragrant flowers
11 Calendula *Calendula officinalis* A bed of bright orange marigold flowers
12 Thymes *Thymus* species A bed of mixed thymes
13 Pots of lemon verbena *Aloysia triphylla* Provide leaves with refreshing scent
14 Pinks *Dianthus* cultivars A border of fragrant clove pinks

15 Golden-rayed lilies *Lilium auratum* Lavish, scented flowers with distinctive markings on each petal

Features
Path covered in ornate paving tiles for extra color
Water channel lined with rich blue tiles to enhance the apparent depth of the water
Pavilion provides shade and color as well as a retreat

Theme garden ideas

The more you involve yourself with herbs, the more ways you will find for selecting and displaying these plants. Practical uses apart, theme gardens that place herbs in a historical context are always interesting to plan, as the significant role played by herbs in ancient cultures and more recent history makes fascinating research.

Archeologists believe that certain plants were used to season food over 50,000 years ago. Certainly, by the Neolithic period over 9,000 years ago, people had discovered how to extract oil from flax, olives, sesame seeds and the castor plant. For those interested in the continuity of plant use through the ages, an herb garden based on a particular era can be immensely rewarding, especially if you plan it in a style to match the period. Here are some ideas to start you off.

A ROMAN COOK'S HERB GARDEN

A translation from a recipe book written by the Roman epicure Apicius in the first century A.D. gives an insight into the fascinating combinations of herbs used in Roman cuisine. For example, a recipe for a sauce includes a mixture of cumin, celery seed, thyme, savory, mint and pine nuts.

A Roman-style herb garden would suit a sunny courtyard filled with terra-cotta pots, formal raised beds, a vine-clad pergola and a suitable statue.

Some of the herbs used in Roman cooking are: anise, arugula, basil, bay, capers, caraway, catmint, celery seed, coriander, costmary, cumin, dill, elecampane, garlic, hyssop, mustard, myrtle, oregano, parsley, pennyroyal, pepper, rue, safflower, saffron, savory, Welsh onion and wormwood.

A MONASTIC HERB GARDEN FOR LIQUEURS

In their commitment to self-sufficiency, monks produced a range of spirit-based drinks flavored by a sweetened infusion or a distillation of herbs. In the past, these liqueurs, called variously balms, cremes and elixirs, were used as medicines, tonics and love potions. Their digestive properties make liqueurs popular after-dinner drinks today.

The monks' recipes have always been guarded vigorously: benedictine, first produced in 1510, is one of the most secret, along with chartreuse, created in 1607. However, any of the following herbs can add good flavor to spirits: angelica, anise, balm, caraway, coriander, elecampane, fennel, hyssop, mint, speedwell, sweet cicely, sweet flag root, sweet woodruff, tansy, thyme, violets and wormwood.

A MEDICINAL HERB GARDEN

Hundreds of plants have been used medicinally in different cultures throughout history. Some are now considered highly poisonous, while new research is confirming the powerful healing properties of others. Apart from their many and ancient applications, medicinal herbs are frequently extremely decorative, striking plants, that add enormous interest to a garden regardless of whether you use them yourself.

A traditional idea is to plant the herbs out in beds according to the ailments they treat, as in the infirmary gardens of medieval monasteries. You could have a bed of herbs for coughs, colds and sore throats; a bed for herbs to help insomnia; a bed for herbs that aid digestion; and one for tonic herbs. When you have a choice of herbs, you can quickly see which are ready for picking. Consult the chapter about herbal medicine (pp. 238–250) before attempting any remedies, or just grow the herbs for show. Include a seat, as sitting out in an herb garden is an excellent convalescent activity.

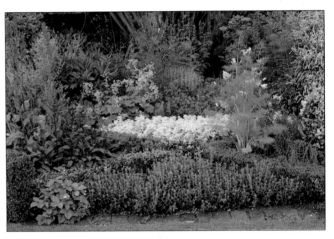

A bed of medicinal herbs forms an attractive corner.

AN ASTROLOGICAL HERB GARDEN

Throughout history, the rhythms of nature have intrigued mankind to the degree that various observers have developed different systems of classification according to the movements of the moon and the stars. In his herbal of 1645, Culpeper attributed each herb to a ruling heavenly body and considered it effective to treat people and diseases of the same zodiacal sign. A suitable plan for an astrological garden would have two interlocking triangles arranged to make a six-pointed star enclosed in a circle. The three points of any triangle could link signs of the same element.

HERBS AND STAR SIGNS

Aquarius elderberry, fumitory, mullein
Pisces lungwort, meadowsweet, rosehip
Aries cowslip, garlic, hops, mustard, rosemary
Taurus coltsfoot, lovage, mints, thyme
Gemini caraway, dill, lavender, parsley, vervain
Cancer agrimony, balm, daisies, hyssop, jasmine
Leo bay, borage, chamomile, marigold, poppy, rue
Virgo fennel, savory, southernwood, valerian
Libra pennyroyal, primrose, violets, yarrow
Scorpio basil, tarragon, wormwood
Sagittarius feverfew, houseleek, mallow, sage
Capricorn comfrey, sorrel, Solomon's seal

NORTH AMERICAN INDIAN HERBS

Research indicates that the Indian tribes of North America have used over 600 native plants in food, medications and decorations. Plants used by the Northern Cree of my native Alberta include sweet gale (to dye porcupine quills), horsetail (to polish arrow heads), bearberry (leaves were smoked and berries were used in necklaces and rattles), lupine (leaves used in incense), wild mint (used to flavor dried meat and take the scent of humans from animal traps), sphagnum moss (made disposable diapers) and wild rose (flowers and fruits used in food and medications). These would all be suitable plants for a woodland or wildflower garden area.

LITERARY HERB GARDENS

The Bible and the works of Chaucer and Shakespeare are rich in references to herbs. Shakespeare in particular wrote with knowledgable delight of over 80 herbs and wildflowers. Clearly he was familiar with their usage and their symbolic associations. A design for a Shakespeare garden should follow the formal Elizabethan style, with clipped knots of evergreen shrubs and a fairy bower planted with fragrant, pretty herbs. The following plants are all mentioned in at least one of Shakespeare's plays and provide an interesting and colorful selection.

balm, bay, borage, box, clover, columbine, cowslip, daffodil, daisies, fumitory, harebell, lady's smock, larkspur, lavender, mustard, myrtle, narcissus, ox-eye daisies, oxslips, pansy, pinks, poppies, primrose, musk rose and sweetbrier roses, rosemary, rue, salad burnet, strawberry, thyme, violet, winter savory, woodbine, wormwood and yarrow.

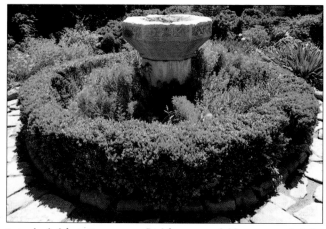

A circular bed featuring an ornamental font surrounded by an aromatic hedge in the Shakespeare section of Washington Cathedral's herb garden.

A WITCH'S HERB GARDEN

Witchcraft is a subject that fascinates many people, and fortunately we live in an age when we can look with lighthearted curiosity at the uses made of some of the more potent and poisonous plants in the past. The fact that up to six million women have been murdered in witch hunts through the ages is a brutal scar in the history of man and the Church's struggle to maintain power.

Just as there were thought to be good and bad witches, the herbs they used were also considered as offensive and defensive. The nine Anglo-Saxon sacred herbs (chamomile, chervil, crab apple, fennel, mugwort, nettle, plantain, sainfoin, watercress) were believed to repel evil attacks. Angelica was considered the sovereign remedy against enchantments and potions. Clovers, whether three-leaved or four-leaved, were thought to have protective powers, even to the degree of releasing people from military service. Dill, garlic, houseleek and mugwort were used to protect people from spells, the devil and lightning.

A GARDEN FOR HONEY BEES

For maximum nectar production and pollination, an herb garden for bees should be in full sun and have herbs planted in groups of five or more. Erect a trellis, or some form of windbreak, if the site is not sheltered, or bees will be buffeted by the wind. A hedge of holly and ivy acts as an effective windbreak and supplies nectar flowers in both spring and autumn. Clovers, lime and fruit trees, oil-seed rape, sainfoin, mustard, charlock, willow herb and dandelion are the most important nectar plants for bees. Select herbs that will provide nectar and pollen for the longest period. The following plants would supply nectar almost all year round and are listed in order of flowering:

winter aconite, crocus, lamiums, forget-me-not, rosemary, catmint, Jacob's ladder, borage, melilot, summer and winter savory, thymes, viper's bugloss, catnip, alliums, chamomile, alkanet, anise, hyssop, chicory, flax, sage, smallage (wild celery), fennel, poppies, safflower, teasel, valerian, verbena, woad, basil, calendula, horehound, musk mallow, marjorams, verbascum, goldenrod, mints, sunflower.

Although a bee skep is a traditional ornament in an herb garden, it is unrealistic to keep working hives within the garden boundary: bees ignore plants within a radius of approximately 50 feet from the hive as this area may be contaminated by the bees' own cleansing flights.

A MEDITATION GARDEN

The next herb garden I would like to make is one designed for contemplation. Any private herb garden is a suitable place, but I wish to design one that will focus the mind on specific ideas. It would take the form of an eight-pointed star or an eight-sided figure with its entrance forming one side. Each of the remaining seven sections would encapsulate a different idea: a day of the week; a color of the spectrum and perhaps a type of fragrance. The central area would be covered to make a dry sanctuary.

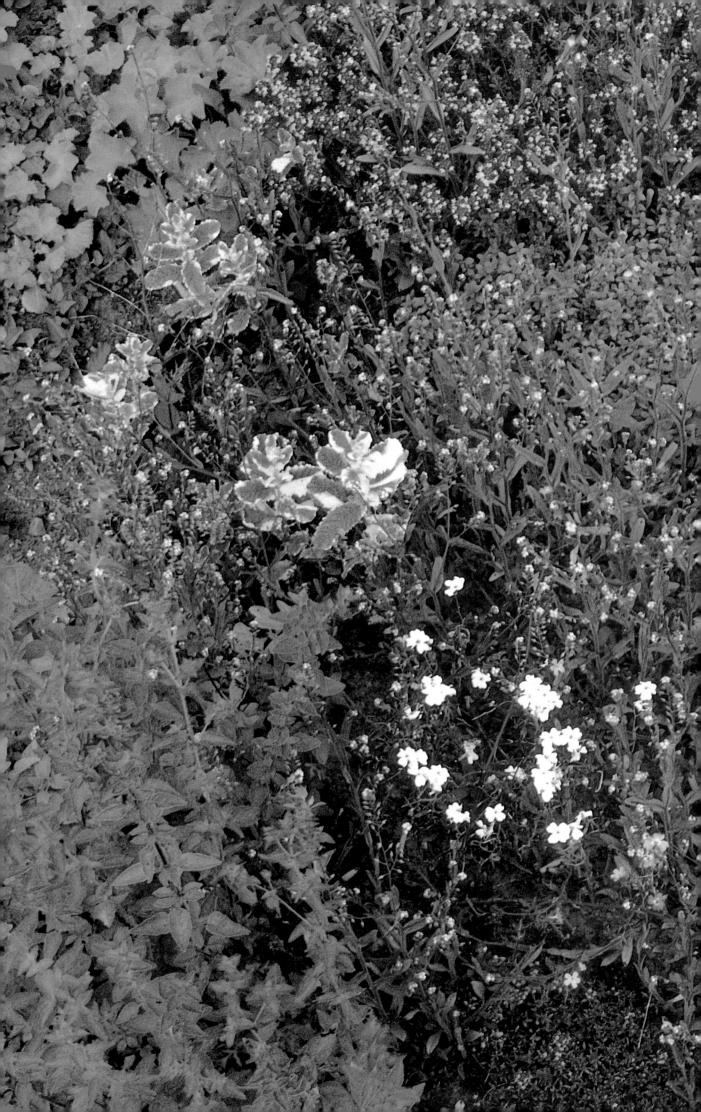

HERBAL INDEX

Inspired by the herbals of John Gerard and
Nicholas Culpeper, published over 300 years ago,
the following pages form a contemporary guide
to over 100 of today's most useful, interesting
and easy-to-grow herbs.

Herbs are listed alphabetically by their botanical
names. Any that have been reclassified recently
include the alternative (in parentheses). The family
name is supplied in italics after the common name.

Each herb has been photographed and
described in detail to facilitate identification.
When a number of species or varieties exists, a
selection illustrates the range available.

Details are provided of each herb's lifespan,
height and required growing conditions. Botanical
terms have been kept to a minimum throughout;
those that are used are explained in the glossary on
p. 279. There is also a wealth of historical and
practical information about each herb: methods of
cultivation, harvesting and preserving, and
suggestions for use. To follow up these ideas,
consult the later chapters and the index.

Four feature sections illustrate and describe plants
less often considered as herbs. These are backed
up by the Catalogue of Herbs on pp. 271–78.

**Note: Read pp. 238–250 before making any
medicinal preparations. If you are uncertain about a
plant, do not use it. Never take anything in excess,
and consult a qualified practitioner
whenever you have any doubts.**

A colorful selection of herbs, including mints, marjorams and thymes.

Achillea millefolium

Yarrow/Milfoil *Compositae*

This unassuming plant conceals great powers. One small leaf will speed decomposition of a wheelbarrow full of raw compost; yarrow's root secretions will activate the disease resistance of nearby plants; and it intensifies the medicinal actions of other herbs. Yarrow is also a potent healer. The name *Achillea* may stem from the battle of Troy, when Achilles healed many of his warriors after being instructed in yarrow's ability to staunch blood flow.

Long considered sacred, yarrow stems were used by the Druids to divine seasonal weather in Europe, while in China yarrow stems were used to foretell the future with the assistance of the I *Ching* (the Book of Changes or Yarrow Stalk Oracle).

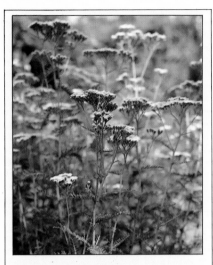

Seed
Small, gray-brown, flat and tear-shaped.

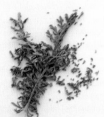

Dried leaves
These exude a mild, sagelike flavor for use as a medicinal and cosmetic tea.

Flower
Small, dull white, sometimes pink, flattish clusters with pungent scent appear from summer to autumn.

Dried stems
50 straight stems of even length are "thrown" by masters of the I Ching before consulting this oriental ancient guide to the future.

Stem
Hollow, ridged, branching near top, and green.

Leaf
Narrow, aromatic, feathery, deeply cut and dark grayish-green; rich in vitamins and minerals.

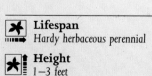 **Lifespan**
Hardy herbaceous perennial

Height
1–3 feet

CULTIVATION
Site Sunny. Tolerates light shade.
Soil Moderately rich and moist.
Propagating Sow or divide invasive roots in spring or autumn.
Growing Thin or transplant to 12 inches apart. Deadhead for second blooming. Yarrow is not suitable for growing indoors.
Harvesting Gather leaves and flowers in late summer.
Preserving Dry leaves and flowers.

USES
Decorative
● *Flower* Display dried heads.

Culinary
● *Leaf* Finely chop slightly bitter, peppery young leaves into salads and soft cheese dips. Use to garnish.

Household
● *Whole plant* May help nearby plants to resist disease and deepens their fragrance and flavor. Infuse to make a copper fertilizer.
● *Leaf* Speed decomposition by adding one small finely chopped fresh leaf to each wheelbarrow-load of compost.

Cosmetic
● *Flower* Infuse fresh flowers for a facial steam and tonic lotion. Use the infusion as a basis for a face pack for greasy skin or in a relaxing bath.
● *Leaf* Press fresh leaves onto a shaving cut.

Medicinal
● *Leaf* Chew fresh leaf to aid toothache. Infuse as a tea for digestive problems, and to regulate menstrual flow, induce perspiration, cleanse the system and cure a cold. Make a decoction for wounds, chapped skin and rashes. Use as a mouthwash for inflamed gums.

Note: *Extended use of yarrow leaves may make the skin sensitive to light.*

Alchemilla vulgaris

Lady's mantle/Dewcup Rosaceae

From "little magical one," the Arab *alkemelych* (alchemy), comes *Alchemilla*, so-called because of this herb's healing reputation and the dew that collects in each enfolding leaf. The crystal drops of dew have long inspired poets and alchemists and were part of many mystic potions. So powerful a herb was acquired by the Christian Church, which named it "Our Lady's mantle." Its protective role was reflected in its nickname, "a woman's best friend," as it was thought to regulate periods, ease the menopause and clear inflammations of the female organs. One German herbalist claims prolonged use of lady's mantle tea could cut gynecological operations by one-third. *A. vulgaris* is an aggregate name for about 21 subspecies which seen. to have similar medicinal properties.

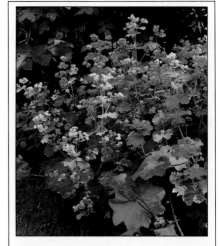

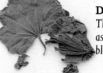

Dried leaves
These make a cosmetic astringent and staunch bleeding.

Lifespan
Hardy herbaceous perennial

Height
6–20 inches

Flower
Loose clusters of small greenish-yellow flowers appear in summer.

A. alpina
Alpine lady's mantle
Small, yellow-green clusters borne in late summer and silver-edged leaves with white, silky undersides. Ht: 6 inches.

Leaf
Soft, blue-green and almost circular with seven to 11 rounded, toothed lobes joined by deep folds.

Stem
Hairy, slightly flattened, ridged, branching and green; usually bends outward as flowers develop.

Young plant
A mass of fibrous roots develop into a short, dark rhizome; leaf stalks emerge directly from base.

CULTIVATION
Site Full sun or partial shade.
Soil Rich, moist, alkaline loam.
Propagating Sow or divide lady's mantle in spring or autumn.
Growing Thin or transplant to 2 feet apart. Small plants can be grown indoors.
Harvesting Select large leaves as needed. They are best during flowering period.
Preserving Dry leaves.

USES
Decorative
● *Whole plant* Attractive in hanging baskets.
● *Flowers and leaves* Add to posies.

Culinary
● *Leaf* Tear young leaves, with their mildly bitter taste, into small pieces and toss in herb salads.

Household
● *Leaf* Boil for a green wool dye.

Cosmetic
● *Leaf* Infuse dried leaves as an astringent and as a facial steam for acne. Apply infusion in a cold compress for inflamed eyes and as a tonic to reduce large pores and acne. Use in creams to soften dry, rough skin. To lighten freckles, rinse with juice extracted from leaves.

Medicinal
● *Whole plant (Green parts only)* Infused as a tea to drink during pregnancy and for 10 days after giving birth to help womb contract, and to regulate monthly cycle. After the age of 40, drink infusion for 10 days each month to relieve menopausal discomfort. Also used as a mouth rinse after tooth extraction and for diarrhea.
● *Leaf* Decoct for a compress for healing wounds and reducing inflammation. *A. alpina* has same constituents; may be more powerful.

Allium species

Alliums Liliaceae

One of the most popular and widespread culinary flavorings is the onion family. The value of these alliums is reflected in the Latin *unio*, "one large pearl," and the Chinese name "jewel among vegetables." Alliums also have marvelous health-giving properties. The stronger the smell, the more effective their healing powers. Pyramid builders and Roman soldiers on long marches were fed on a daily ration of garlic, whose power even extended to protection from black magic, as vampire films continue to remind us. Today, garlic is a major flavoring in many cuisines.

Chives were recorded 4,000 years ago in China and appreciated there by the traveller Marco Polo. He reported their culinary virtues to the West, where they rapidly became indispensable. Chinese chives have a garlic flavor, and the Chinese grow several forms: one for its leaves; one, 'Tenderpole,' for its long-stemmed flower buds – good stir-fried or as a garnish; and one to blanch (using clay pots or straw "tents" to produce yellow, sweetly flavored bundles). These blanched chives are featured in a popular meal available on trains and street stalls in China: little finger-length pieces are served with rice and slivers of pork, often in prepacked containers with chopsticks.

Another important allium species in China and Japan is the Welsh onion (Welsh meaning "foreign"), which provides a continuous supply of bunching onions and leaves throughout the year.

A. tuberosum
Chinese chives
White, starry, sweet-scented flowers late summer, flat green leaves, mild garlic flavor and tuberous root.

A. fistulosum
Welsh onion
White flowers in summer and strong-flavored evergreen leaves.

Seed
Black, faceted and tear-shaped, fractionally larger than a chive seed.

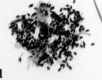

Seed
Black, faceted and tear-shaped, $\frac{1}{8}$ inch long, with mild onion flavor.

Dried leaves
Require low temperature drying to retain color; best suited to cooked recipes.

Leaves
Variable grass (leaf) sizes depend on plant's age, soil fertility and seed source.

A. schoenoprasum
Chives
Cylindrical leaves and a mild onion flavor. Globular mauve flowers midsummer.

✳ **Lifespan**
Hardy perennial bulbs

✳ **Height**
8 inches–3 feet

A. cepa
Everlasting onion
"Ever-ready"
perennial producing
sharp-flavored
"spring" onions.
Rarely flowers.

A.c. var. *proliferum*
Tree onion/
Egyptian onion
Small pickling
onions grow on stem
tips. May need
staking. Ht: 3 feet.

A. sativum
Garlic
White flowers and
flat solid leaves with
culinary bulb.

A.
scorodoprasum
Rocambole/
Giant garlic
Mild garlic-
flavored bulb.
Mauve flowers
develop edible
aerial bulbs.

Garlic cloves
Highly flavored
segments of a bulb.

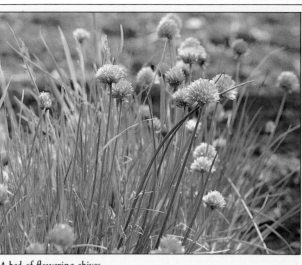

A bed of flowering chives.

CULTIVATION

Site Sunny; tolerates partial shade.
Soil Rich, moist and well drained; tolerates poorer soil.
Propagating Take offsets or divide bulb in autumn or
spring; plant garlic cloves $1\frac{1}{2}$ inches deep; sow seed in
spring (not available for everlasting and tree onion).
Growing Transplant or thin to 9 inches apart; garlic
to 6 inches apart. Water in dry spells and enrich soil
annually (or monthly, when cutting chives). Remove
flowers for better flavor. Divide and replant clumps every
3–4 years. Pot in autumn for indoor supply.
Can be grown indoors.
Harvesting (Chives) Cut leaves, leaving 2 inches for
regrowth. Pick flowers as they open. (Garlic) Dig bulbs in
late summer; handle gently to avoid bruising.
Preserving Refrigerate chive leaves in a sealed plastic bag
to retain crispness for 7 days, or freeze (in ice cubes, for
convenience) or dry them. Dry flowers and bulbs. Make
garlic oil, and garlic and chive vinegars.

USES

Decorative
● *Whole plant* (Tree onion) Cultivate as a novelty plant.

Culinary
● *Flower* (Chives) Sprinkle florets on salads.
● *Leaf* (Chives) Eat in salads, sandwiches and soups and
as a garnish. Make butter or cream cheese (allow 1 hour
for flavor to infuse). To reconstitute dried chives, moisten
with salad dressing or lemon juice.
● *Bulb* (Garlic) Use sparingly; rub clove around salad
bowl or fondue dish to improve flavors. Chew parsley
or cardamom seed to counteract garlic breath. (Tree,
everlasting and Welsh onion) Pickle in wine vinegar.

Household
● *Whole plant* (Chives) Grow as deterrent for aphids,
apple scab and mildew. (Garlic) Plant under peach trees
to control leafcurl and near roses to enhance scent.
● *Leaf* (Chives) Infuse as a spray for aphids, apple scab
and mildew. (Garlic) Spray potato blight with a freshly
made infusion.

Medicinal
● *Whole plant* All alliums contain some iron and vitamins
and are a mild antibiotic. (Chives) Sprinkle on food to
stimulate appetite and promote digestion. Take as a mild
laxative. (Garlic) Use as an antibiotic, to cleanse blood,
reduce blood pressure and clear catarrh; take as protection
against common colds, worms, dysentery and typhoid.

Aloe vera (A. barbadensis)

Aloe vera Liliaceae

One of Cleopatra's secret beauty ingredients was reputed to be aloe vera, and it is still chosen by contemporary cosmetic firms for face and hand creams, suntan lotions and shampoos. Aloe vera has also attracted the interest of many governments for its ability to heal radiation burns, and the U.S. government is said to be stockpiling the herb for use in the event of a nuclear disaster. It is the fresh sap from this remarkable herb that can heal skin and soothe burns; old sap, however, deteriorates rapidly when isolated.

A beautiful violet dye is produced from aloe plants native to the island of Socotra in the Indian Ocean, and it was thought to be the desire for this product that motivated Alexander the Great to conquer the island in the fourth century B.C. Some 1,400 years later, Muslim traders reported that the island was still the only source of the herb, although it is now known to grow in Africa, China, India and Central America. There are about 350 aloe species.

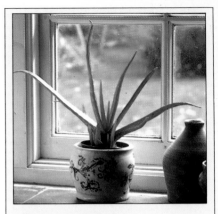

Leaf
Long, very fleshy, tapering, pointed, pale green blades, often with spiny teeth along margins.

Split leaves
Inside each leaf is a clear gelatinous sap, which has an immediate soothing effect on burns and forms a clear protective seal, allowing healing to take place rapidly.

Plant base
Stemless base, which eventually produces a flowering stem, with spikes of narrow, trumpet-shaped, yellow or orange flowers, and offshoots for propagation.

Root
Strong, light brown and fibrous.

 Lifespan
Tender evergreen perennial

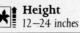 **Height**
12–24 inches

CULTIVATION
Site Full sun or light shade in frost-free location.
Soil Gritty and well drained.
Propagating Sow in spring at 70 °F. Remove any offshoots during summer; then dry for 2 days before planting in 2 parts compost to 1 part sharp sand.
Growing Maintain 41 °F minimum. Aloe vera is an excellent indoor plant.
Harvesting Cut leaves as needed. Best from plants at least 2 years old.
Preserving No method known at present, although a product called Aloe Vera gel is available. This contains 99.9 percent aloe vera and is sold in a dark glass bottle with instructions to keep refrigerated.

USES
Decorative
● *Whole plant* (A. variegata) Use as an ornamental pot plant.

Household
● *Leaf* Socotrine aloes is prepared from *Aloe perryi* on the island of Socotra and gives a rich violet dye.

Cosmetic
● *Leaf* Use the leaf sap to make a soothing and healing moisturizing cream, especially good for dry skin. Mix into shampoos to help dry or itchy scalp. Add to suntan lotions for its cooling and healing effect.

Medicinal
● *Leaf* Crush sap from fresh leaves or slice them and apply as a poultice for chapped skin, dermatitis, eczema and burns. For small burns, break off a leaf segment and apply its sap to the burn. For large burns, split and open out a leaf; place sap against damaged skin and lightly bandage in place. Renew as necessary.

Note: *Always seek medical attention for serious burns.*

Aloysia triphylla (Lippia citriodora)

Lemon verbena *Verbenaceae*

Lemon verbena's immediate attraction lies in its leaves, which have a clean, sharp, lemony fragrance that gives unexpected pleasure with each contact. Despite such an appeal, there is remarkably little history and legend attached to this plant, which is a native of South America. Lemon verbena was, however, brought to Europe in the seventeenth century by the Spanish, who grew it for its perfume oil. Although it is not hardy, a straw-covered pruned plant with deep roots should survive some frost. New growth can appear very late, so never discard a plant until late summer.

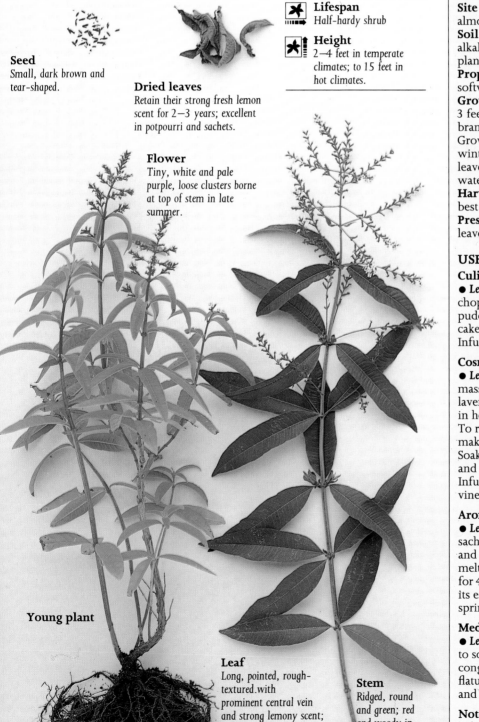

Seed
Small, dark brown and tear-shaped.

Dried leaves
Retain their strong fresh lemon scent for 2–3 years; excellent in potpourri and sachets.

Lifespan
Half-hardy shrub

Height
2–4 feet in temperate climates; to 15 feet in hot climates.

Flower
Tiny, white and pale purple, loose clusters borne at top of stem in late summer.

Young plant

Leaf
Long, pointed, rough-textured with prominent central vein and strong lemony scent; arranged on stem in threes.

Stem
Ridged, round and green; red and woody in second season.

CULTIVATION

Site Full sun. Needs shelter in almost frost-free position.
Soil Light, well drained and alkaline. Poor soil produces stronger plants able to survive cold winters.
Propagating Sow in spring. Take softwood cuttings in late spring.
Growing Thin or transplant to 3 feet apart. Prune drooping branches to encourage new growth. Grow lemon verbena indoors in winter, though it may drop its leaves. Prune and spray with warm water in spring to revive plant.
Harvesting Pick leaves anytime: best when flowers begin to bloom.
Preserving Dry leaves. Use fresh leaves to flavor oil and vinegar.

USES

Culinary
● *Leaf* Infuse as herb tea. Finely chop young leaves for drinks, fruit puddings, confectionery, apple jelly, cakes and homemade ice cream. Infuse in finger bowls.

Cosmetic
● *Leaf* Macerate in almond oil for a massage; for interesting blends, add lavender or rosemary. Use this oil in homemade lotions and creams. To reduce puffiness around eyes, make an infusion and allow to cool. Soak cotton wool in the infusion and place over eyes for 15 minutes. Infuse and add to a bath. Make floral vinegar to soften and freshen skin.

Aromatic
● *Leaf* Use in potpourri, linen sachets, sofa sacks and herb pillows and to scent ink and paper. Infuse in melted candle wax at about 180 °F for 45 minutes to scent candles. Use its essential oil in perfumes and to sprinkle over potpourri.

Medicinal
● *Leaf* Infuse as a mildly sedative tea to soothe bronchial and nasal congestion, to reduce indigestion, flatulence, stomach cramps, nausea and palpitations.

Note: *Long-term use of large amounts of leaf may cause stomach irritations.*

Althaea officinalis

Marsh mallow Malvaceae

This is indeed the original source of the confectionery of this name. Marsh mallow's powdered root contains a mucilage that thickens in water and was heated with sugar to create a soothing sweet paste. However, today's spongy cubes share only sugar in common with the original recipe.

Marsh mallow is one of over 1,000 species in the *Malvaceae* family, all of which contain a healing mucilage, and its genus name, *Althaea*, is from the Greek *althe*, to cure. Long used as a healing herb, marsh mallows were eaten by the Egyptians and Syrians, and mentioned by Pythagoras, Plato and Virgil. The plant was enjoyed by the Romans in barley soup and in a stuffing for suckling pig, while classical herbalists praised its gentle laxative properties.

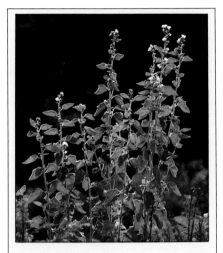

Seed
Light brown and disk-shaped, slotted upright in a ring called a "cheese."

Flower
Pink or white blooms, $1\frac{1}{2}$ inches across, with purple stamens, borne in late summer to early autumn.

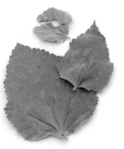

Dried leaves
These contain mucilage and can be infused and drunk for internal inflammation or used externally as an eye compress.

Leaf
Large, velvety, toothed, tear-shaped and gray-green, containing mucilage.

Lifespan
Hardy herbaceous perennial

Height
6 feet

Stem
Velvety, round and light green.

Dried root
Contains a highly valued thickening and softening mucilage.

Root
Thick, long, yellow-brown and tapering, with white fibrous flesh. To release mucilage, steep second- or subsequent-year roots in cold water for 8 hours.

CULTIVATION

Site Full sun.
Soil Moist, moderate fertility.
Propagating Sow in spring. Divide base or try stem cuttings in spring.
Growing Thin or transplant to 1 foot apart; in second season, thin again to 2 feet apart. Not suitable for growing indoors.
Harvesting Collect seeds when ripe. Pick leaves as required and dig up roots in autumn.
Preserving Dry seeds and leaves. Scrape and dry roots or make into syrup (see p. 242).

USES

Decorative
● *Leaf* Add to posies.

Culinary
● *Seed* Eat fresh "cheeses" alone or sprinkled like nuts on salads.
● *Flower* Toss on salads.
● *Leaf* Mix young leaves into salads. Add to oil and vinegar. Steam and serve as a vegetable.
● *Root* Boil to soften, then fry.

Cosmetic
● *Leaf and root* Boil leaves or use the liquid from steeped root, warmed or cold, as a soothing mucilage for dry hands, sunburn and dry hair, and in facial steams, masks and lotions. Make into an eye compress to soften skin around eyes.

Medicinal
● *Root* Infuse as a tea for coughs, diarrhea and insomnia. Add to ointment for burns. Put in a poultice for inflammations. Used in Persia to reduce inflammation in teething babies and to stimulate growth of late teeth. Boil root, skim off the starchy byproduct on the water surface and use as a gentle soap for problem skins, including psoriasis. Marsh mallow root powder has been used as a binding agent in pill manufacture.

Anethum graveolens

Dill Umbelliferae

"Woe unto you, scribes and Pharisees, hypocrites! for ye pay tithe of mint and dill and cumin, and have omitted the weightier matters of the law" (Matt.23:23). This biblical reference shows that herbs had a high and sufficiently stable value to be used as tax payment. Well before that, the ancient Egyptians had recorded dill as a soothing medicine, and the Greeks knew "dill stayeth the hickets" (hiccups). During the Middle Ages, it was one of the St John's Eve herbs, to be prized as protection against witchcraft. Magicians used dill in their spells, while lesser mortals infused it in wine to enhance passion. Early settlers took dill to North America, where it became known as "meetin' seed," because children were given dill seed to chew during long sermons.

Seed
Aromatic, flattish, oval, with brown, ribbed center and buff wings; contains silicic acid, calcium, phosphorus and other valuable mineral salts.

Dried leaves
These retain only a little flavor so use generously when cooking and add at the last minute.

Flower
Tiny, highly aromatic, yellow blooms, arranged in flat clusters 8 inches across, appear in midsummer.

Leaf
Aromatic, feathery, threadlike and blue-green.

Stem
Hollow, ridged, branching and blue-green; usually one main stem per plant.

Lifespan
Hardy annual

Height
2–5 feet

CULTIVATION
Site Full sun. Protect from wind.
Soil Rich and well drained.
Propagating Sow in situ from spring until midsummer. Do not plant near fennel, as they cross-pollinate and flavors muddle. Self-seeds. Seeds viable for 3–10 years.
Growing Thin to 9–12 inches apart. Can be grown indoors.
Harvesting Gather leaves when young. Pick flowering tops just as fruits begin to form. To collect seed, after flowering head turns brown, hang the whole plant over a cloth.
Preserving Dry or freeze leaves. Dry ripe seed. Make dill vinegar with flowering heads or seed.

USES
Culinary
● *Seed* Use whole or ground in soups, fish dishes, pickles, cabbage, apple pies, dill butter, cakes and breads (see p. 164). Serve seed as a digestive at the end of a rich meal.
● *Flowering top* Add one flower head per jar to pickled gherkins, cucumbers and cauliflowers (see p. 188) for a flavor stronger than dill leaves but fresher than seeds.
● *Leaf* Add finely chopped to soups, potato salads, cream cheese, eggs, salmon and grilled meats, and use as a garnish. Boil with new potatoes.

Cosmetic
● *Seed* Crush and infuse as a nail-strengthening bath. Chew to sweeten breath.

Medicinal
● *Seed* Use in a salt-free diet, as it is rich in mineral salts. Make dill water for indigestion, flatulence, hiccups, stomach cramps, insomnia and colic: infuse $\frac{1}{2}$ ounce bruised seeds in 1 cup boiling water, then strain. Take 1 tablespoon per adult or 1 teaspoon for babies. Repeat as needed. Infuse as a tea to stimulate milk of nursing mothers.

Angelica archangelica

Angelica Umbelliferae

An ancient and highly aromatic plant, angelica is praised in the folklore of northern European countries as a panacea for all ills. Its name is thought to derive from the fact that, in the old calendar, it usually came into bloom around the feast day of the Archangel Michael, the Great Defender, who appeared in a vision to explain its protective powers against evil.

Angelica is a moisture-loving native of damp meadows and river banks. Its large leaves have a tropical appearance and can give the garden a lush atmosphere.

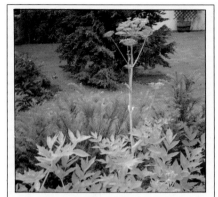

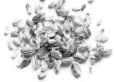

Seed
Buff, $\frac{1}{4}$ inch long, produced in profusion, ripening late summer of third year.

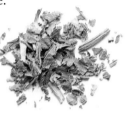

Dried leaves
These are indispensable for herb teas.

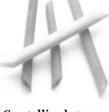

Crystallized stem
Choose fresh, young, green stems of pencil thickness for crystallizing.

Leaf
Large, glossy, divided and bright green.

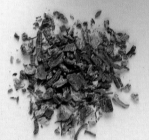

Dried root
Angelica root has the longest-lasting aroma of any part of the plant.

Stem
Thick, hollow and ridged.

Lifespan
Three-year hardy herbaceous "biennial" (extendable to four years if emerging flower spikes are removed)

Height
3–8 feet

Root
Thick, ridged, aromatic taproot, usually with two or three major side roots.

CULTIVATION

Site Light shade. Benefits from a mulch when in full sun.
Soil Deep and moist.
Propagating Allow plants to self-seed or sow fresh in early autumn. Take care when buying angelica seed; it loses most of its viability within three months.
Growing Seedlings should be transplanted in spring before the taproot becomes established. Leave about a square yard between plants.
Harvesting Cut stems before midsummer for crystallizing. Harvest leaves before flowering. Collect ripe seed in late summer. Dig up root in autumn of first year.
Preserving Dry leaves and root. Crystallize stems.

USES

Decorative
● *Flower* Display dried seed heads for a striking winter decoration.
● *Leaf* Long-stemmed leaves look attractive in a vase.

Culinary
● *Seed* Mix with stems and use to flavor drinks, including gin, vermouth and chartreuse.
● *Leaf* Stew with acidic fruits to reduce sugar requirement. Serve fresh chopped leaves mixed with mint and mayonnaise (see p. 182).
● *Stem* Crystallize for decoration.

Cosmetic
● *Leaf* Use for a relaxing bath.

Aromatic
● *Seed* Burn in a chafing dish to perfume a room.
● *Leaf* Use in potpourri.
● *Root* In spring, make an incision at the crown to yield an aromatic gum. Use as a fixative in potpourri.

Medicinal
● *Leaf* Make tea from fresh or dried leaves as a tonic for colds and to reduce flatulence. Crushed leaves freshen the air in a car and help prevent travel sickness.

Anthriscus cerefolium

Chervil Umbelliferae

In the past, the modest chervil has often been overlooked. It now enjoys increasing popularity as people discover its special, delicate parsleylike flavor with a hint of myrrh. It is one of the traditional *fines herbes*, indispensable in French cuisine, and is a fresh green asset to any meal.

A graceful clump of chervil plants will retain more flavor in its feathery foliage if grown in light shade. Viewed in an herb garden by moonlight, the clusters of tiny white flowers are like fairy dust during spring and late summer.

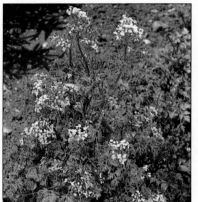

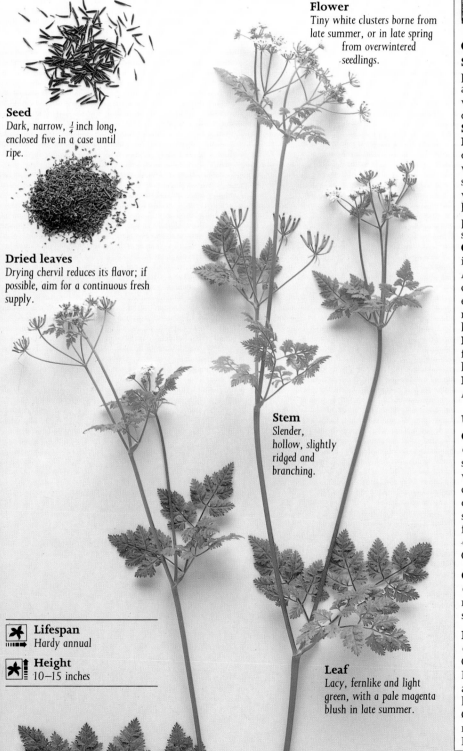

Seed
Dark, narrow, ¼ inch long, enclosed five in a case until ripe.

Dried leaves
Drying chervil reduces its flavor; if possible, aim for a continuous fresh supply.

Flower
Tiny white clusters borne from late summer, or in late spring from overwintered seedlings.

Stem
Slender, hollow, slightly ridged and branching.

Leaf
Lacy, fernlike and light green, with a pale magenta blush in late summer.

Lifespan
Hardy annual

Height
10–15 inches

CULTIVATION

Site Light shade in summer (ideally plant under a deciduous plant so autumn seedlings can enjoy full winter sun). In hot conditions, it quickly runs to seed.

Soil Light and well drained.

Propagating Ripe seed germinates quickly and can be used six to eight weeks after gathering. For a regular supply, sow monthly except in winter. Scatter on soil, press in lightly. Left to self-seed, chervil provides one early and one late summer crop.

Growing Thin seedlings to 6–9 inches apart; do not transplant. Although chervil is hardy, some cloche protection is needed to ensure leaves in winter. Chervil makes a good indoor plant, given light shade and humidity.

Harvesting Gather leaves before flowering, once the plant reaches a height of 4 inches.

Preserving Freeze or dry leaves. Also good added to vinegar.

USES

Culinary
● *Leaf* Use generously in salads, soups, sauces, vegetables, chicken, white fish and egg dishes. Add chervil freshly chopped near the end of cooking to avoid flavor loss. In small quantities, it enhances the flavor of other herbs.
● *Stem* Chop and use raw in salads. Cook in soups and casseroles.

Cosmetic
● *Leaf* Use in an infusion or face mask to cleanse skin, maintain suppleness and discourage wrinkles.

Medicinal
● *Leaf* Eat raw for additional vitamin C, carotene and some minerals. Infuse in tea to stimulate digestion and alleviate circulation disorders, liver complaints and chronic catarrh. Chervil is traditionally taken for its restorative qualities after Lent on Holy Thursday.

Apium graveolens

Smallage/Wild celery Umbelliferae

Smallage was used to crown the victors of the Greek Nemean games, held in honor of Zeus. The son of the Nemean king was subsequently killed by a snake concealed in smallage, and so it was then carried as a funeral wreath. The Greeks also used this herb medicinally, and the Romans exploited its culinary properties: stems were puréed with pepper, lovage, oregano, onion and wine; leaves were used with dates and pine nuts as a stuffing for suckling pig. Much later, in the nineteenth century, the American Shakers grew smallage for their nostrums and other medicinal compounds.

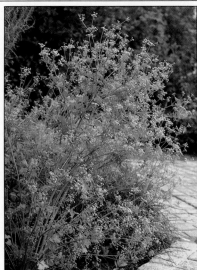

Seed
Tiny, brown, oval
and aromatic.

Flower
Small, greenish-cream clusters
produced in late summer
of second year.

Dried leaves
These have a slightly stronger
aromatic flavor than
cultivated celery and are
useful in soups, stocks,
stuffings and stews.

Leaf
Fan of aromatic,
loosely toothed,
shiny light green leaflets,
forming upright rosette
in first year; darker
green on rising stem in
second season.

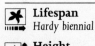 **Lifespan**
Hardy biennial

Height
1–3 feet

Stem
Faceted, ridged,
branching and green;
flowering stem grows
in second season.

CULTIVATION
Site Sunny with midday shade. Shelter from strong winds.
Soil Rich, moist and well drained.
Propagating Sow under heat in early spring or outdoors in late spring. Germination is slow.
Growing Transplant or thin to 16 inches apart. Smallage is not suitable for growing indoors.
Harvesting Pick leaves in late summer or as needed. Collect seeds when ripe.
Preserving Dry seed. Dry or freeze leaves or infuse in vinegar.

USES
Culinary
● **Seed** Grind as an ingredient of celery salt. Add to soups, curries, casseroles and pickles. Use as a salt substitute in a salt-free diet.
● **Leaf** Chop small amounts into salads, cream cheese, poultry stuffings, and use as a garnish. Add a handful of finely chopped leaves to milk for poaching fish and shellfish. Stir into thick vegetable soups and stews during last 3 minutes of cooking to retain flavor and nutritive value.

Medicinal
● **Seed** Decoct as a sedative to calm nerves, promote restfulness, ease flatulence and some kidney disorders.
● **Leaf** Rich in vitamins, mineral salts and other active ingredients of nutritive value. Smallage is reported to contain a hormone which has an effect similar to insulin, and is considered a useful seasoning for diabetics. Infuse as a tonic and appetizer and to ease indigestion and colic.
● **Leaf and stem** Extract juice and drink as a urine stimulant.

Armoracia rusticana

Horseradish Cruciferae

Originally, horseradish was cultivated chiefly as a medicinal herb. Now it is considered a flavoring herb. In the late sixteenth century, its culinary use was developed by the Germans and Danes in a fish sauce. Around 1640, this usage spread westward to Britain, where horseradish sauce has since become strongly associated with roast beef. Its sharp pungency frequently has a dramatic effect and has been known to clear sinuses in one breath – the volatile flavoring oil is released by grating the root. The oil evaporates rapidly, so horseradish is not successful in cooked dishes.

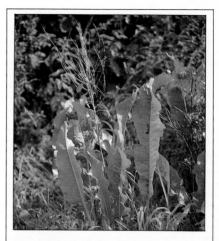

Leaf
Large, elliptical, pointed, scallop-edged and bright green, with pungent aroma when bruised.

Dried leaves
These yield a yellow dye with a chrome mordant; may be used to dress skin wounds.

Stem
Thick, deeply ridged and round.

Root
Long, invasive and yellow with hot, pungent-tasting white flesh. Fresh root contains calcium, sodium, magnesium and vitamin C, and has antibiotic qualities that are useful for preserving food and protecting the intestinal tract.

✳ Lifespan
Hardy perennial

✳ Height
2–3 feet

CULTIVATION
Site Open sunny position.
Soil Light, well-dug, rich and moist soil preferred.
Propagating Sow seed, divide roots or take root cuttings (thongs) in spring. Choose roots about ½ inch thick. Cut into pieces 6 inches long, and plant vertically in soil, at a depth of 2 inches.
Growing Thin out or transplant to 12 inches apart. Do not grow indoors.
Harvesting Dig up roots as needed or in autumn. Pick young leaves.
Preserving Store roots in sand; or wash, grate or slice and dry; or immerse whole washed roots in white wine vinegar. Dry leaves.

USES
Culinary
● *Leaf* Add young leaves to salads.
● *Root* Make horseradish sauce to accompany roast beef, smoked or oily fish. Grate into coleslaw, dips, pickled beets, cream cheese, mayonnaise and avocado fillings.

Household
● *Whole plant* Grow near potatoes for more disease-resistant tubers.
● *Root* Infuse, dilute four times and spray apple trees against brown rot.
● *Leaf* Chop finely into dogfood to dispel worms and improve body tone. Boil for a deep yellow dye.

Cosmetic
● *Root* Slice and infuse in milk for a lotion to improve skin clarity. Express juice, mix with white vinegar and use to lighten freckles.

Medicinal
● *Root* Include grated root in diet to stimulate digestion, eliminate mucus and waste fluids. Take as a syrup for bronchitis and coughs. Grate into a poultice and apply to chilblains, stiff muscles, sciatica and rheumatism.

Note: *Avoid continuous large doses when pregnant or suffering from kidney problems.*

Artemisia species

Artemisias Compositae

Artemisia was the sister and wife of the Greek/Persian King Mausolus and ruled after his death in 353 B.C. In his honor she built a magnificent tomb called the Mausoleum, which was one of the seven wonders of the ancient world. She was also a famous botanist and medical researcher, and this genus of 200 mostly aromatic plants was named in her honor.

The medicinal values of artemisias were discovered by people living in semiarid and temperate regions where the plants are found. In the ancient Greek text of Dioscorides, wormwood is mentioned for its internal worm-expelling property. Indians from New Mexico to British Columbia use similar varieties to treat bronchitis and colds. The Chinese still use a leaf of wormwood rolled up in the nostril to stop nosebleeds. Many artemisias are also visually appealing. Their silver leaves are stunning when reflected in moonlight, and they also enhance any dried herb arrangement.

Mugwort, though less aromatic and attractive than other artemisias, features in the magical lore of Europe, Asia and China. In the pre-Christian "Lay of the Nine Herbs," the first incantation for protection is to mugwort, the "mother of herbs":

Have in mind, Mugwort, what you made known,
What you laid down, at the great denouncing.
Una your name is, oldest of herbs,
Of might against thirty, and against three,
Of might against venom and the onflying,
Of might against the vile She
who fares through the land.

Leaf
Aromatic, deeply indented and gray-green, covered with fine silky hairs.

Leaf
Aromatic, threadlike, gray-green and semievergreen.

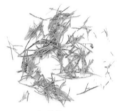

Dried leaves
Use as a sweet-scented insect repellent and in potpourri.

Seed
Tiny, taupe color, tear-shaped; contained in slightly flattened, gray, cylindrical fruit.

**A. abrotanum
Southernwood/
Old Man**
The sweetest perennial artemisia with its hint of lemon – evocative of childhood gardens.

Stem
Slightly ridged and green when young; smooth, woody and tan when mature.

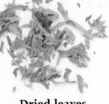

Dried leaves
These retain their aroma. Both leaves and flowering tops have medicinal and household uses.

Stem
Aromatic, downy, ridged and gray-green.

Leaf
Indented and mid-green, with dense, cottony silver underside.

Stem
Slightly hairy, ridged, reddish and herbaceous.

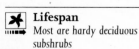 **Lifespan**
Most are hardy deciduous subshrubs

Height
2–4 feet

**A. absinthium
Wormwood**
The most bitter herb after rue. 'Lambrooke Silver' has more silvery leaves; 'Faith Ravens' has leaves that are more divided.

**A. vulgaris
Mugwort**

OTHER SPECIES

A. pontica
Roman wormwood
Spreading rootstalk and strongly aromatic, feathery silver foliage. Used to flavor vermouth.

A. lanata
(A. pedemontana)
Tufted, 4 inches high mat-forming evergreen clumps with silky, finely cut silver leaves.

A. arborescens
Tree artemisia
Half hardy, with finely cut, tufted, semievergreen silky foliage. Ht: 3½ feet.

A. campestris sp. borealis
(A. canadensis)
Delicate, silver, filamentlike, semi-evergreen leaves with weak scent.

A. ludoviciana
'Silver King'
Silver king artemisia
Herbaceous; spreading rootstalk and willow-like, very silvery leaves.

A. lactiflora
White mugwort
Herbaceous form with plumes of fragrant cream flowers in late summer and deeply cut mid-green leaves, 6 inches long. Ht: 5 feet.

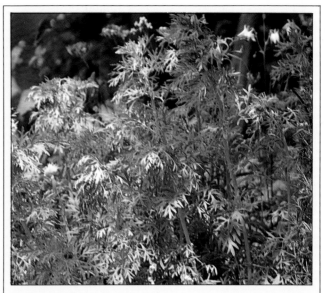

A bed of tall, silver-green wormwood.

CULTIVATION

Site Full sun.
Soil Light, dry, well drained. However, *A. lactiflora* requires moist soil and will tolerate some shade.
Propagating Sow when available. Take semihardwood cuttings in late summer.
Growing Thin out or transplant shrubby artemisias to 18 inches–3 feet apart. Do not plant wormwood next to fennel, sage, caraway, anise and possibly other culinary and medicinal herbs, as rain washes a growth-inhibiting toxin out of the leaves that affects nearby plants. For winter protection, prune all forms except southernwood in autumn. Prune southernwood in summer. Artemisias are not suitable for indoor culture.
Harvesting Pick flowering tops and leaves in mid- to late summer for medicinal use.
Preserving Dry leaves and flowering tops.

USES

Decorative
● *Leaf* (Southernwood) Plant for a neat hedge. (Wormwood) Grow for a fast temporary hedge. Pick all silver forms for bouquets, wreaths and nosegays.

Culinary
● *Leaf* (Mugwort) Use in stuffings for roast goose.

Household
● *Leaf* Powder or infuse to make a moth repellent. Deter onion and carrot fly with branches laid between onion and carrot rows. When walked on, wormwood's pungent aroma masks carrot scent. Infuse to make a strong domestic disinfectant; mix a weaker infusion for an effective insecticide on older plants. Grow southernwood or wormwood near hen houses for protection against lice; near cabbages to deter cabbage butterfly; and near fruit trees to deter fruit tree moth. Hang leaves in a granary to dispel beetles.

Medicinal
● *Leaf* (Southernwood) Infuse as a tea for a tonic. (Mugwort) Dried leaves (moxa) are made into small cones for use in moxibustion (the Chinese practice of leaves smoldering on the skin to give deep penetrating heat) to soothe rheumatism. Use aromatic species for a disinfectant and antiseptic.

Note: *Wormwood is toxic and should not be taken internally.*

Artemisia dracunculus

Tarragon Compositae

To be connected with dragons is an honor worthy of this important culinary herb, its name tarragon deriving from the French *estragon* and the Latin *dracunculus*, a little dragon. The dragon connection may have come from tarragon's fiery tang or from its serpent-like roots. "Dragon" herbs were believed to cure the bites of venomous creatures, but tarragon's primary use today is culinary. It will also sweeten the breath, act as a soporific, and, if chewed before taking medicine, dull the taste, according to the thirteenth-century Arabian botanist, Ibnal Baithar. Two varieties of tarragon are available: French, which has the refined flavor indispensable to classic French cuisine but needs winter protection when growing; and Russian, which survives both colder and hotter climates but has a coarser flavor. French tarragon should be divided and replanted every third year to avoid deterioration, whereas the flavor of Russian tarragon improves the longer it grows in one place.

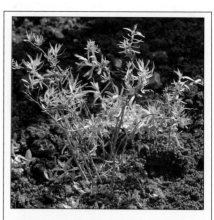

Flower
May develop little, ball-shaped, greenish-white flowers. Only Russian tarragon sets seed in temperate climates.

Dried leaves
These retain a little flavor if carefully dried, but often hay-like overtones develop.

A. dracunculoides
Russian tarragon
Bitter flavor, lacking aniseed subtleties and aroma. Narrower and paler leaves than French tarragon. Ht: 5 feet.

A. dracunculus
French tarragon

Stem
Ridged, round, branching and light green, becoming brown and brittle near base.

Leaf
Glossy, long, narrow and green, with oil glands on the underside which release a bitter-sweet, warm, peppery scent with an anise undertone.

✱ Lifespan
Hardy to a few degrees of frost; perennial

✱ Height
2–3 feet

Root
Light brown, brittle, fleshy, spreading rhizome with hairlike roots.

CULTIVATION
Site Sunny and sheltered.
Soil Rich, light and dry.
Propagating Divide roots in spring. Take stem cuttings in summer. (Russian tarragon) Sow in spring.
Growing Thin or transplant to 12–18 inches apart. Cut back in autumn. Protect in winter with straw or similar mulch. Tarragon is suitable for growing indoors.
Harvesting Pick leaves anytime, but in late summer for main crop. If cutting branches, sever maximum of two-thirds of branch to allow for regrowth, unless it is the end of the growing season.
Preserving Freeze leaves or dry quickly at 80 °F. Infuse leaves in oil or vinegar.

USES
Culinary
● **Leaf** Use sparingly for a warm, subtle, highly desirable flavor, which diffuses quickly through other ingredients (see p. 165). Tarragon is an important part of *fines herbes*, together with chervil and parsley. Use it to make tarragon vinegar and vinegar blends, for Béarnaise, tartar and hollandaise sauces. Add shredded leaf to avocado fillings, mayonnaise for fish dishes, salad dressings, light soups, tomatoes, omelettes and scrambled eggs. Make an herb butter for vegetables, steaks, chops and grilled fish. Rub tarragon onto roast chicken or mix with chicken stuffing. Add to preserves, pickles and mustards. Freeze in ice cubes for interesting flavor in cold drinks. (Russian tarragon) Used by Persians on grilled meat.

Medicinal
● **Leaf** Tarragon leaves are rich in iodine, mineral salts, vitamins A and C. Infuse as an appetite stimulant, digestive and general tonic. In the past, it was used against scurvy.
● **Root** Used to cure toothache.

Borago officinalis

Borage *Boragninaceae*

The common thread running through historical descriptions of borage is its ability to make men and women glad and merry, to comfort the heart, dispel melancholy and give courage. The Celtic name *borrach* meant courage and the Welsh name *Llawenlys* translates as herb of gladness. According to Dioscorides and Pliny, borage was the famed *nepenthe* of Homer, a herb wine that brought absolute forgetfulness.

The flowers are a beautiful pure blue often chosen by Old Masters to paint the Madonna's robe. Flowers were embroidered on fine medieval tapestries and on scarves for tournament jousters. They were included in the page borders of herbals and Books of Hours. For courage, they were floated in the stirrup-cups given to Crusaders at their departure. The noble qualities of borage may derive from its high content of calcium, potassium and mineral salts, and research suggests borage works on the adrenal gland, where courage begins.

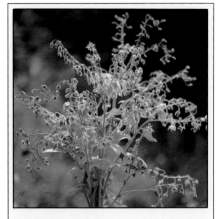

CULTIVATION
Site Open sunny position.
Soil Light and dry, well drained.
Propagating Seed on site or singly in pots in spring for summer flowers; autumn for spring flowers. Self-sows freely on light soils.
Growing Set out 12 inches apart. Plant among roses or summer prune to keep tidy. Possible to grow small plants indoors.
Harvesting Pick flowers and leaves.
Preserving Dry flowers; freeze in ice cubes; crystallize.

USES
Decorative
● *Flower* String together as a necklace. Add to summer arrangements.

Culinary
● *Flower* Sprinkle in salads and as a garnish; crystallize for cake decorations.
● *Young leaf* Add to cold drinks (claret cup, Pimm's No.1) for their cucumber flavor and cooling effect. Chop finely in salads, yogurt, soft cheese, pickles and sandwiches. Cook as spinach or with spinach. Add to ravioli stuffing.

Household
● *Flower* Attracts bees to gardens.
● *Whole plant* Plant near strawberries, as they stimulate each other's growth. May control tomato worm if planted near tomatoes. When burned, the nitrate of potash content will emit sparks and slight explosive sounds, like fireworks.

Cosmetic
● *Leaf* Add to a face pack for dry skin. Mix with barley and bran in a bath bag to cleanse and soften skin.

Medicinal
● *Leaf* Use in a salt-free diet as rich in mineral salts. A poultice soothes inflammation and bruises.
● *Seed* Early research suggests the presence of gamma-linoleic acid (see evening primrose, p. 102).

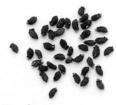

Seed
Largish, brown-black, tri-sided and lozenge-shaped; often viable for up to eight years.

Flower
Sky blue (sometimes pink, rarely white), five-petalled stars with prominent black stamen tips nod downward in clusters at the tip of the stem.

Leaf
Dark gray-green, oval-pointed, textured, covered with prickly white hairs. Cucumber-scented juice when crushed.

Stem
Sturdy, hollow, round, branching, with prickly white hairs. Cucumber-scented juice.

Flower heads
Pick off by grasping the black stamen tips and gently separating the flower from its green back.

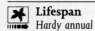
Lifespan
Hardy annual

Height
1 foot–2 feet 6 inches

Herbs for flowers and foliage

Over the last 200 years, many herbs, particularly the medicinal plants, dropped out of common usage but continued to be grown in gardens. This may have been for reasons of nostalgia or traditional associations, but more likely because they are pretty garden plants that are easy to care for. Eventually their herbal connections were forgotten; now many people are surprised to discover what useful attributes some of their favorite flowers have. It is fortunate that the cultivation of these herbs continued; occasionally a new discovery is made and a once forgotten herb is suddenly in demand. Feverfew is one such case. After research into migraines publicized its ability to reduce pain, a few gardeners were able to offer seedlings for large-scale cultivation.

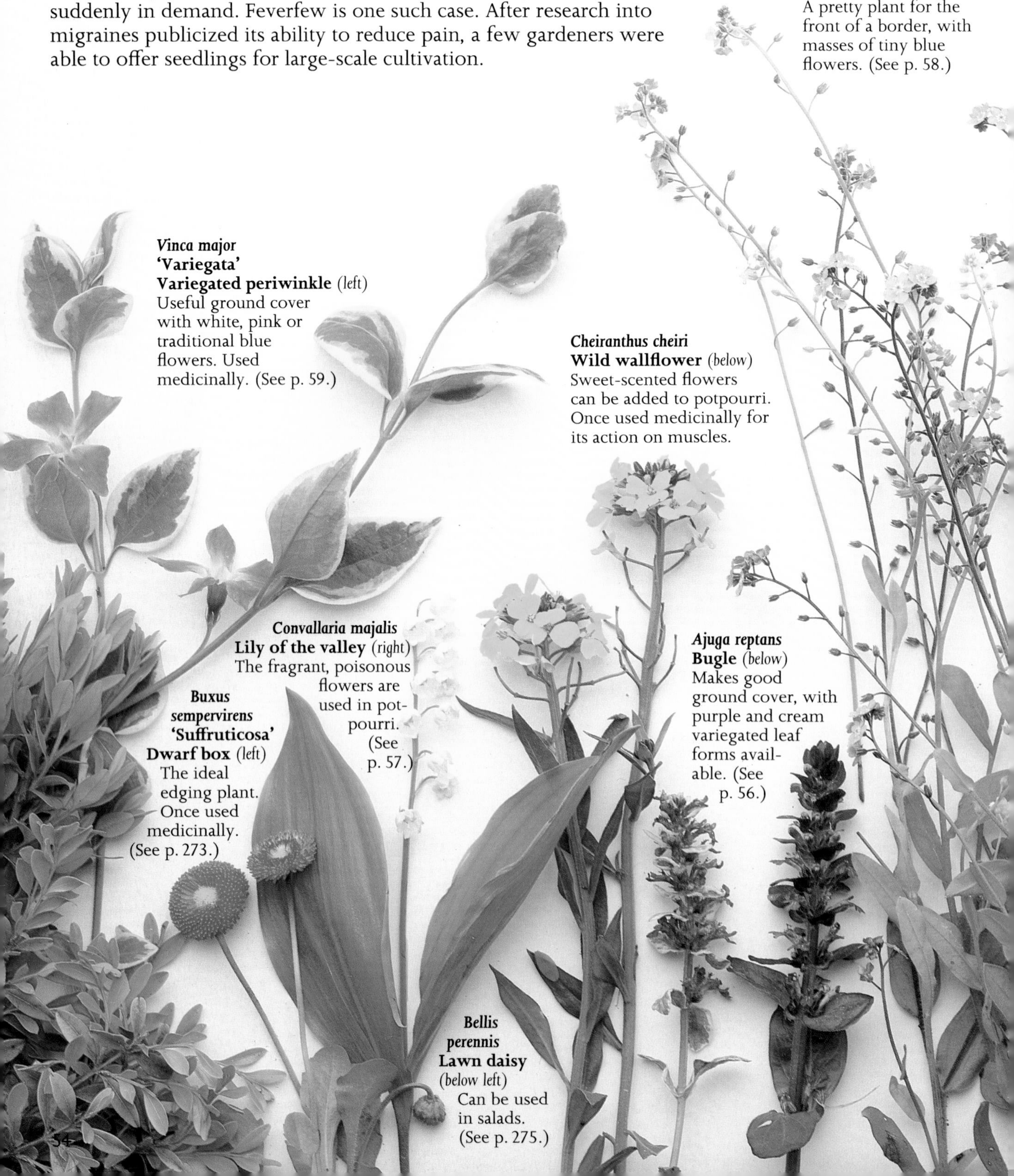

Myosotis sylvatica
Forget-me-not (below)
A pretty plant for the front of a border, with masses of tiny blue flowers. (See p. 58.)

Vinca major
'Variegata'
Variegated periwinkle (left)
Useful ground cover with white, pink or traditional blue flowers. Used medicinally. (See p. 59.)

Cheiranthus cheiri
Wild wallflower (below)
Sweet-scented flowers can be added to potpourri. Once used medicinally for its action on muscles.

Convallaria majalis
Lily of the valley (right)
The fragrant, poisonous flowers are used in potpourri. (See p. 57.)

Buxus sempervirens
'Suffruticosa'
Dwarf box (left)
The ideal edging plant. Once used medicinally. (See p. 273.)

Ajuga reptans
Bugle (below)
Makes good ground cover, with purple and cream variegated leaf forms available. (See p. 56.)

Bellis perennis
Lawn daisy
(below left)
Can be used in salads. (See p. 275.)

54

Hedera helix
Ivy (*right*)
There are many attractive leaf forms
available. The ancient Greeks
thought ivy prevented
intoxication; it is now
used cosmetically.

Aquilegia vulgaris
Columbine (*right*)
The essence of a
cottage garden. Its
flowers, leaves, seeds
and root were once
used medicinally.
(See p. 56.)

Lamium maculatum
Dead nettle (*below*)
Attractive ground cover with white,
pink, peach or mauve flower
forms, and variegated
or silver leaves.
(See p. 58.)

Cardamine pratensis
Lady's-smock (*below*)
Also called cuckoo-
flower, because it
flowers when the
cuckoo returns.
Flower supplies food
for butterflies.
(See p. 57.)

Pulmonaria officinalis
Lungwort (*below*)
The decorative spotted
leaves were once thought
to resemble lungs, and so
were used for lung ailments.
(See p. 59.)

55

Herbs for flowers and foliage

Ajuga reptans
Bugle <small>Labiatae</small>

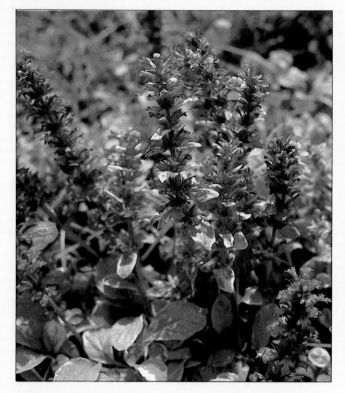

A low-growing, creeping perennial, cultivated mainly for its decorative foliage. The oval leaves are dark-green with a purplish tinge, although both multi-colored and variegated forms are available. It bears blue tubular flowers on short spikes from late spring throughout the summer. Some forms produce pink or even white flowers. Bugle is an excellent ground-cover plant, growing to a height of 4–6 inches. It needs partial shade, making it suitable for planting under taller flowering shrubs, near hedging or a trellis.

CULTIVATION
Sow seed in moist, fertile soil in autumn or spring. Propagate by dividing runners and planting out in autumn or spring at 1 foot intervals, to allow space for spreading.

USES
A reliable garden plant because of its eager growth and pretty flowers and foliage. In the past, bugle was a very popular herbal remedy. Among its many applications, it was made into an ointment for bruises, and a lotion of bugle, honey and alum was recommended for mouth sores. An infusion of dried leaves and boiling water is thought to lower blood pressure and stop internal bleeding. It is also believed to have a mildly narcotic effect.

Aquilegia vulgaris
Columbine <small>Ranunculaceae</small>

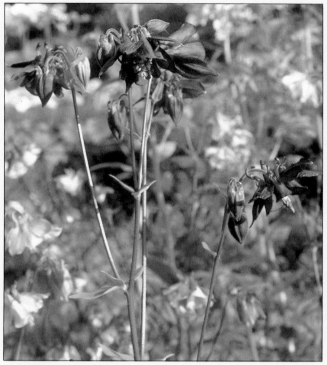

This dainty and elegant border perennial has been a garden favorite for over 300 years. It grows to a height of 2–3 feet with thin, erect flower stems that are topped by a loose head of drooping, funnel-shaped flowers in late spring and early summer. The old-fashioned columbine produces blue, pink, or white flowers, but cultivated forms are available in a variety of eyecatching colors. Each of the flower's five petals has a prominent spur, resembling an eagle's talon. Hence the plant's botanical name *aquilegia* from the Latin word *aquila*, meaning "eagle." In spring the gray-green, ferny leaves are tinged with pink. While columbine tolerates a sunny, open area of the garden it is happiest in partial shade.

CULTIVATION
Sow seeds at 1 foot intervals during spring, in the flowering site, or divide clumps in autumn or spring. Soil should be fertile and fairly alkaline. Water well in dry weather, and cut the stems down after flowering.

USES
Today the columbine owes its place in the herb garden solely to its beauty and grace. Once made into an astringent lotion, it is now known to be slightly poisonous and so is no longer used.

Cardamine pratensis
Lady's-smock Cruciferae

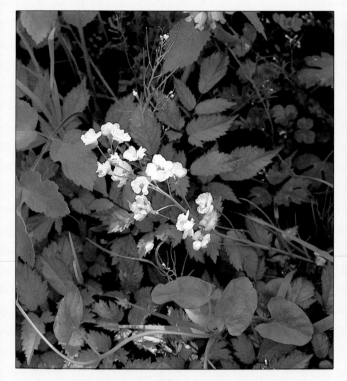

Once commonly found growing wild in moist meadowland, lady's-smock is seen less frequently now that fewer meadows are left undrained. The slender flower stalks can grow to 16 inches in height and have dark-green oval leaves that resemble the leaves of bittercress, to which it is related. It bears flowers of such a pale pink or lilac that they appear white at first glance. A double-flowered form is available which has a longer flowering period. It is also known as the cuckoo-flower because it flowers at the same time of the year as the cuckoo is heard. Plant lady's-smock in the shade of a tree, a wall or a fence where the ground is damp.

CULTIVATION
Sow seeds in early autumn in moist soil, and water in well. Propagate by placing a leaf, taken from the base of the stem, on moist compost, where it will soon grow roots. Divide clump in spring or autumn.

USES
Lady's-smock will grow vigorously in a damp, shady part of the garden. In the eighteenth century it was recommended for scurvy, and has since been found to contain vitamin C. It also has expectorant properties, making it a useful ingredient in cough remedies. The leaves taste rather like watercress and make a welcome addition to a springtime salad.

Convallaria majalis
Lily of the valley Liliaceae

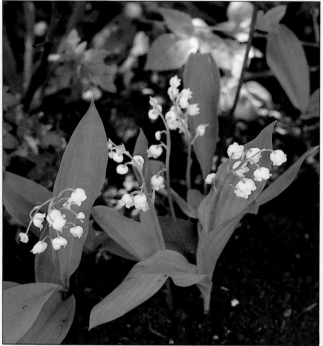

A hardy perennial that grows from creeping, horizontal rhizomes, or underground stems, lily of the valley is an important plant in the herb garden as much for its characteristic sweet scent as for the beauty of its small, white, bell-shaped flowers which appear in late spring. The flowers are borne on a slender, arched stem about 6–8 inches high between a pair of large, lance-shaped, mid-green leaves. Lily of the valley grows well in moist soil in the dappled shade of deciduous trees.

CULTIVATION
Divide clumps in early autumn, then plant 6 inches apart in well-drained soil with plenty of compost added. Place the clumps so that the point where the leaves emerge from the rhizomes is just below the surface of the soil.

USES
A plant that spreads quickly in the right conditions, its leaves provide dense ground cover until winter. The flowers have traditionally formed part of a bridal bouquet. An infusion made from the whole plant can act as a diuretic as well as slowing the pace of the heart. It is said to be a safer though weaker cardiac tonic than foxglove, but it should only be used by medical personnel.

Herbs for flowers and foliage

Lamium maculatum and species
Dead nettle Labiatae

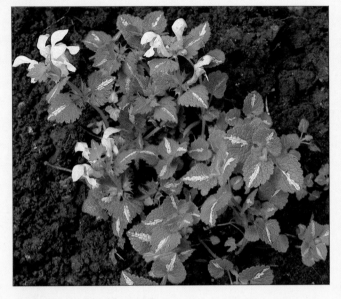

Myosotis sylvatica
Forget-me-not Boraginaceae

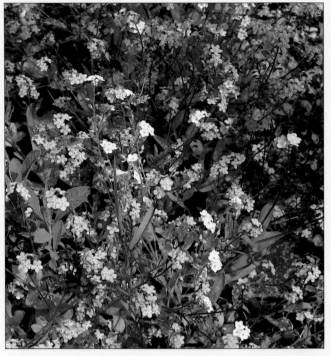

So-named because of its strong resemblance to the stinging nettle, the dead nettle is totally unrelated and its leaves have no sting. It can be distinguished from the stinging nettle, even before its clusters of tubular white, yellow, pink or purple flowers appear, by its squarer, hollow stem. The leaves are heart-shaped at the base, and those of the purple dead nettle have a purple tinge, with an irregular white stripe in some species. Because in England it first flowers around the day dedicated in the old calendar to the Archangel Michael, 8 May, the dead nettle is also commonly called archangel. It is an important nectar plant for bees, particularly the white dead nettle which, in some areas, can be found in flower in late autumn.

CULTIVATION
Dead nettles grow well in most soils. Sow seeds for white and purple species in spring, for yellow species in autumn, and barely cover with soil. Or divide yellow dead nettle plants in early spring. White and purple species prefer full sun, although the yellow dead nettle will tolerate deep shade. Avoid planting in herbaceous borders, where it may spread too vigorously. Cut after flowering for good leaf cover.

USES
An adaptable plant, which provides long-flowering ground cover for wild areas of the garden. It has long been thought to have astringent properties. A decoction of the flowers was sometimes prescribed as a blood purifier. Bruised leaves applied to the skin were said to staunch bleeding, while dried leaves were made into a tea to encourage perspiration. The leaves have occasionally been used in soups or eaten as vegetables in parts of France and Sweden.

An edging or rock-garden plant, the forget-me-not provides a dense carpet of blue, fragrant flowers mid- to late spring. It has oblong, tapering mid-green leaves below open sprays of small salver-shaped flowers. Easy to grow, the forget-me-not thrives in the shade of other springtime flowers such as tulips or wallflowers. Myosotis sylvatica, a short-lived perennial, can grow to a height of 12 inches, so makes a striking display in a bed of its own and is attractive viewed by moonlight.

CULTIVATION
Sow seeds in late spring. Plant out 6 inches apart in autumn in any well-drained soil. Do not allow the soil to dry out.

USES
An asset to any springtime border, with its vivid blue flowers and delicate fragrance. Myosotis is used in a homeopathic remedy for respiratory problems, particularly in Europe, where it is sometimes made into a syrup for pulmonary disorders. The juice of the forget-me-not was believed to harden steel. In flower language, a man who gave a woman a bunch of roses entwined with forget-me-nots and lemon grass is offering her words of love.

Pulmonaria officinalis
Lungwort Boraginaceae

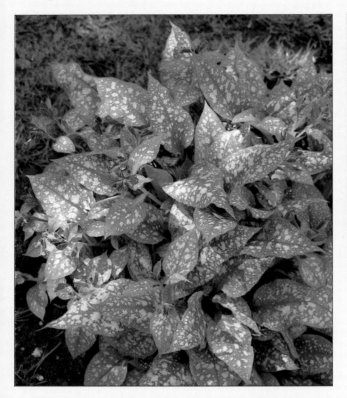

Lungwort is a hardy herbaceous perennial, often cultivated for its ornamental, white-spotted oval leaves. Growing to a height of about 12 inches, it bears clusters of funnel-shaped flowers in mid- to late spring. As they open, the flowers change from pink to purplish-blue. An old cottage-garden favorite, commonly known as Jerusalem cowslip, lungwort thrives in the shade of trees and shrubs.

CULTIVATION
Seed can be sown outdoors in any soil in spring, but better plants are produced by dividing and replanting roots in a shady position during late autumn months. Water frequently in dry weather, and cut the stems back in autumn.

USES
The leaves of this rapidly spreading plant provide ideal ground cover for shady parts of the garden. Its name derives from the fact that its leaves resemble lungs and lungwort has long been thought to be effective in pulmonary disorders. Chesty coughs, wheezing and shortness of breath were thought to benefit from an infusion of the dried leaves. It is now sometimes prescribed by herbalists for diarrhea.

Vinca major
Greater periwinkle Apocynaceae

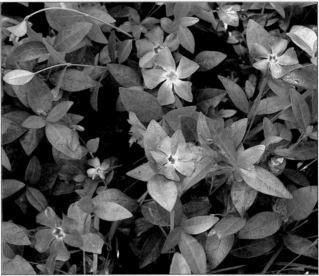

An evergreen, spreading perennial, the greater periwinkle's large, glossy, egg-shaped leaves occur in pairs on the stem. From midspring to early summer it bears purplish-blue, tubular flowers, each with five petals that open out flat. Sometimes more flowers appear in early autumn. The plant extends itself by long, trailing and rooting stems, making it invasive if planted in a border. The botanical name *vinca* comes from the Latin *vincaper vinca*, meaning "to bind," and these roots make it an excellent choice for sloping ground, where they serve to bind the soil.

CULTIVATION
Periwinkles will grow in any ordinary, well-drained soil. Take stem sections 6 inches long and plant in partial shade in early autumn or early spring. Or divide and replant in the autumn. *Vinca minor* is a more hardy species.

USES
Most attractive year-round ground cover for partially shaded areas of the garden, with the bonus of perhaps two flowerings a year. An old name for the periwinkle was sorcerer's violet, when it was an important constituent of charms and love philters, and was believed to have the power to exorcize evil spirits. Wrapped around the affected part of the body, the periwinkle was also believed to cure cramps. Its astringent and tonic properties were thought to staunch hemorrhaging, and an ointment of bruised leaves and lard was used for treating inflammatory skin conditions. However, today herbalists use the greater periwinkle mainly in the treatment of diabetes. It is related to the plant known as rose periwinkle, which is being used in the treatment of leukemia, but it should not be used in home remedies.

Mustard *Cruciferae*

Known since prehistoric times, mustard's uses have always been manifold: the writer Pliny, in the first century A.D., listed 40 remedies with mustard as chief ingredient. The Romans also named this herb: from *mustus*, the new wine they mixed with the seed, and *ardens* for fiery. They served mustard with every imaginable dish. Its leaves are so fast growing that it was said you could grow the salad for dinner while the meat was roasting. Belief in its aphrodisiac powers ensured mustard's inclusion in love potions. Black mustard seed has the strongest flavor, brown is easier to harvest, and white mustard seed is the most preservative.

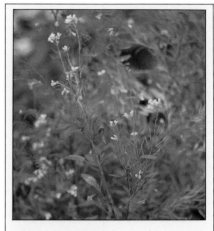

Flower
Yellow, four-petalled blooms, in small clusters, borne in midsummer; contain mild mustard flavor.

Seed (Brown mustard)
Small, mid- to dark brown, bitter-tasting spheres in upright, smooth pods. Flavor is released only when ground and mixed with a liquid. Brown mustard is less pungent than black mustard.

Seed (White mustard)
Light cream, spherical seeds, which taste bitter, in horizontal, hairy pods. Slightly hairy, light green leaves.
Ht: 12–18 inches.

Stem
Smooth, round, hard, branching and mid-green.

B. juncea
Brown mustard
Ht: 2–4 feet

Leaf
Oval, pointed and dark green with mid-green undersides and pungent flavor. Lower leaves are toothed.

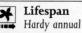 **Lifespan**
Hardy annual

Height
1–8 feet

CULTIVATION
Site Sunny. Benefits from light shade in summer to prevent bolting.
Soil Fertile and well drained.
Propagating Sow in spring for seed crop, or every 3 weeks throughout year for salad greens.
Growing Thin to 6 inches for seed crop. It is not necessary to thin salad crops. Can be grown indoors.
Harvesting Gather flowers as they open. Pick seed pods before they open in late summer. Cut salad leaves 8–10 days after sowing. Pick single leaves on older plants.
Preserving Dry seed in pods or infuse in vinegar. Dry leaves.

USES
Culinary
● *Seed* (Black or brown mustard) Make into mustard sauce: add ground seed or powder to cold water to activate enzymes; leave paste for 10 minutes before use. (White mustard) Use in pickles, as a strong preservative, and in mayonnaise as an emulsifier.
● *Flower* Sprinkle on sandwiches. Toss into salads.
● *Leaf* Mix young leaves into salads.

Household
● *Seed* To clean odorous cooking pots: put in a few bruised seeds, swish with water and rinse well.

Cosmetic
● *Seed* Rub pulverized seed onto hands as a deodorizer; rinse off after 2 minutes.

Medicinal
● *Seed* Take 1 tablespoon crushed in warm water to induce vomiting. Use powdered to make a poultice to draw blood to skin or lungs, and to relieve pain and inflammation in rheumatism, arthritis, congested lungs and chilblains. Add to a foot bath to warm and deodorize feet and relieve colds.

Note: *Mustard seed can irritate tender skins.*

Calendula officinalis

Calendula/Marigold Compositae

One of the most versatile herbs, calendula is popular as a cheerful cottage garden flower; for its use in cosmetic and culinary recipes; as a dye plant and for its many healing properties.

As this hardy annual seems to be in flower continuously, it attracted a botanic name which reflects the belief that it was always in bloom on the first day of each month (Latin: *kalends*). The regular supply of petals and young leaves contributed to its frequent use. Ancient Egyptians valued it as a rejuvenating herb. Hindus used it to decorate temple altars and Persians and Greeks garnished and flavored food with its golden petals. In Europe it has long been used to flavor soups and stews, and to color butter and cheese.

It is a soothing antiseptic and an excellent skin healer, especially for cracked skin and chapped lips. In the American Civil War, doctors on the battlefield employed the leaves to treat open wounds.

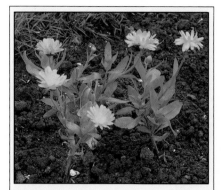

CULTIVATION
Site Sunny position.
Soil Fine loam but tolerates most soils, except waterlogged.
Propagating Sow seed in spring in situ or singly in pots.
Growing Plant out 12–18 inches apart. Deadhead for continuous flowers.
Harvesting Pick flowers when open, leaves when young.
Preserving Dry petals at low temperature to preserve color, or macerate in oil.

USES
Decorative
● **Flower** Dry petals to add color to potpourri.

Culinary
● **Flower** Use petals lavishly to give saffron color and a light tangy flavor (not saffron flavor) to rice, fish and meat soups, soft cheese, yogurt, butter, omelettes, milk dishes, cakes and sweet breads. Add 1 teaspoon petals to fish and venison. Garnish meat platters, pâté, fruit salad.
● **Leaf** Sprinkle in salads and stews.

Household
● **Flower** Boil for a pale yellow dye.

Cosmetic
● **Flower** Add petals to creams and baths for cleansing, healing and softening the skin.

Medicinal
● **Flower** Soothing, healing and antiseptic. Use in ointments for leg ulcers, varicose veins, bedsores and bruises. Take in an infusion to aid digestion and promote bile production in the liver (helpful for alcoholics). Make into a healing mouthwash for gums after tooth extraction. Calendula oil is extracted from the petals by maceration. It is healing and rejuvenating, used in many skin preparations and in aromatherapy. In particular, soothes inflammations, chilblains, cracked nipples from breast-feeding (and it's nontoxic for baby).

Flower
2–3 inches across, golden yellow-orange petals sometimes fluted, radiating from a pronounced center.

Seed
Beige, ¼ inch long, shaped like a curved apostrophe with a knobbly backbone.

Petals
Bright orange petals have the highest concentration of active ingredients.

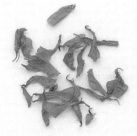

Dried petals
These keep their color well and have many uses.

Leaf
Mid-green, hairy base leaves are paddle-shaped, stem leaves are lance-shaped.

Stem
Green, succulent, angular, branching; covered with fine hairs.

Lifespan
Hardy annual

Height
12–20 inches

Carum carvi

Caraway Umbelliferae

Definitely a herb with a pedigree, caraway has been found in the remains of Stone Age meals, Egyptian tombs, and ancient caravan stops along the Silk Road. The Arabic word for the seed, *karawya*, gives us the present name, and Isaiah speaks of its culture in the Bible. In Shakespeare's *Henry IV*, Falstaff is offered a "pippin (apple) and dish of caraways," this being a traditional finish to an Elizabethan feast. Caraway has always been popular in Germany, and when Queen Victoria married Prince Albert, Britain renewed its interest in his favorite seed.

Such an ancient herb is not without its magical properties. Caraway gave protection from witches and was believed to be able to prevent departures, so it was used in love potions.

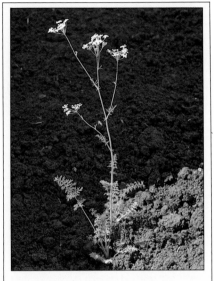

Flower
Minute white flowerheads borne in midsummer.

Stem
Slender, furrowed, smooth and branching.

Seed
Two aromatic, $\frac{1}{4}$ inch long, narrow seeds grow in each capsule, which explodes when ripe. Each is dark brown, crescent shaped with pale ridges. Darkest seed from northern Europe, especially Holland, said to be best quality.

Leaf
Finely cut and feathery.

Root
Thick and tapering.

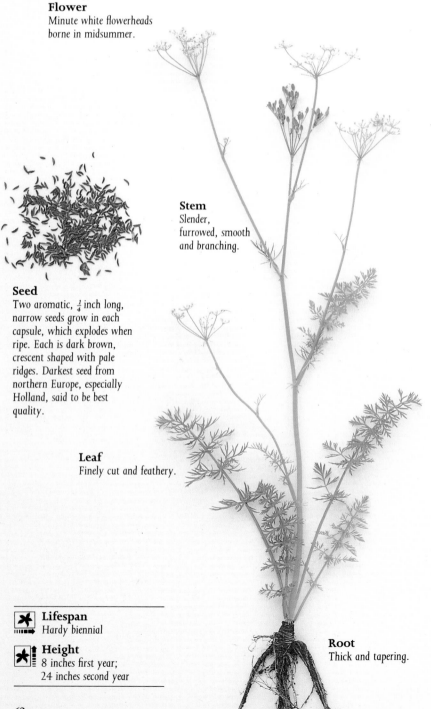

Lifespan
Hardy biennial

Height
8 inches first year; 24 inches second year

CULTIVATION
Site Full sun.
Soil Rich loam.
Propagating Sow outside in late spring or early autumn, in shallow drills in permanent position.
Growing Thin out to 8 inches apart, when large enough to handle. Caraway can be grown indoors in a sunny position.
Harvesting Gather leaves when young. Pick seed heads in late summer or when seeds are brown. Dig up roots in second year.
Preserving Hang seed heads upside down over an open container.

USES
Culinary
● *Seed* Sprinkle over rich meats, pork, game and Hungarian beef goulash to aid digestion. Add to cabbage water to reduce cooking smells. Use to flavor soups, breads, cakes, biscuits, apple pie, baked apples and cheese. Serve in a dish of mixed seeds at the end of an Indian meal. Encrust with white sugar to make caraway comfits. Its essential oil is used in liqueurs such as kümmel, and in confectionery.
● *Leaf* Chop young leaves into salads and soups.
● *Roots* Cook as a root vegetable.

Household
● *Seed* Pigeon fanciers claim that tame pigeons will never stray if there is baked caraway dough in their cote.

Cosmetic
● *Seed* Use essential oil in mouthwashes and colognes.

Medicinal
● *Seed* Chew raw or infused seed to aid digestion, promote appetite, sweeten the breath and relieve flatulence. Safe for children.

Cedronella canariensis (C. triphylla)

Balm of Gilead Labiatae

The name of this herb conjures up biblical images of aromatic resins and healing oils. The true balm of Gilead is a rare desert shrub, *Commiphora opobalsamum*, a gift from the Queen of Sheba to Solomon. The tree is guarded and export prohibited. To share this name, and possibly scent, is the lure of *Cedronella canariensis*, which has a strange "masculine" fragrance – the kind of musky scent that gives depth to perfumes. The tree *Populus balsamifera* is also called balm of Gilead. This has leaf buds which exude a rich balsamic scent and have been used medicinally to treat coughs and sore throats.

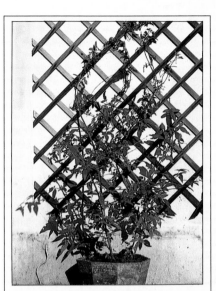

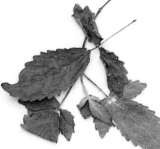

Dried leaves
Add to spicy or "woody" potpourri mixtures for their musky scent.

Flower
Two-lipped pink clusters, from late summer to early autumn.

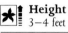 **Lifespan**
Half-hardy semievergreen shrub

Height
3–4 feet

Stem
Prickly, square, ridged, mid-green, occasionally red-tinged at leaf joints, becoming woody in second season.

Leaf
Three-lobed, toothed, pointed and mid-green with paler underside and aromatic, musky lemon-camphor scent.

CULTIVATION
Site Full sun.
Soil Well-drained, medium loam.
Propagating Sow in spring (and note that seedlings resemble nettles). Take stem cuttings in early autumn.
Growing Thin out or transplant to 18 inches apart. Balm of Gilead makes an excellent conservatory plant, but a 9–10 inch pot is needed for it to reach its full size.
Harvesting Pick leaves just before flowers open or in autumn before pruning. (*Populus balsamifera*) Gather buds (see p. 274).
Preserving Dry leaves. (*Populus balsamifera*) Dry buds.

USES
Decorative
● *Whole plant* Makes an elegant greenhouse plant with its long-lasting pink flowers.

Aromatic
● *Leaf* Infuse or macerate in alcohol with other perfume ingredients to add a musky scent. Use dried leaves in spicy or "woody" potpourris. (*Populus balsamifera*) Boil buds in water to extract their covering, which contains a rich balsamic resin. Use whole buds in potpourri.

Medicinal
● *Leaf* (*Populus balsamifera*) Buds are considered to be a stimulant and tonic, antiseptic and expectorant. When used internally, they are said to treat bronchitis, coughs and laryngitis and, when used externally in creams, may relieve arthritic pain, cuts and bruises. The buds contain the aspirin substance, salicin, which is useful for minor aches and pains.
● *Stem* (*Commiphora opobalsamum*) The resin, which is seldom available in a pure state, was in the past credited with near-miraculous powers.

Chamaemelum nobile (Anthemis nobilis)

Perennial chamomile Compositae

The Egyptians dedicated chamomile to the sun and worshiped it above all other herbs for its healing properties, while Greek physicians prescribed it for fevers and female disorders. Among the Nine Sacred Herbs of the *Lacnunga*, an ancient Anglo-Saxon manuscript, chamomile is the "Maythen." Moreover, chamomile has inspired a proverb about energy in adversity, "like a chamomile bed, the more it is trodden the more it will spread."

Chamomile is also valued for its sweet apple-scented leaves. In a popular gardening book of 1638, William Lawson wrote of the "large walks, broad and long, like the Temple groves in Thessaly, raised with gravel and sand, having seats and banks of Camomile – all this delights the mind and brings health to the body." The relaxing aroma was also inhaled as snuff or smoked to relieve asthma and cure insomnia. At beauty salons, chamomile tea is often served to relax facial muscles.

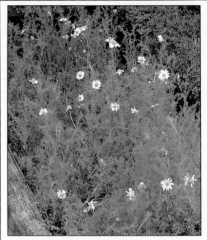

A bed of perennial chamomile in flower.

CULTIVATION

Site Full sun.
Soil Light and well drained.
Propagating (All except 'Treneague') Sow in spring. (Perennials) Divide in spring or autumn. Take 3 inch cuttings from side shoots in summer.
Growing For a chamomile lawn or seat, plant 4–6 inches apart. (M. recutita) Plant 9 inches apart. (A. tinctoria) Plant 18 inches apart.
Harvesting Gather leaves anytime. Pick flowers when fully open.
Preserving Dry flowers and leaves.

USES

Household
● *Whole plant* Grow this "physician" plant near a failing plant to revive it. Infuse and spray on seedlings to prevent "damping off" and on compost to activate decomposition.
● *Flower* (A. tinctoria) Boil for a strong yellow-brown dye (see p. 199).

Cosmetic
● *Flower* (C. nobile, M. recutita) Infuse as a facial steam and as a hand soak to soften and whiten skin. Make an eye bath or tea bag compress to reduce inflammation and eliminate fatigue shadows. Add infusion for a reviving bath. Boil flowers for 20 minutes, and use regularly as a rinse to lighten and condition fair hair.

Aromatic
● *Flower and leaf* Use in potpourri and herb pillows.

Medicinal
● *Flower* (C. nobile, M. recutita) Infuse flowers as a tea for a general tonic and sedative (good for restless children and nightmares). Apply a compress to treat wounds and eczema. Use in a bath to relieve sun- or wind burned skin.

Seed
Beige, narrow and tiny.

Dried flower
Yellow center contains the active ingredients.

Dried leaves
These retain their apple scent and are used in potpourri and herb pillows.

Flower
Scented, solid, conical, golden-yellow center with white petals, to 1 inch across; appears in summer and autumn.

C.n. var. flore-pleno Double-flowered chamomile
Apple-scented leaves and double cream flowers.

Leaf
Apple-scented, finely cut and bright green.

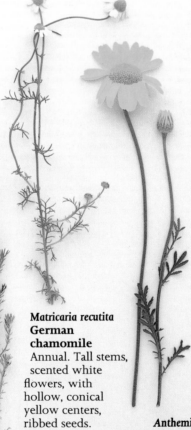

C.n. 'Treneague'
Nonflowering, mat-forming clone, with apple-scented leaves. Ht: 2 inches.

Stem
Lax, ridged, round and light green.

Matricaria recutita German chamomile
Annual. Tall stems, scented white flowers, with hollow, conical yellow centers, ribbed seeds. Ht: 2 feet.

Root
Creeping rootstock spreads plant, creating desirable carpeting surface.

Anthemis tinctoria Dyer's chamomile
Golden flowers, yielding yellow-brown dye, borne all summer. Ht: 2½ feet.

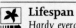 **Lifespan**
Hardy evergreen perennial

Height
8 inches in full sun; 12 inches in light shade

Chenopodium bonus-henricus

Good King Henry *Chenopodiaceae*

Good King Henry was a most popular herb from Neolithic times until the last century. Its curious name is not taken from the English king Henry VIII, with his many wives, but rather comes from Germany, where it distinguishes the plant from the poisonous mercury, which is known as "bad Henry."

Both Good King Henry and fat hen (*C. album*) have nutritious leaves. The seeds of fat hen, which are rich in fat and albumen, were a food supplement for primitive man, and fat hen was found in the stomach of preserved Iron Age Tollund Man. American wormseed (*C. ambrosioides*) is sometimes used to expel worms, but only under strict medical supervision, as large doses are poisonous. It is also known in China as "fragrant tiger bones."

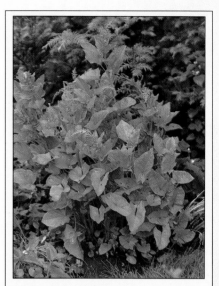

Flower
Tiny greenish-yellow flowers borne in early summer on 2 inch spikes where leaf joins stem.

Seed
Tan colored, rough, round and knobbly.

Leaf
Arrow-shaped and dark green with white mealy undersides.

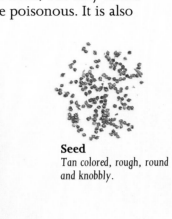

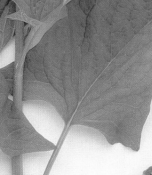

Variegated leaves
Such forms occasionally appear among seedlings.

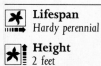
Lifespan
Hardy perennial

Height
2 feet

Stem
Tall, slender, ridged and green.

CULTIVATION

Site Prefers full sun but will tolerate light shade.
Soil Rich loam, deeply dug and well drained.
Propagating Sow in spring; cover seed with $\frac{1}{4}$ inch of soil. Divide roots in autumn.
Growing Thin or transplant seedlings to 1 foot apart. Water in dry weather; fertilize during summer. Unsatisfactory indoors.
Harvesting Allow plants 1 year to develop, then gather leaves as required and pick flowering spikes as they begin to open.
Preserving Freeze only when an ingredient in a cooked dish.

USES

Culinary
● *Seed* (Fat hen) Grind into flour and make into gruel.
● *Flower* Steam spikes and toss in butter like broccoli.
● *Leaf* Eat young leaves raw in salads, cooked in casseroles, stuffings and soups, and puréed in savory pies.
● *Shoot* On rich soil, cut shoots of pencil thickness and 5 inches tall; boil, peel and eat as asparagus.

Household
● *Whole plant* Use to fatten poultry.
● *Seed* Used commercially in the manufacture of shagreen, an artificially granulated untanned leather, often dyed green.

Medicinal
● *Leaf* Eat raw or cooked as a source of iron, vitamins and minerals. A poultice and ointment cleanses and heals skin sores.
● *Root* Used in a veterinary cough remedy for sheep.

Chrysanthemum balsamita (Tanacetum balsamita)

Alecost/Costmary Compositae

According to Gerard, the sixteenth-century herbalist, alecost was "cherished for its sweete flowers and leaves." Its balsamic leaves and flowering tops were also important in brewing to help clear and preserve ale and to impart an astringent, minty bitterness. Alecost was taken by settlers to America, where the Puritans carried a leaf in their bibles as a fragrant bookmark and to allay appetites during long sermons, giving alecost the nickname "bible leaf." The word "cost" derives from *costum*, the Latin for a spicy oriental herb, so alecost means a spicy herb for ale, and costmary is Mary's (or women's) spicy herb, as it was used to ease childbirth.

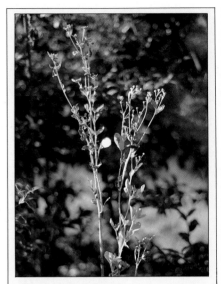

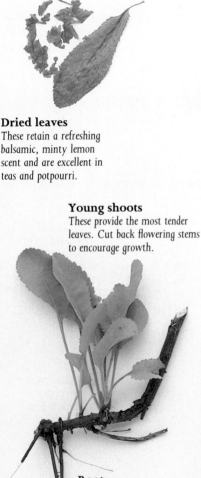

Dried leaves
These retain a refreshing balsamic, minty lemon scent and are excellent in teas and potpourri.

Young shoots
These provide the most tender leaves. Cut back flowering stems to encourage growth.

Flower
Small heads of insignificant yellow blooms borne in late summer; may also have outer row of white petals if grown in full sun.

Root
Light brown creeping rootstalk with fine root hairs.

Leaf
Up to 12 inches long, spearmint-scented, finely toothed, oval, pointed and silvery green.

Stem
Fibrous, ridged, round to flattish, pale green becoming gray-brown, with a woody appearance near base; rises from the creeping roots.

Lifespan
Hardy herbaceous perennial

Height
2–3 feet 6 inches

CULTIVATION
Site Prefers full sun.
Soil Rich, dryish and well drained.
Propagating Divide roots in spring or autumn. Seed is not viable in cool climates.
Growing Transplant to 2 feet apart. Small alecost plants can be grown indoors.
Harvesting Pick leaves anytime or for most aroma, as flowers open.
Preserving Dry leaves.

USES
Culinary
● *Leaf* Use in only small amounts as it has a sharp tang. Add finely chopped leaves to carrot soup, salads, game, poultry stuffing and fruit cakes. Try with melted butter on peas and new potatoes. Use to clear, flavor and preserve beer.

Household
● *Leaf* Add to linen bags to repel insects. Infuse to make a "sweet water" and use in the final rinse of linen to impart fragrance. Popular medieval strewing herb for its insect-repelling properties and lasting scent. (*C. balsamita* 'Tomentosum' or Camphor plant) Use as an insect repellent for fabrics and place in rooms for a stronger camphor scent.

Cosmetic
● *Leaf* Infuse as a scented rinse water for hair or skin.

Aromatic
● *Leaf* Use in potpourri and herb bags to intensify other herb scents.

Medicinal
● *Leaf* Infuse as a tonic tea for colds, catarrh, upset stomachs and cramps, and to ease childbirth. Lay crushed leaf on bee stings to relieve the pain. Add to a salve for burns and stings.

Chrysanthemum cinerariifolium (Pyrethrum cinerariifolium)

Pyrethrum Compositae

Although to some the name pyrethrum includes all the single-flowered chrysanthemums, it is in fact only the flowers of C. cinerariifolium that contain a natural insecticide, also called pyrethrum. Because it is nontoxic to mammals and nonaccumulative, pyrethrum is also used to kill pests living on the skin of man and animals. Another advantage is suggested by the traveller Chang Yee: "It is a strange coincidence that the leaves can be used for wiping the fingers after eating crabs, to wipe away the smell. Crabs, chrysanthemums, wine and the moon are the four autumn joys of our scholars, artists and poets." Garland chrysanthemum or "chop suey greens" (C. coronarium) is popular in oriental cuisine, and C. indicum is a valued tonic and part of the Taoist elixir of immortality.

Flower
Single "daisy" heads, with long white fluted petals and flat yellow centers, appear in midsummer. They have a pungent aroma when crushed.

Seed
Beige, narrow, ribbed "fruit," blunt one end, containing a single seed.

Stem
Slender, ribbed, branching and gray-green, each bearing a single terminal flower.

Leaf
Finely divided and gray-green with silver edge created by white down on underside; has a pungent aroma similar to tansy.

Flowerhead
The flower is used in powdered form to make contact insecticides. The active ingredients are pyrethrin and cinerin.

Lifespan
Hardy herbaceous perennial

Height
30 inches

CULTIVATION
Site Sunny and open.
Soil Alkaline and well drained.
Propagating Sow in late spring to summer. Divide roots in spring.
Growing Thin or transplant to 6–12 inches apart. Do not grow as an indoor plant.
Harvesting Gather open flowers.
Preserving Dry. Store away from light to preserve insecticide.

USES
Decorative
● **Flower** Cut for a long-lasting flower arrangement.

Culinary
● **Leaf** (C. coronarium) Sow seed thickly and cut leaves young, like cress. Use raw in salads or stir-fried.
● **Flower** (C. coronarium) This is the edible yellow chrysanthemum of Chinese recipes. Add to oriental dishes. (C. leucanthemum) Toss white petals into salads.

Household
● **Flower** Sprinkle dried powdered flowers to deter all common insect pests: bedbugs, cockroaches, flies, mosquitoes, aphids, spider mites and ants. (Note, it also kills helpful insects and fish.) Wear gloves when processing flowers as prolonged contact may cause allergies. Dust or make a paste with water to repel fleas and lice.

The active ingredients in the powder are not water soluble. To make a spray, steep 4 ounces of pyrethrum powder in $\frac{2}{3}$ cup of denatured alcohol, then dilute with 13 gallons of water. Alternatively, buy a proprietary liquid pyrethrum and follow manufacturer's instructions. Spray insecticide on herbs at dusk, so plants and bees will be safe by morning. (Solution decomposes rapidly, especially in bright sunlight.)

Note: When the active ingredient pyrethrin or cinerin is extracted, it is toxic to humans and animals.

Cichorium intybus

Chicory/Succory Compositae

According to folk tales, the flowers of chicory are a beautiful clear blue because they are the transformed eyes of a lass weeping for her lover's ship, which never returned. These blue flowers can be changed to bright red by the acid of ants: place a flower in an ant hill and watch the color show.

Chicory is often grown in floral clocks for the regular opening of its flowers and their closing five hours later. These opening times relate to latitude, but the leaves always align with north. Gardeners interested in metaphysics credit this plant with life-giving forces.

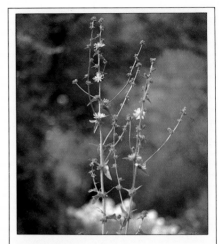

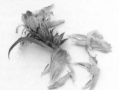

Dried petals
Attractive in potpourri.

Flower
Clear blue fluted petals; two or three flowers borne at each leaf joint mid-summer to midautumn.

Chicons
These are blanched heads produced by forcing roots in warmth and darkness. They are also known as Belgian endives.

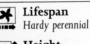

Lifespan
Hardy perennial

Height
3–5 feet

Stem
Hollow, furrowed, green with small hairs; bitter milky juice inside.

Leaf
Mid-green with hairy underside; coarsely toothed at the base; smaller, arrow-shaped leaves further up the stem.

Root
Long taproot, occasionally branching; bitter milky fluid inside.

CULTIVATION
Site Sunny and open.
Soil Light, preferably alkaline soil. Dig deeply for good roots.
Propagating Sow in early summer, selecting Witloof variety for chicons and Magdeburg or Brunswick varieties for "coffee" roots.
Growing Thin or transplant to 18 inches apart. Chicory is not suitable for growing indoors. To grow chicons, dig up roots in autumn, cut leaves to 1 inch and trim 1 inch off root. Bury well in sandy compost and water. Exclude light and move into a cellar or garage. Chicons are ready to eat in 3–4 weeks.
Harvesting Gather leaves when young. Dig up roots in first autumn and chicons in winter.
Preserving Dry root and leaves.

USES
Culinary
● **Flower** Use in salads; pickle buds.
● **Leaf** Seedlings can be cut and eaten fresh.
● **Root** When young, boil and serve with a sauce. Use as a coffee substitute: dig up thick, cultivated roots, wash, slice, dry in gentle heat; roast and grind.
● **Chicon** Toss in salads; braise in butter as a vegetable dish.

Household
● **Whole plant** Grow for fodder and in nutritious pasture mixtures.
● **Leaf** Boil for a blue dye.

Medicinal
● **Leaf** May be used for jaundice and spleen problems. A poultice soothes inflammation.
● **Root** Infuse dried root to make a tonic, mild laxative and diuretic. A decoction may alleviate gallstones, kidney stones and inflammation of the liver or urinary tract.

Coriandrum sativum

Coriander Umbelliferae

Cultivated as a medicinal and culinary herb for at least 3,000 years, coriander is mentioned in Sanskrit texts, on Egyptian papyri, in *Tales of the Arabian Nights* and in the Bible, where manna is compared with coriander seed. Coriander was brought to northern Europe by the Romans, who, combining it with cumin and vinegar, rubbed it into meat as a preservative. The Chinese once believed it conferred immortality, and in the Middle Ages it was put into love potions as an aphrodisiac. All coriander parts have a pungent aroma; one Peruvian tribe is so fond of the leaf that they exude its scent. That of the mildly narcotic seed changes considerably when it ripens to a sweet spicy flavor, which is best after a few months. Coriander's use in exotic cuisines has rekindled its popularity today.

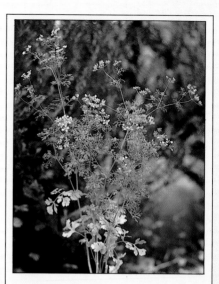

Seed
Small, round and beige, with a light brown, ribbed spherical seed case; aromatic.

Flower
Loose, flat, white or pale pinkish-mauve heads borne from early to midsummer.

Upper leaf
Finely cut, threadlike and bright green, with a strange pungent scent.

Lower leaf
Finely scalloped and broad, with same strange scent as upper leaves, but tasting like an aromatic parsley.

Lifespan
Annual

Height
2 feet

Stem
Round, branching and pale green, finely grooved.

CULTIVATION
Site Full sun.
Soil Rich and light.
Propagating Sow in autumn, to overwinter in mild climates, or early spring in final position, away from fennel, which seems to suffer in its presence.
Growing Thin to 8 inches apart. Coriander can be grown indoors but its scent is unpleasant.
Harvesting Pick young leaves anytime. Collect seeds when brown but before they drop. Dig up roots in autumn.
Preserving Dry seeds, store whole or infuse to make a coriander vinegar. Freeze leaves, or place their stems in water and cover with a plastic bag to retain their freshness.

USES
Culinary
● *Seed* Use in tomato chutney, ratatouille, frankfurters and curries; also in apple pies, cakes, biscuits, and marmalade. Add whole seeds to soups, sauces and vegetable dishes.
● *Leaf* Add fresh lower leaves to curries, stews, salads, sauces and use as a garnish (see also p. 164).
● *Stem* Cook with beans and soups.
● *Root* Cook fresh root as a vegetable. Add to curries.

Household
● *Whole plant* Sow close to aniseed to speed up the latter's germination and growth.

Aromatic
● *Seed* Use in potpourri.

Medicinal
● *Seed* Chew or infuse as a tea for an aperitif, digestive tonic and mild sedative. Add essential oil to ointments for painful rheumatic joints and muscles. Used to flavor various medicines.

Dianthus caryophyllus

Clove pink Caryophyllaceae

This herb was a flower of divinity to the Greeks, who dedicated it to the "sky father" and called it *dianthus*, meaning Zeus's flower. To the Romans, it was *flos Jovis*, Jove's flower. In the making of coronets and garlands, in which both these cultures delighted, pinks were given place of honor. These flowers of love were also floated in the drinks of engaged couples, and in medieval art they indicated betrothal. Pinks have long been used to flavor dainty dishes with their spicy fragrance: flowers were crystallized, and petals were used in soups, sauces, syrups, cordials and wine. In 1699, John Evelyn suggested that the petals could be mingled with other salad ingredients but had "a more palatable relish infused in vinegar."

Seed
Small, dark brown, flattish and round.

Flower
Single or double, white, pink or purple flowers, with very sweet, clovelike perfume, borne in summer.

D. carthusianorum
Bright pink clusters above low mound of grasslike, ridged green leaves. Ht: 18 inches.

D. plumarius 'Doris'
One of the Allwoodii scented pinks. Pale salmon-pink flowers. Ht: 6–12 inches.

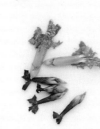

D. deltoides
Maiden pink
Small carmine flowers over mats of dark green foliage. Ht: 8 inches.

Leaf
Long, narrow and blue-green.

Dried flowers
These can be used in potpourri, and in cooking, when petals should be separated and the bitter white heel removed.

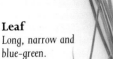

Stem
Smooth, round, blue-green, thickening at leaf joints.

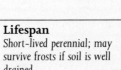
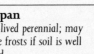
Lifespan
Short-lived perennial; may survive frosts if soil is well drained

Height
1–3 feet

D. 'Inchmery' has double flowers.

CULTIVATION
Site Open sunny position.
Soil Well drained and alkaline.
Propagating Sow seed or take stem cuttings in spring. Divide roots or layer in late summer.
Growing Thin or transplant to 1 foot apart. Can grow indoors.
Harvesting Pick open flowers.
Preserving Air dry flowers or put in silica gel. Infuse in almond oil for sweet oil or in wine vinegar for floral vinegar. Crystallize petals.

USES
Decorative
● **Flower** Pretty and long-lasting.

Culinary
● **Flower** Remove bitter white heel. Add petals to salads, fruit pies and sandwiches. Use to flavor sugar, jam, vinegar and wine. To make a syrup: pour 1 fluid ounce boiling water on 1 ounce fresh petals, steep for 12 hours. Strain, add $1\frac{1}{4}$ cups sugar, stir and bottle.

Household
● **Flower** Provides nectar for bees.

Aromatic
● **Flower** Use dried in potpourri.

Medicinal
● **Flower** Infuse petals in wine as a nerve tonic.

Note on species
D. caryophyllus, an Elizabethan gillyflower, is about 2 feet high with erect stems and rose-purple flowers which have the richest, spicy sweet scent. The parent of carnations, it is doubtful if the true species is now available commercially.
D. plumarius, cottage pink, is the parent of most "old-fashioned pinks." The Allwoodii pinks are a cross between D. caryophyllus and D. plumarius. All clove-scented varieties can be used herbally.

Eupatorium purpurea

Sweet Joe Pye *Compositae*

A glorious feature of the herb garden in late summer, the vigorous purple stems of sweet Joe Pye display clouds of rose-pink flowers. This herb was named after a North American Indian called Joe Pye, who cured a grateful New Englander of typhus. The Indian used this plant to induce profuse sweating, which broke the fever. Its Latin name *Eupatorium* is derived from Eupator, a first-century B.C. king of Pontus, famed for his herbal skills. Other species, E. *cannabinum* and E. *perfoliatum*, are similar in appearance and have medicinal properties.

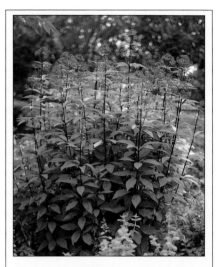

Flower
Tubes of rose-pink overlapping petals appear in clusters in late summer.

Seed
Brown, narrow, pointed, tufted, $\frac{1}{8}$ inch long.

Root
Thick and purplish-brown, with cream flesh and smaller roots. Dried root is used medicinally.

Leaf
Up to 1 foot long, lance-shaped and green, in whorls; when bruised, emits a faint scent of apple peel.

Stem
Aromatic, thick, round and purple, with vertical line markings toward base.

 Lifespan
Hardy herbaceous perennial

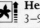 **Height**
3–9 feet

CULTIVATION

Site Partial shade or sun.
Soil Any rich, alkaline soil. (E. *cannabinum*) Prefers marshy soil.
Propagating Sow fresh seed in autumn. Divide in spring or autumn.
Growing Thin or transplant to 3 feet apart. Sweet Joe Pye is not suitable for indoor cultivation.
Harvesting Pick leaves anytime. Dig up roots in autumn; remove small side roots. Collect seed heads when petals have dropped.
Preserving Dry leaves, roots and seed heads.

USES

Decorative
● *Whole plant* Makes a magnificent specimen in herb garden borders. The sturdy erect stems withstand storms well.

Household
● *Seed* Crush unripe and ripe seed heads and boil for a pink-red dye.
● *Leaf* (E. *cannabinum*) Dried leaves were said by Culpeper to drive away wasps and flies if burned in a room.

Medicinal
● *Flowering top and leaf* (E. *cannabinum*) When dried, these were used as a tonic for biliousness and as a laxative, but this is now felt by some to be too toxic. (It is not related to the cannabis plant.)
● *Root* Use dried root in small doses as a tincture or infusion to induce perspiration, relieve gout and rheumatism, and promote the flow of urine (specifically to help remove stones in the bladder caused by excess uric acid – hence one of its nicknames, "gravel root"). Infusion may be used as an astringent tonic and stimulant.

Filipendula ulmaria (Spirea ulmaria)

Meadowsweet *Rosaceae*

Meadowsweet was the favourite strewing herb of Queen Elizabeth I, and the herbalist Gerard believed it outranked all other strewing herbs because its leaves delighted the senses without causing headaches. Meadowsweet was so frequently in demand for strewing at church weddings and for making into bridal garlands that it was given another name, "bridewort." Other qualities unknown to us once made this plant – together with mistletoe, watermint and vervain – most sacred to the Druids. There is also a gold variegated leaf form, and *F. vulgaris*, which grows to 3 feet but has larger flowers.

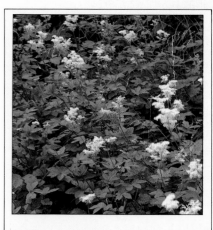

Flower
Cream-colored clusters of tiny blossoms with sweet almond fragrance throughout summer.

Seed
Light brown and crescent-shaped, $\frac{1}{8}$ inch long.

Dried flowers
Sweet almond fragrance improves with age; used for tea and potpourri.

Dried leaves
Smell of hay with a hint of wintergreen.

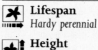

Lifespan
Hardy perennial

Height
4–6 feet

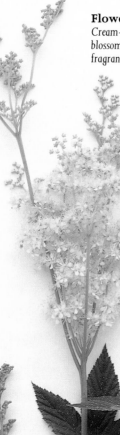

Leaf
Wrinkled, deeply indented and dark green with gray-green undersides; exudes pleasant wintergreen fragrance.

Root
Pinkish-red, sweetly aromatic and creeping.

Stem
Hollow, furrowed, branching and reddish.

CULTIVATION

Site Sun or partial shade.
Soil Moist, fertile and alkaline.
Propagating Sow in spring; divide meadowsweet in autumn.
Growing Thin or transplant to 12 inches apart. Not suitable for growing indoors.
Harvesting Gather young leaves before flowers appear, and pick flowers when new.
Preserving Dry leaves and flowers.

USES

Decorative
● **Flower** Use in bouquets.

Culinary
● **Flower** Flavors herb beers, mead and wines. Gives slight almond flavor to jams and stewed fruit.
● **Leaf** Add to soup for an interesting flavor. Use in meadowsweet beer: boil 2 ounces each of meadowsweet, betony, raspberry leaves and agrimony, in 2 gallons of water for about 15 minutes. Strain and add 2 pounds of white sugar, stirring to dissolve. Bottle when nearly cool.

Household
● **Flowering top** Use to scent linen. Boil for a greenish-yellow dye.
● **Leaf and stem** Boil for a blue dye.
● **Roots** Boil for a black dye.

Cosmetic
● **Flower** Soak in rainwater for an astringent, tonic, complexion water.

Aromatic
● **Flower** Dry for potpourri.
● **Leaf** Gather for strewing and adding to potpourri.

Medicinal
● **Flower buds** First discovered source of salicylic acid in 1835, from which aspirin was later synthesized.
● **Flower** Drink as a tea to help rid body of excess fluid and to alleviate heartburn, for feverish colds and mild diarrhea. Can also be used as a mild sedative and painkiller.

Foeniculum vulgare

Fennel *Umbelliferae*

Fennel is one of our oldest cultivated plants and was much valued by the Romans. "So gladiators fierce and rude/ mingled it with their daily food. And he who battled and subdued/ a wreath of fennel wore" (Henry Wadsworth Longfellow). In an age of banquets, Roman warriors took fennel to keep in good health, while Roman ladies ate it to prevent obesity. Every part of the plant, from the seed to the root, is edible. It was one of the nine herbs held sacred by the Anglo-Saxons for its power against evil. Charlemagne declared in 812 A.D. that fennel, with healing properties also to its credit, was essential in every imperial garden.

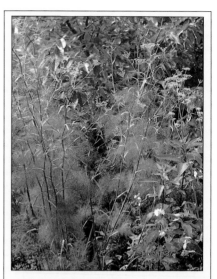

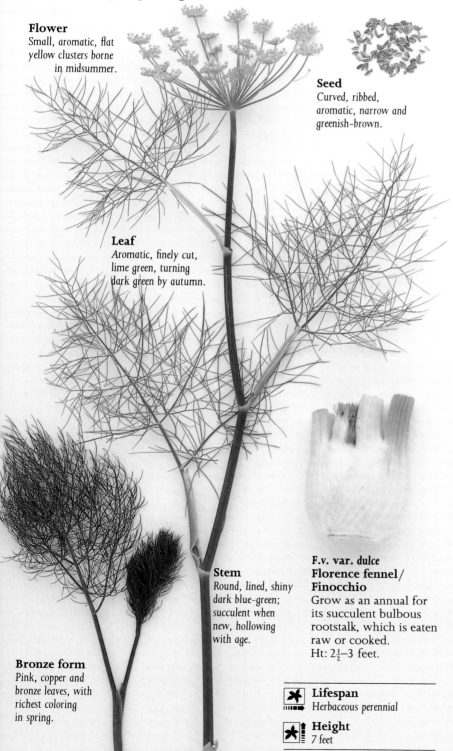

Flower
Small, aromatic, flat yellow clusters borne in midsummer.

Seed
Curved, ribbed, aromatic, narrow and greenish-brown.

Leaf
Aromatic, finely cut, lime green, turning dark green by autumn.

Bronze form
Pink, copper and bronze leaves, with richest coloring in spring.

Stem
Round, lined, shiny dark blue-green; succulent when new, hollowing with age.

**F.v. var. dulce
Florence fennel/
Finocchio**
Grow as an annual for its succulent bulbous rootstalk, which is eaten raw or cooked.
Ht: 2½–3 feet.

Lifespan
Herbaceous perennial

Height
7 feet

CULTIVATION
Site Full sun (to ripen seed).
Soil Well-drained loam. Avoid clay.
Propagating Sow in late spring to early summer. (Self-seeds when established.) Divide in autumn.
Growing Thin or transplant to 20 inches apart. Do not grow near dill, as seeds will cross-pollinate, or coriander, as it reduces fennel's seed production. Remove seed heads if not required to give better leaf production. Fennel is not suitable for growing indoors.
Harvesting Pick young stems and leaves as required. Collect ripe seed. Dig up "bulbs" in autumn.
Preserving Freeze leaves or infuse in oil or vinegar. Dry seed.

USES
Decorative
● *Whole plant* Attractive in borders.

Culinary
● *Seed* Use in sauces, fish dishes, and bread; sprout for winter salads.
● *Leaf* Finely chop over salads and cooked vegetables. Add to soups and to stuffings, for oily fish.
● *Stem* Add young stems to salads.
● *Bulb* (Florence fennel) Slice or grate raw into sandwiches or salads. Cook as a root vegetable.

Cosmetic
● *Seed* Decoct as an eye bath or as a compress to reduce inflammation. Chew to sweeten breath.
● *Seed and leaf* Use in facial steams and baths for deep cleansing.

Medicinal
● *Seed* Infuse as a tea to aid digestion and constipation. Chew to allay hunger and ease indigestion. Recent research indicates fennel reduces the toxic effects of alcohol on the body.

Note: *Do not take excessive doses.*

Fragaria vesca

Wild strawberry Rosaceae

"Doubtless God Almighty could have made a better berry but doubtless God never did." Dr Butler's praise sums up most people's feelings about strawberries. Growing in cool, secret woodlands, strawberries are often associated with fairy folk, and in Bavaria a basket of fruit is sometimes tied between a cow's horns to please the elves so that they bless the cow with abundant milk. Woodland strawberries were recommended by Sir Hugh Platt in his *Garden of Eden* (1653), as most likely to prosper in gardens. While discussing plants that scent the air, Francis Bacon noted that "the strawberry leaves dying ... yield a most excellent cordial smell."

Strawberries are one of the fruits dedicated to the Virgin Mary, and, astrologically, to the planet Venus. In Lapland, they are mixed with reindeer milk and blueberries to make a Christmas pudding. Their one unhappy association is with the fateful handkerchief that Shakespeare's Othello gave Desdemona, which was "spotted" with strawberries.

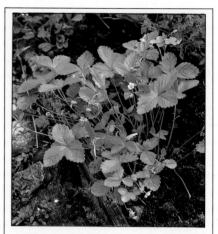

Seed
Tiny, mid-brown, shiny and tear-shaped.

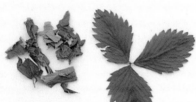

Dried leaves
Dry thoroughly as wilting process creates a toxin that disappears on drying; contain tannin, vitamin C and a lemon-scented essential oil.

Flower
White petals and yellow center appear from early spring until first frosts.

Leaf
Deeply veined, toothed, three-lobed and bright green with white felted underside; rich in vitamin C.

Stem
Hairy, ridged, round and green to reddish.

Fruit
Pips, containing seeds, are scattered over each fleshy, red fruit (the tasty strawberry) throughout summer and autumn.

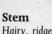 **Lifespan**
Hardy evergreen

Height
10 inches; good ground cover

Root
Short, woody rootstalk with numerous rootlets. Rooting stems (runners) are produced from stem area.

CULTIVATION
Site Cool, sun or shade, sheltered.
Soil Alkaline, moist, well drained.
Propagating Sow in spring at a temperature of 65 °F. In spring, sever the daughter plants produced on runners and transplant to 12 inches apart.
Growing Apply a potash fertilizer as fruits begin to form. Can be grown indoors.
Harvesting Pick fruit as ripe. Collect leaves as required. Dig up roots in autumn.
Preserving Freeze or bottle fruit. Dry leaves.

USES
Culinary
● *Leaf* Infuse with other herb teas to add "bite." Use bruised leaves to flavor meat stock.
● *Fruit* Eat fresh with cream. Use for jam, cakes, pies and syrups or to flavor liqueurs and cordials.

Cosmetic
● *Leaf* Decoct as an astringent for oily skin.
● *Fruit* Rub on teeth to remove tartar and reduce stains; leave juice on teeth for 5 minutes, then clean using warm water with a pinch of bicarbonate of soda. Apply cut strawberry to washed face to ease slight sunburn. Mash or extract juice and add to face packs to whiten skin and lighten freckles.

Aromatic
● *Leaf* Use dried in potpourri.

Medicinal
● *Leaf* Infuse as a tea for anemia, nervousness, diarrhea, other gastrointestinal and urinary disorders and as a tonic for kidneys.
● *Root* Decoct as a tonic and diuretic.
● *Fruit* Eat as an iron supplement, mild laxative and for rheumatic gout. Drink to cool fevers.

Note: *Strawberries can cause an allergic reaction in some people.*

Galium odoratum (Asperula odorata)

Sweet woodruff Rubiaceae

This pretty little woodland plant will, when added to a wine cup, "make a man merrie," wrote Gerard. Sweet-smelling garlands of woodruff were hung in churches, strewn on domestic floors, sprinkled into potpourri and linen and stuffed into mattresses, spreading its cordiality around the household. The coumarin in the leaves develops its sweet hay scent only when the plant is dried, so sweet woodruff is invaluable from the appearance of its first flowers for the traditional German May Bowl punch, through to Christmas, when it is used in herb pillows.

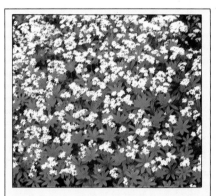

Lifespan
Hardy perennial

Height
12 inches; good ground cover

Flower
Brilliant white, loose clusters of star-shaped flowers appear in late spring.

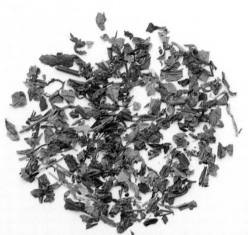

Dried leaves
Smell like new-mown hay and act as a fixative in potpourri.

Leaf
The shiny green circular spokes of the leaves give the plant its "ruff" name.

Stem
Slender, squarish and smooth.

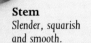

Root
Small, red-brown creeping rootstalk with hairlike roots.

CULTIVATION
Site Semishade, particularly good under trees. Leaf color fades in bright sun.
Soil Prefers moist, porous loam but will survive on less rich soil.
Propagating Sow seeds when ripe in late summer in moist shaded soil. Propagation, however, is easiest by dividing the creeping rootstock after flowering is finished.
Growing Transplant in spring, 6–9 inches apart. Sweet woodruff is not suitable for growing indoors.
Harvesting Pick leaves and flowering stems.
Preserving Store leaves whole to preserve scent.

USES
Decorative
● **Flowering stem** Use in garlands.

Culinary
● **Leaf** Make "an exhilarating drink to lift the spirits and create a carefree atmosphere": dry a small handful of fresh woodruff leaves in a warm cupboard for 3 hours. Remove stems and put leaves in a large bowl. Pour over juice of one lemon and half a bottle of Rhine wine to cover the leaves. Put in a warm place for 3–4 hours. Add 4–6 tablespoons of sugar and one and a half bottles of Rhine wine. Chill. Just before serving, add a bottle of sparkling white wine or champagne. For a stronger drink, add a measure of brandy. Float wild strawberries on the top.

Household
● **Leaf** Put dried leaves under carpets and among linens to deter moths and other insects.

Aromatic
● **Leaf** Add dried leaves to potpourri and herb pillows.

Medicinal
● **Leaf** Bruise fresh leaves and apply to wounds. Infuse dried leaves to make a refreshing and relaxing tea, which can relieve stomach pains.

Helianthus annuus

Sunflower Compositae

This remarkable flower, which was cultivated by American Indians some 3,000 years ago, has always been revered as an emblem of the sun. In the fifteenth century, Aztec sun priestesses were crowned with sunflowers, carried them in their hands and wore gold jewelry with sunflower motifs. Sunflowers were introduced into Europe by Spanish explorers in the sixteenth century. Large-scale cultivation began in Russia, where the seeds are sold on street corners and offered in large bowls at railway restaurants.

All parts of sunflower are usable. The pith, for example, is one of the lightest substances known and is used in scientific laboratories. The Chinese have used it as moxa in acupuncture, and in the making of delicate silks and coarse ropes, having cultivated sunflowers for hundreds of years. The plant's ability to absorb water from soil has been utilized in the reclamation of marshy land in the Netherlands.

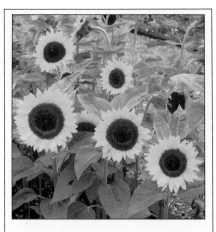

Flower
Yellow petals surround a purple-brown central disk, borne from late summer until frosts.

Seed (shell)
Oval, flattish, thin covering, $\frac{1}{2}$ inch long, with gray, white and brown stripes.

Seed (kernel)
Light gray, flattish and oval inside shell; rich in vitamins B1, B2, niacin, iron, phosphorus, potassium, sulfur, vegetable fats and proteins.

Seed head
Edible seeds form stunning geometric concentric patterns.

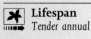 **Lifespan**
Tender annual

Height
3–10 feet

Leaf
Large, rough, toothed, heart-shaped and mid-green with three prominent veins.

Stem
Thick, hairy, light green and high in potash. Pith is valued for its cellular lightness. Dried stems are very hard and make excellent fuel.

CULTIVATION
Site Full sun.
Soil Any well-drained loam.
Propagating Sow seeds in their shells in spring. Avoid planting near potatoes as growth becomes stunted.
Growing Thin or transplant to 12–18 inches apart. Not suitable for growing indoors.
Harvesting Pick leaves and flower buds as required. Cut flower heads when they droop. Hang until seeds fall. Gather stems in autumn.
Preserving Dry leaves and seed.

USES
Decorative
● *Whole plant* Grow as a colorful windbreak or focal point.

Culinary
● *Seed* Shell and eat kernel raw, or roast: brown 1 ounce of seed with shells in $\frac{1}{2}$ teaspoon oil, drain and toss in salt. Add sprouted seeds to salads and sandwiches, when $\frac{1}{4}$ inch long, before they become bitter. Cook with sunflower oil.
● *Flower* Eat raw buds in salad, or steam and serve like artichokes.

Household
● *Whole plant* Grow as a moisture-absorbent plant near a house to deter rising damp and drain ground.
● *Seed* Feed whole seed to chickens to increase egg laying.
● *Flower* Boil for a yellow dye.
● *Leaf* Can be smoked, dried.
● *Stem* Use fibrous pith for textiles and paper-making. Burn and scatter ashes as potash fertilizer.

Cosmetic
● *Seed* Pressed oil contains vitamin F and other substances that benefit the skin.

Medicinal
● *Seed* Eat a handful or take 15 oil drops three times a day, or boil seed for 20 minutes and take as a tea to relieve coughs and inflammation of the kidneys.

Helichrysum angustifolium

Curry plant *Compositae*

This plant from southern Europe is a relatively new addition to herbal lists. Curry plant's initial attraction lies in the intense silver of its evergreen leaves, which make it and its dwarf form, *H.a.* var. *nana*, a good choice for formal edgings and knot gardens. However, it is the sweet curry scent of its leaves which is so unusual and has caused its recent rise in popularity, especially among adventurous cooks. Visitors to my garden who accidentally brush against curry plant often look around for a picnic group to track down the source of the spicy aroma.

The genus *Helichrysum* also includes *H. bracteatum*, whose everlasting flowers, though scentless, are often added to potpourri and dried arrangements for their decorativeness.

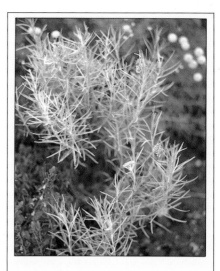

Dried flowers
These everlasting flowers retain their color well for potpourri and flower arrangements.

Dried leaves
These add a mild curry flavor to soups and casseroles.

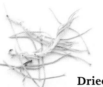

Flower
Tiny, mustard-yellow clusters, with sweet mild curry scent, borne in late summer.

Leaf
Narrow, needle-like and silvery-gray with sweetish curry scent.

Stem
Downy, round and white, becoming green then woody in second season.

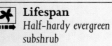

Lifespan
Half-hardy evergreen subshrub

Height
18 inches

CULTIVATION
Site Full sun.
Soil Rich and well drained.
Propagating Take stem cuttings in spring or autumn.
Growing Plant 12 inches apart. Prune lightly in early autumn or spring. In areas with light frost, curry plants may die back temporarily. Protect leaves with 5-inch sleeve of straw set between chicken wire. In areas where temperature drops below 22 °F, bring curry plants indoors for winter protection.
Harvesting Pick leaves anytime. Gather flowers as they open.
Preserving Dry leaves and flowers.

USES
Decorative
● *Whole plant* Provides decorative silver edging in formal beds and knot gardens. (*H.a.* var. *nana*) This half-hardy dwarf form, 8 inches high, makes a pretty edging and knot garden plant and is attractive in sink gardens.
● *Flower* (*H. bracteatum*) Dry petals to add color to potpourri, and whole flowers for arrangements, garlands and wreaths.
● *Leaf* Add sprigs to nosegays, garlands and wreaths.

Culinary
● *Leaf* Add a sprig to soups, stews, steamed vegetables, rice dishes and pickles for a mild curry flavor. Remove sprig before serving.

Hesperis matronalis

Sweet rocket *Cruciferae*

This pretty cottage flower has maintained its position in the herb garden because of its sweet-scented flowers as well as its medicinal properties. A native of Italy, it can be found growing wild in much of Europe and northern America as a garden escapee.

Its massed flowers, a glorious sight in midsummer, are sometimes called dame's violet or vesper flower, since its perfume is strongest in the evening. The young leaves are occasionally eaten as a salad herb, but they are more bitter than arugula, or salad rocket (see p. 135).

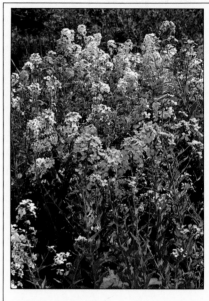

Flower
Sweetly fragrant, purple, mauve and white flowers appear in midsummer. Most fragrant in evenings.

Seed
Brown, narrow and pointed, $\frac{1}{8}$ inch long.

Stem
Slender and carries flowers in second year.

Leaf
Spear-shaped and dark green.

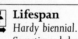

Lifespan
Hardy biennial. Sometimes behaves as a perennial, sending out new shoots from old roots

Height
3 feet

CULTIVATION
Site Full sun or light shade.
Soil Prefers rich loam in beds or light woodland.
Propagating Sow outdoors in late spring.
Growing Thin seedlings or transplant in autumn to 18 inches apart. Sweet rocket is too tall to grow indoors.
Harvesting Gather leaves when young for eating but at flowering time for medicinal properties. Collect flowers as they open.
Preserving Dry leaves and flowers.

USES
Decorative
● **Flower** Pick for a pretty, sweet-scented summer bouquet.

Culinary
● **Flower** Toss in salads. Use as a decoration for desserts.
● **Leaf** Add chopped young leaves sparingly to salads.

Aromatic
● **Flower** Add dried flowers to potpourri for their pastel color and sweet scent.

Medicinal
● **Leaf** Dried leaves were once popular for preventing and curing scurvy. A strong dose may cause vomiting.

Humulus lupulus

Hops Cannabaceae

In the first century A.D., the Roman writer Pliny described hops as a popular garden plant and vegetable: in spring, young shoots were sold on markets, to be eaten like asparagus. By the ninth century, this plant was used in brewing throughout most of Europe for its clearing, flavoring and preserving qualities. However, in Britain, brewers continued to rely on herbs such as ground ivy and alecost (costmary) until the sixteenth century, under the curious belief that hops engendered melancholy. Even in 1670, John Evelyn explained that "hops . . . preserve the drink indeed, but repay the pleasure in tormenting diseases and a shorter life."

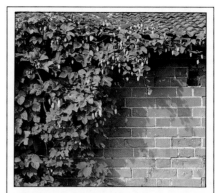

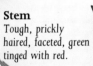

Leaf
Large, roughly textured, toothed, heart-shaped and mid-green, with three or five lobes.

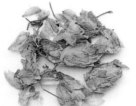

Dried flowers
Use ripe, unpollinated female flowers to clear, preserve and flavor ale with a bitter taste; can also be used medicinally and around the house.

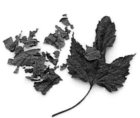

Dried leaves
Boil for a brown dye. Sometimes added to hop pillows for bulk, but they do not contain the same medicinal properties as hop flowers.

Stem
Tough, prickly haired, faceted, green tinged with red.

H.l. 'Aureus'
Soft golden leaves, best grown in full sun. Dried flowers and leaves are believed to have the same properties as the species.

Flower
Yellowish-green, cone-like female blooms borne in late summer, ripen into larger globes of pale papery bracts containing powdery glands, which have many uses. Male flowers appear on separate plants.

Lifespan
Hardy deciduous perennial climber

Height
23 feet

CULTIVATION
Site Sunny open position.
Soil Fertile and deeply dug.
Propagating Reproduce female plants only. Divide roots and separate rooted stems and suckers in spring. Take cuttings in early summer. Avoid sowing, as plant gender is unknown for 2–3 years.
Growing Grow 3 feet apart against support. Hops can be grown indoors but they seldom flower.
Harvesting Pick young sideshoots in spring. Gather young leaves as required. Pick ripe flowers in early autumn. Collect stems in late autumn.
Preserving Dry leaves and stems. Dry and use female flowers within a few months, otherwise the flavor will become unpleasant.

USES
Decorative
● *Whole plant* (H.l. 'Aureus') Makes a leafy screen or focal point trained on a tripod or frame.
● *Flowers* Attractive in dried arrangements and garlands.

Culinary
● *Flower* Use dried ripe female flowers to flavor, clear and preserve beer. Parboil male flowers and toss into salads.
● *Leaf* Blanch young leaves to remove bitterness. Add to soups.
● *Shoot* Steam young side shoots and serve like asparagus.

Household
● *Leaf* Boil for a brown dye.
● *Stem* Weave into baskets and other wickerwork. Used to make durable cloth and paper.

Cosmetic
● *Flower* Infuse and add to a relaxing bath.

Medicinal
● *Flower* Sprinkle with alcohol and add to pillows to induce sleep. Infuse as a mild sedative tea for digestive problems and as an antiseptic. Add flowers to any other tea and drink as a digestive aid and appetite stimulant.

Flowering herbs

As with the early flowering herbs on p. 54, the herbal properties of these plants were for a long time largely forgotten; but they continued to be grown as attractive garden plants. Now many of these herbs are being rediscovered, particularly for their medicinal properties: agrimony, for example, is used to treat sore throats, childhood diarrhea and cystitis. With the renewed interest in herbal decorations and potpourri, the scented flowers of mock orange and honeysuckle are doubly valued; with a return to herbal cosmetics, lupine seeds are added to face masks and scrubs. All the plants shown below have interesting uses, past and present, and all of them add decorative color, shape and fragrance to the garden.

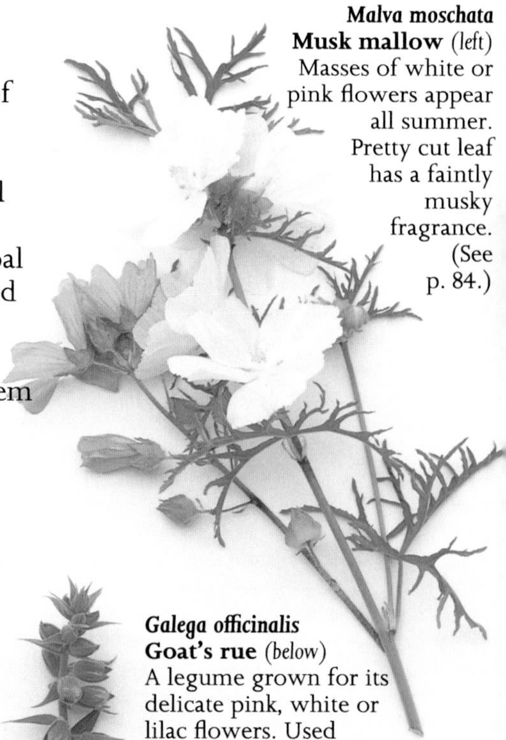

Malva moschata
Musk mallow (left)
Masses of white or pink flowers appear all summer. Pretty cut leaf has a faintly musky fragrance. (See p. 84.)

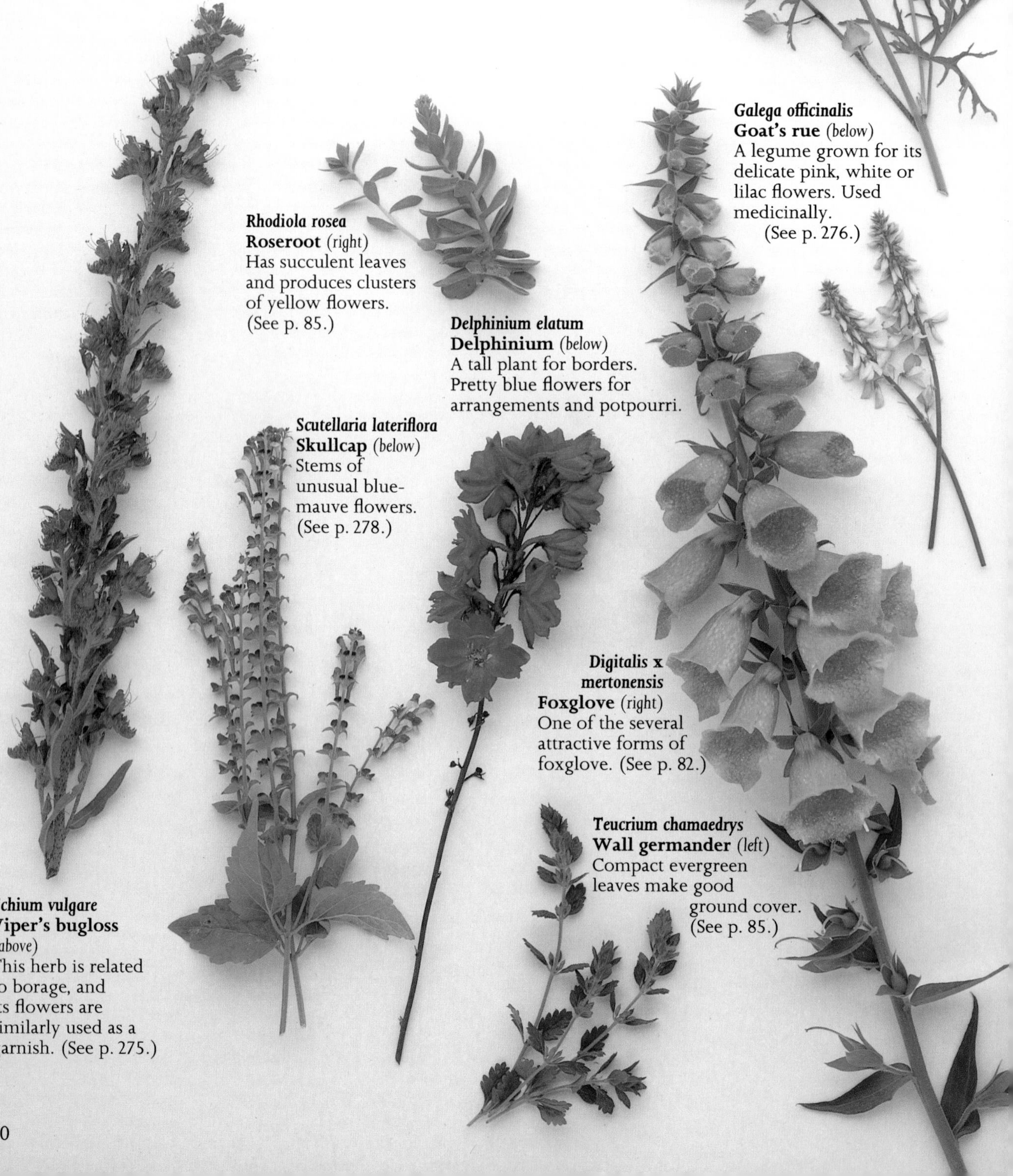

Rhodiola rosea
Roseroot (right)
Has succulent leaves and produces clusters of yellow flowers. (See p. 85.)

Galega officinalis
Goat's rue (below)
A legume grown for its delicate pink, white or lilac flowers. Used medicinally.
(See p. 276.)

Delphinium elatum
Delphinium (below)
A tall plant for borders. Pretty blue flowers for arrangements and potpourri.

Scutellaria lateriflora
Skullcap (below)
Stems of unusual blue-mauve flowers. (See p. 278.)

Digitalis x mertonensis
Foxglove (right)
One of the several attractive forms of foxglove. (See p. 82.)

Teucrium chamaedrys
Wall germander (left)
Compact evergreen leaves make good ground cover. (See p. 85.)

Echium vulgare
Viper's bugloss
(above)
This herb is related to borage, and its flowers are similarly used as a garnish. (See p. 275.)

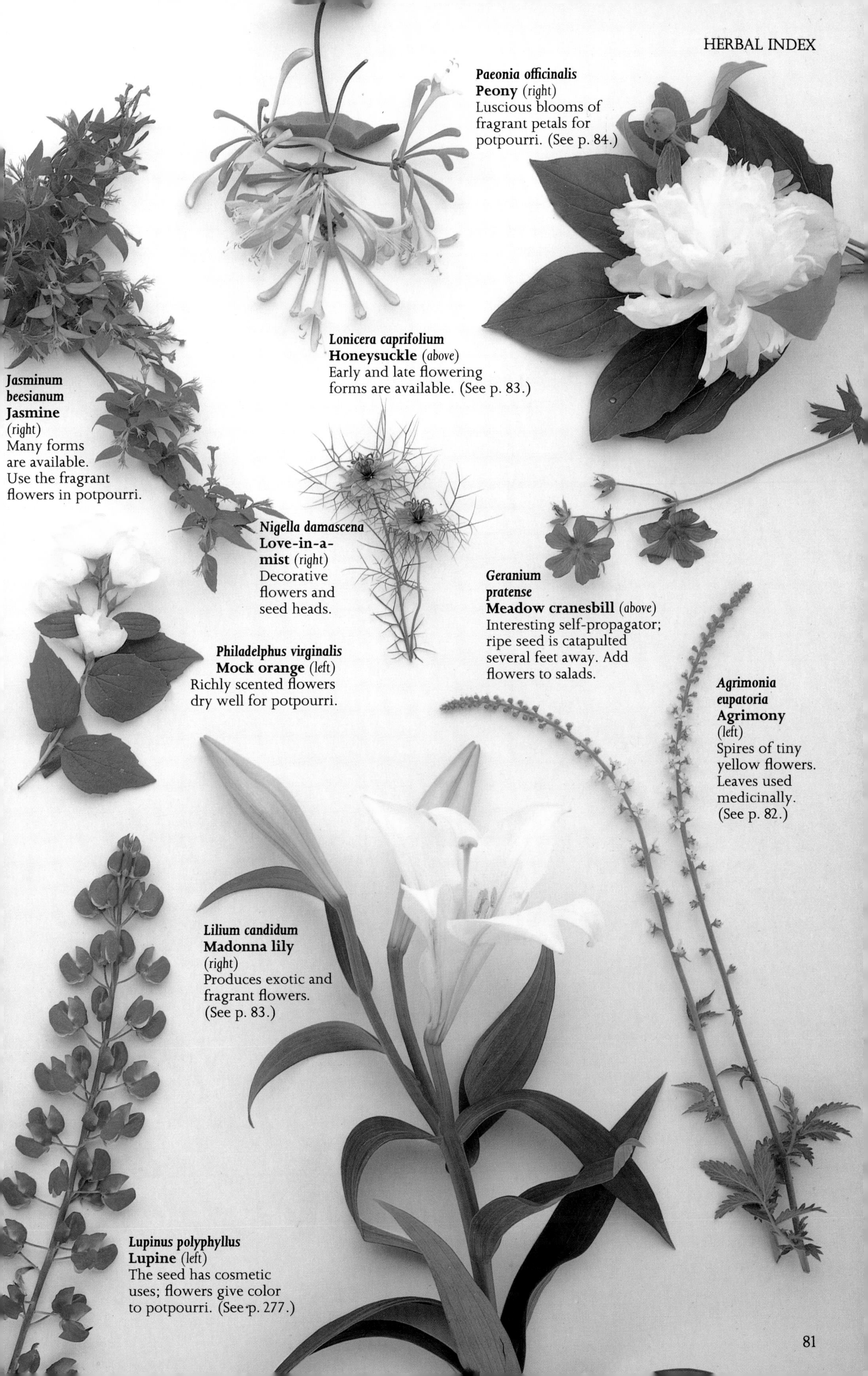

Paeonia officinalis
Peony (right)
Luscious blooms of
fragrant petals for
potpourri. (See p. 84.)

Lonicera caprifolium
Honeysuckle (above)
Early and late flowering
forms are available. (See p. 83.)

Jasminum
beesianum
Jasmine
(right)
Many forms
are available.
Use the fragrant
flowers in potpourri.

Nigella damascena
Love-in-a-
mist (right)
Decorative
flowers and
seed heads.

Geranium
pratense
Meadow cranesbill (above)
Interesting self-propagator;
ripe seed is catapulted
several feet away. Add
flowers to salads.

Philadelphus virginalis
Mock orange (left)
Richly scented flowers
dry well for potpourri.

Agrimonia
eupatoria
Agrimony
(left)
Spires of tiny
yellow flowers.
Leaves used
medicinally.
(See p. 82.)

Lilium candidum
Madonna lily
(right)
Produces exotic and
fragrant flowers.
(See p. 83.)

Lupinus polyphyllus
Lupine (left)
The seed has cosmetic
uses; flowers give color
to potpourri. (See p. 277.)

Flowering herbs

Agrimonia eupatoria

Agrimony   *Rosaceae*

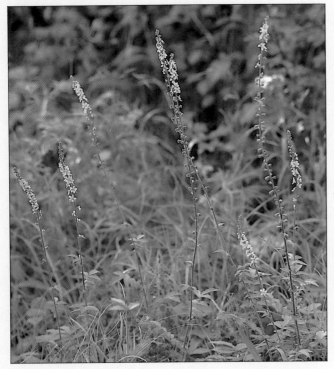

A graceful perennial suitable for a sunny border, agrimony is sometimes known as church steeples because of its thin, tapering spikes of small, star-shaped yellow flowers. The mid-green leaves have serrated edges and grow in alternate large and small pairs. The flowers, which are borne throughout the summer, have an apricot scent, particularly attractive to bees and other insects. The flower spike can grow to over 2 feet high.

CULTIVATION
Sow seed in late winter or spring, or, for better results, in late summer or early autumn in well-drained soil.

USES
In Anglo-Saxon times agrimony was virtually regarded as a heal-all with almost magical powers. Its name is thought to be a corruption of the Greek *Argemone*, used by Dioscorides to describe plants that healed eye disorders. It contains tannin, which as well as being recommended for dressing leather is good for skin eruptions, and it yields a yellow dye. Today it is made into an apricot-scented herb tea, and an infusion of agrimony is often prescribed for gastro-intestinal complaints, coughs, cystitis and as a gargle for sore throats. It may be used in an eyebath to add sparkle to tired eyes.

Digitalis purpurea

Foxglove   *Scrophulariaceae*

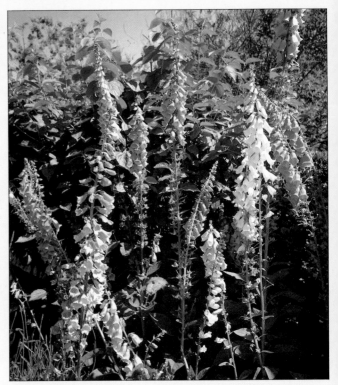

In some conditions the foxglove is a perennial, but it is usually best treated as a biennial. Tall spikes, growing 3–5 feet long, bear tubular, bell-like flowers throughout the summer. The flowers of the common *Digitalis purpurea* are purple or reddish, but hybrids are available in a variety of colors. The large, downy, mid-green leaves have slightly indented edges. Those of the common foxglove are oval, while *D. × mertonensis* (p. 80) has lance-shaped leaves and more luxuriant, showy flowers. Happy in full sun or partial shade, the foxglove makes a colorful and dramatic background to smaller border plants.

CULTIVATION
Sow seed in spring or early summer the year before the plant is to flower. The foxglove prefers well-drained, acid soil. Water well in dry weather and remove the central spike after flowering to increase the size of flowers on the side-shoots.

USES
For over 200 years *D. purpurea* has provided the main drug for treating heart-failure. It is also a powerful diuretic. Although a synthetic form of the drug has been developed, the plant is still grown commercially for the drug industry.

Note: *Foxgloves are poisonous and should not be eaten or used domestically.*

Lilium candidum
Madonna lily Liliaceae

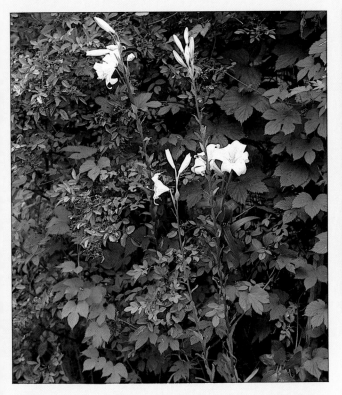

A favorite plant even as far back as ancient Greek and Roman times, the madonna lily, with its pure white flowers, was dedicated to the Virgin Mary in the early days of Christianity. The 3 inch long, trumpet-shaped flowers, borne in midsummer, have a sweet, penetrating fragrance. The erect flower stem grows to a height of 4–5 feet, with pale-green, lance-shaped leaves growing from it. After the stem dies down in autumn, it produces a rosette of basal leaves. Once established in a site where it is happy, preferably on a sunny sheltered slope, the madonna lily will flourish if left relatively undisturbed.

CULTIVATION
Plant bulbs in early autumn in well-drained, alkaline soil. Unlike many lilies, the madonna lily roots only from the base of its bulb, which needs to be covered in no more than 2 inches of soil. Do not allow to dry out. It can be difficult to establish.

USES
Plant along a garden path or within sight of a favorite bench to appreciate the madonna lily's striking, exotic-looking flowers and strong perfume. The flowers were once thought to be anti-epileptic and, steeped in spirit, provided a soothing lotion for bruises. The bulbs, collected in late summer, contain a rich mucilage which is used in cosmetics and added to an ointment for treating corns and burns. In some Eastern countries the bulbs are cooked and eaten.

Lonicera caprifolium
Honeysuckle Caprifoliaceae

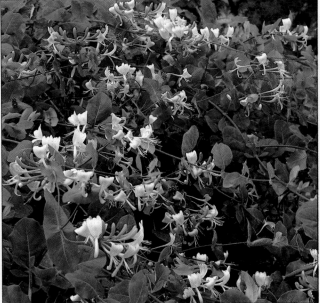

Also known as woodbine, the honeysuckle is a perennial twining climber which, given suitable support, can reach a height of 20 feet. Like the more common *Lonicera periclymenum*, *L. caprifolium* (above) can be found growing wild. It is distinguishable by its light-green oval leaves which sometimes merge across the stem rather than growing in pairs one on either side. The pink-tinged, creamy-white flowers, basically tubular with diverging lips, are borne in close pairs from midsummer to early autumn. Poisonous small orange berries appear after the flowers. The berries were once fed to chickens, and the Latin name *caprifolium*, meaning "goat's leaf," may reflect the belief that honeysuckle leaves are a favorite food of goats and resemble goat's ears.

CULTIVATION
Take cuttings from non-flowering shoots in summer and root in cuttings compost. Plant out during the autumn or winter, preferably in light shade. For areas with cold winters, *L. sempervivum* is a hardier species.

USES
Extremely tolerant, honeysuckle will flourish vigorously in the most unpromising sites. In leaf for most of the year, it can be used to cover an unsightly wall or provide a rich summer-evening fragrance in an arbour. Perfume can be obtained from the flowers, which add scent and interesting shapes to potpourri. They are also useful, as an infusion or syrup, for treating coughs, catarrh and asthma. The plant has diuretic and laxative properties and also contains salicylic acid, from which aspirin was once produced. Large doses cause vomiting.

Flowering herbs

Malva moschata
Musk mallow Malvaceae

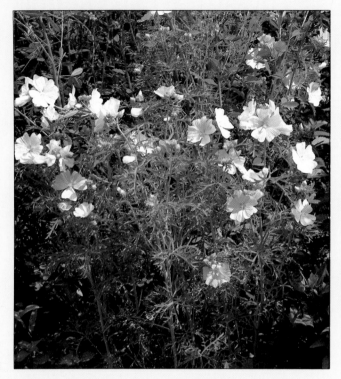

A pretty, bushy border perennial, the musk mallow grows to a height of about 2 feet. Spikes of large, single pink or white flowers are borne in abundance on its thick, erect stems from midsummer to early autumn. Even when the plant is not in flower, ample decoration is provided by its mid-green leaves, kidney-shaped near the base and divided on the stem. The leaves emit a musky aroma in warm weather or when gently pressed.

CULTIVATION
Sow seed in early autumn or spring, or plant rooted cuttings during autumn months, preferably in well-drained, fertile soil. Musk mallow needs staking in moist soil. It likes full sun but will also tolerate semi-shade. Cut down the stems in autumn.

USES
With similar properties to the common mallow (M. sylvestris), its larger flowers and subtle fragrance make the musk mallow the better choice in the herb garden. The leaves can be boiled and eaten as a vegetable. Both the leaves and the roots were once made into ointments and soothing syrups for coughs.

Paeonia officinalis
Peony Paeoniaceae

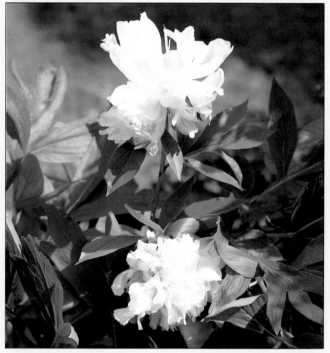

The sumptuous beauty of the peony makes it well worth the initial care needed to establish it in the herb garden. Several large bowls of petals, up to 5 inches across, are borne by each flower stalk in late spring and early summer. Growing to a height of 2 feet, the common peony was once available with only single, purplish-red flowers, but now double white or pink varieties are also to be found. The deeply indented leaves are mid-green. It thrives in an open sunny site, although early-morning sun is best avoided.

CULTIVATION
Single varieties can be grown from seed sown in autumn. The planting site should be dug deep and enriched with compost. Plant with the base of the stem no more than 1 inch deep in early autumn. It will take at least three years to become properly established. Water frequently in dry weather and stake the stems. Deadhead the spent flowers and cut down in autumn.

USES
Many ancient superstitions are connected with the peony. It was thought to be a divine plant that would drive away evil spirits and keep nightmares at bay. The seeds were once used as a spice in cookery. Herbalists prescribed an infusion of the powdered root for the liver and associated complaints. It was also thought to relieve spasms and convulsions and was given to women immediately after childbirth. It is now considered poisonous.

Rhodiola rosea (Sedum rosea)
Roseroot   *Crassulaceae*

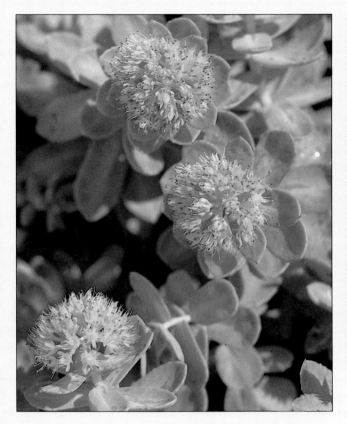

A perennial alpine or rock plant with egg-shaped, silvery-green, succulent leaves grouped closely around its thick stem. The star-shaped yellow flower heads attract bees and butterflies. When dry, the thick roots give off the scent of roses. Some sedums are used successfully to cover a dry wall, but roseroot, which can reach a height of 1 foot, is better suited to a sunny border.

CULTIVATION
Propagate by taking stem cuttings in late summer and inserting them in compost, or divide the roots in spring and plant in full sun in a well-drained, gritty soil. Remove dead flowerheads in spring.

USES
A tough, reliable plant, its flowers provide a splash of summer color. Mentioned in herbals as early as the sixteenth century, the root of the plant was used to make a "poor man's rosewater." Roseroot is little used today except in Greenland, where the leaves are eaten in salads all year round.

Teucrium chamaedrys
Wall germander   *Labiatae*

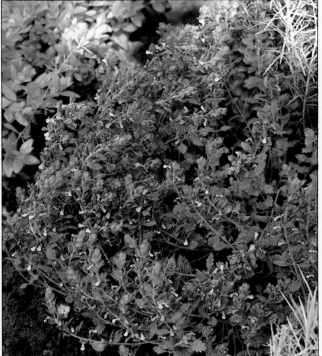

This small, bushy perennial, with its spreading, creeping root, bears tubular, purplish-pink flowers on short terminal spikes from midsummer to early autumn. The shiny evergreen leaves are indented and rather similar to oak leaves. Indeed the word *chamaedrys* means "ground oak." When rubbed, the leaves smell pleasantly spicy. Suitable for a rock garden, it also establishes itself well in the crevices of a dry wall, and is often found growing wild in old ruined buildings. It reaches a height of 1–2 feet and prefers well-drained soil in a sunny position.

CULTIVATION
For decorative wall-covering, sow seeds outdoors in seed trays in early summer and cover lightly with soil. Plant seedlings in the wall. For a rock garden, divide the roots in autumn. Take cuttings in late spring.

USES
Wall germander is a traditional knot-garden plant. The whole herb was collected in midsummer and dried. A decoction of germander was a famous remedy for gout and other pains in the limbs, such as rheumatism. Thought to be a diuretic and stimulating tonic, germander was also recommended for coughs and asthma. It was a popular strewing herb.

Hyssopus officinalis

Hyssop Labiatae

The Greek *hyssopos* may derive from the Hebrew *ezob*, or holy herb, because it was used for purifying temples and the ritual cleansing of lepers: "Purge me with hyssop, and I shall be clean" (Ps. 51: 7). The biblical plant may not in fact have been common hyssop but rather a form of oregano or savory. However, research now favors common hyssop once again, with the discovery that the mold that produces penicillin grows on its leaf. This could have acted as antibiotic protection when lepers were bathed in hyssop.

A wine called *hyssopites*, made from hyssop, was mentioned by the Roman writer Pliny in the first century A.D. This may have influenced the Benedictine monks who, in the tenth century, brought the herb into central Europe to flavor their liqueurs.

Seed
Brown, flattish, tear-shaped, $\frac{1}{8}$ inch long; may have a white tip.

Dried leaves
Used in tiny quantities in cooking; also medicinally and cosmetically.

Purple form

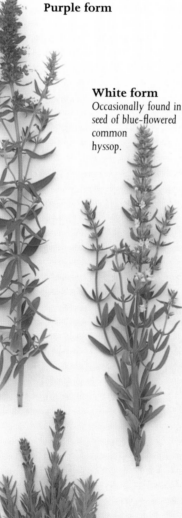

White form
Occasionally found in seed of blue-flowered common hyssop.

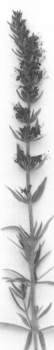

Flower
Rich blue, lipped clusters, in leaf axils up one side of the stems, borne in late summer; loved by bees and butterflies.

Stem
Square, branching and green, turning woody in second year.

Leaf
Narrow, $\frac{1}{4}$–1 inch long, aromatic, slightly hairy, pointed and dark green.

Pink form

H.o. 'Aristatus' Rock hyssop
Compact, with deep blue-purple flowers borne in late summer and narrow, aromatic leaves.

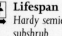 **Lifespan**
Hardy semievergreen subshrub

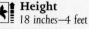 **Height**
18 inches–4 feet

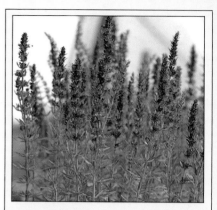

CULTIVATION
Site Full sun.
Soil Light, well drained, alkaline.
Propagating Divide roots in spring. Take stem cuttings from spring to autumn. (Species) Sow in spring.
Growing Transplant or thin to 2 feet apart, or to 1 foot apart, for hedging. Cut back to 8 inches in mild-winter areas after flowering; otherwise in spring. Hyssop can be grown indoors.
Harvesting Pick flowers and young flowering tops as flowering begins. Gather leaves anytime.
Preserving Dry young leaves and flowering tops.

USES
Decorative
● *Whole plant* Grow for hedging and knots, and in borders.

Culinary
● *Flower* Toss in salads.
● *Leaf* Use small amounts. Aids digestion of fatty fish and meat. Add to game (rub on skin), rabbit pie, kidney and lamb stews, rich pâté, vegetable soup and pulses. Serve with cranberries in fruit salads. Sprinkle $\frac{1}{4}$ teaspoon under the crust of peach and apricot pies.

Household
● *Whole plant* Grow near cabbages to lure away cabbage-white butterflies. Plant near vines to increase yield.

Aromatic
● *Flower and leaf* Add to potpourri.

Medicinal
● *Flowering top* Infuse as a tea for throat and lung complaints, bronchial catarrh, and poor digestion and appetite. Use essential oil in aromatherapy for bruises.
● *Leaf* Put leaves in a poultice to heal wounds and bruises.

Note: *Do not take hyssop when pregnant.*

Inula helenium

Elecampane *Compositae*

Helen of Troy was believed to be gathering elecampane when she was abducted by Paris, and its botanic name has captured this association. Its root contains a sweet starchy substance called inulin, which is responsible for elecampane's popularity as a crystallized sweet. According to the Roman writer Pliny, the Empress Julia Augusta "let no day pass without eating some of the roots candied, to help the digestion and cause mirth." In the Middle Ages, apothecaries sold the candied root in flat, pink, sugary cakes, which were sucked to alleviate asthma and indigestion and to sweeten the breath. In ancient China large-leafed plants were grown under scholars' windows so they could listen to different sounds of rain. Elecampane can be used for a similar effect in temperate climates.

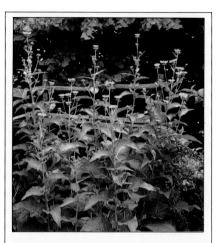

Seed
Mid-brown, torpedo-shaped, $\frac{3}{16}$ inch long, with short tufts of hair at one end, in velvety, dark brown seed heads.

Dried petals
Dry the shaggy, daisy-like, yellow flowers and use the petals in potpourri for color.

Leaf
Up to 18 inches long, pointed, coarsely toothed and green, with downy gray underside.

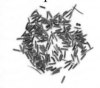

Lifespan
Hardy herbaceous perennial

Height
5–8 feet

Stem
Thick, hairy, ridged, round and green, filled with white spongy pith.

Root
Thick, dark brown, tuberous and aromatic with creamy, edible flesh smelling of bananas.

Dried root
This smells of violets and is used medicinally.

CULTIVATION
Site Prefers sun.
Soil Moist and fertile.
Propagating Sow in spring or divide plant in spring or autumn.
Growing Thin or transplant to 3–4 feet apart. Elecampane may require staking; it can become untidy. Prune in late summer. It is not suitable for indoor cultivation.
Harvesting Dig up second- or third-year roots in autumn.
Preserving Slice and dry root.

USES
Decorative
● *Whole plant* Striking garden plant.
● *Seed* Use velvety seed heads for winter arrangements.

Culinary
● **Root** Eat dried pieces or cook as a root vegetable. Be prepared for its sharp, bitter flavor. Crystallize as a sweet. It was a popular ingredient in Roman times, used to stimulate the appetite and to counteract the effects of rich food. Also used more recently to flavour absinthe.

Household
● **Root** Burn over embers to scent a room. Stephen Blake, in his *Complete Gardener's Practice* of 1664, suggested a more unusual use: To be revenged on a person who steals your flowers, sprinkle dry powdered elecampane root on clove gillyflowers, give to the party, who will delight to smell it, and when they draw the powder into their nostrils they will fall a sneezing until "tears run down their thighs."

Cosmetic
● **Root** Apply a decoction to acne.

Medicinal
● **Root** Decoct as a general tonic, as an expectorant to ease bronchitis and coughs, and as a digestive. Infuse in wine or port for a cordial. Crystallize and eat to relieve indigestion, asthma and coughs.

Lavandula angustifolia (L. officinalis or L. spica)

Lavender Labiatae

Tranquillity and purity are inherent in the unique fragrance of lavender, as reflected by the seventeenth-century angling author Izaak Walton, "I long to be in a house where the sheets smell of lavender." Its fresh clean scent was the favorite bathwater additive of the Greeks and Romans, and its name derives from the Latin lavare, "to wash."

A strewing herb popular both for its insect-repellent properties and its long-lasting fragrance, lavender was also distilled for liberal use in masking household smells and stinking streets. Stories that the glovers of Grasse, who used lavender oil to scent their fashionable leather, were remarkably free of plague, encouraged other people to carry lavender to ward off the pestilence.

Lavender has long been used medicinally. The herbalist Gerard, for example, prescribed it to bathe the temples of those with a "light migram or swimming of the braine." One Sir James Smith also told of an alcoholic tincture created "for those who wished to indulge in a dram under the appearance of elegant medicine."

Its healing powers are now mainly obtained from the essential oil. This is distilled from shining oil glands embedded among the tiny star-shaped hairs which cover the flowers, leaves and stems. The best-quality oil is extracted from L. angustifolia and L. stoechas. L. latifolia yields "spike" oil, used to perfume cheaper goods, while L. intermedia yields "lavandin," a medium-quality oil.

Seed
Four smooth, dark brown nutlets in each fruit.

Dried flowers
These produce a sweet, clean, long-lasting scent.

Flower
Small, highly scented, lavender-blue flowers borne in spikes 2–6 inches long in summer.

L. angustifolia 'Loddon Pink'
A pale pink-flowered lavender that is attractive mixed with other varieties.

L.a. 'Hidcote'
Compact, with dark purple flowers and small silver leaves. Slow growing.

L.a. 'Nana Alba'
White flower spikes, $1\frac{1}{2}$–2 inches long, with compact silver-gray foliage. Ht: 12 inches.

Stem
Square and green, becoming woody in second season.

L.a. 'Twickle Purple'
Compact, with long, soft purple spikes and broad gray-green leaves.

L.a. 'Vera' Dutch lavender
Purple flowers with leaves that are more slender, silver and compact than the species.

L.a. 'Folgate'
Compact with rich purple-blue flowers and narrow, gray-green leaves.

L.a. 'Munstead'
Early variety with lavender flowers and greenish leaves. Ht: 12–18 inches.

Leaf
Narrow, fragrant and gray-green, $\frac{3}{4}$–2 inches long.

Lifespan	Evergreen shrub
Height	18 inches–3 feet

OTHER SPECIES

L.stoechas var. pedunculata
Half-hardy, magenta-pink flowers with purple bracts above and gray-green leaves.

L. lanata
Half-hardy, bright purple flowers and white woolly leaves with balsamic-lavender scent.

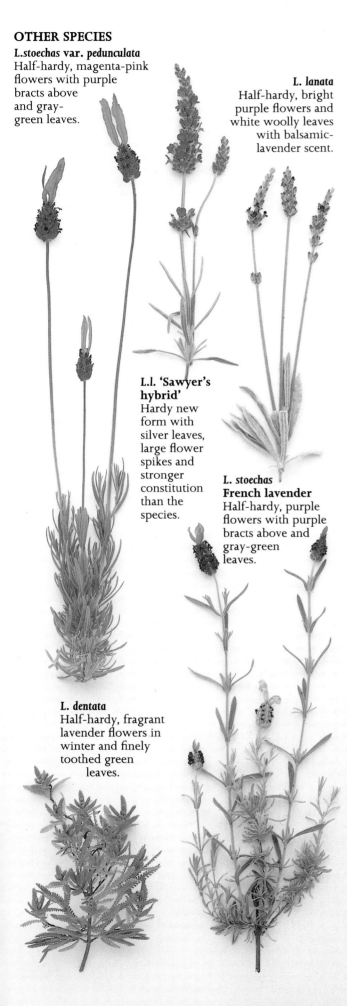

L.l. 'Sawyer's hybrid'
Hardy new form with silver leaves, large flower spikes and stronger constitution than the species.

L. stoechas
French lavender
Half-hardy, purple flowers with purple bracts above and gray-green leaves.

L. dentata
Half-hardy, fragrant lavender flowers in winter and finely toothed green leaves.

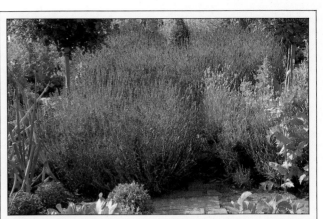

English lavender in flower.

CULTIVATION

Site Sunny and open, to discourage fungus disease.
Soil Well drained, sandy with lime content.
Propagating Take 4–8 inch stem cuttings during autumn or spring, or divide or layer plant. (Species only) Sow from fresh seed in late summer and autumn.
Growing Thin or transplant to 18 inches–2 feet apart, or 12 inches apart for hedges. Remove faded flower stems; prune hedges and straggly plants in late autumn or spring. (L.a. 'Grappenhall') Plant 4 feet apart.
Harvesting Gather flowering stems just as flowers open. Pick leaves anytime.
Preserving Dry flowering stems by laying on open trays or hanging in small bunches.

USES

Decorative
● *Whole plant* Good for hedging.
● *Flower* Hang dried in bunches on its own or with other tiny flowers. Add sprigs to wreaths and nosegays.

Culinary
● *Flower* Use to flavor jams and to make lavender vinegar (see p. 188). Mix small amounts with savory herbs for fragrant stews. Crystallize flowers.
● *Leaf* Bitter; used in southern European cooking.

Household
● *Flower* Put dried flowers in sachets and bundles to scent drawers and to protect linen from moths. Rub fresh flowers on skin, or pin on clothes, to discourage flies.
● *Stem* Use dried as incense or scented firelighters.

Cosmetic
● *Flower* Make tonic water for delicate and sensitive skins to speed cell replacement and for an antiseptic against acne. Add to soap. Use oil in massage for muscular aches, fluid retention and cellulite.

Aromatic
● *Flower* Use in potpourri, herb pillows, linen sachets. Add a few drops of essential oil to final rinse water for scented linen or hair.

Medicinal
● *Flower* Infuse as a tea to soothe headaches, calm nerves, ease flatulence, fainting, dizziness and halitosis. Use neat essential oil as an antiseptic, mild sedative and painkiller, particularly on insect bites, stings and small (cooled) burns. Add six drops to bathwater to calm irritable children, and place one drop on the temple for headache relief. Blend for use as a massage oil in aromatherapy for throat infections, skin sores, inflammation, rheumatic aches, anxiety, insomnia and depression.

Laurus nobilis

Bay/Sweet bay/Laurel Lauraceae

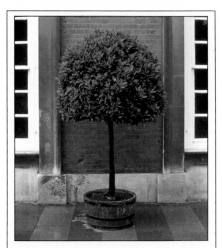

The bay tree was sacred to Apollo, the Greek god of prophecy, poetry and healing. His prophecies were communicated through his priestess at Delphi, who, among other rituals, ate a bay leaf before expounding her oracle. As bay leaves are slightly narcotic in large doses, they may have induced her trance.

Apollo's temple at Delphi had its roof made entirely of bay leaves for protection against disease, witchcraft and lightning. Bay-leaf garlands were subsequently adopted as architectural moldings. A wreath of bay leaves became the mark of excellence for poets and athletes and, to the Romans, bay was a symbol of wisdom and glory. The Latin *laurus* means "laurel" and *nobilis* "renowned"; *laureate* means "crowned with laurels," hence poet laureate and baccalaureate.

Bay was also dedicated to Apollo's son, Aesculapius, the Greek god of medicine, and it has been used against disease, especially plague, for many centuries.

CULTIVATION
Site Full sun. Protect from wind.
Soil Rich, moist and well drained.
Propagating Take 4 inch stem cuttings or layer in late summer. Plant cuttings in heated propagator with high humidity.
Growing Transplant to 4 feet apart, in frost-free area for first 2 years. Bay can be container-grown but bring indoors should the temperature drop below 5 °F.
Harvesting Pick leaves anytime.
Preserving Dry leaves. Use to flavor vinegar.

USES
Decorative
● *Whole plant* Clip for topiary.
● *Leaf* Make into wreaths.

Culinary
● *Leaf* Include in bouquet garni for stews, soups and sauces. Add to marinades, stock, potato soup, stuffing, pâté, curry, game and poached fish liquid. Remove leaf before serving. Boil in milk to flavor custards and rice pudding. Use as a garnish. Place in rice storage jar to flavor rice.

Household
● *Whole plant* Used as a strewing herb by highest-ranking officials.
● *Leaf* Place in flour bin and around dried figs as a weevil deterrent.

Cosmetic
● *Leaf* Add decoction to bathwater to relieve aching limbs.

Aromatic
● *Branch* Hang to freshen air.
● *Leaf* Crumble into potpourri.

Medicinal
● *Leaf* Infuse as a digestive aid and to stimulate the appetite. Massage blended essential oil around sprains and into rheumatic joints.

Note: *All laurels except sweet bay are poisonous.*

Dried leaves
Use within a few days of drying to capture optimum flavor. Old dried leaves lack pungency.

Leaf
Fragrant, leathery, pointed, oval, glossy dark green, with olive-green underside and bitter flavor.

L.n. 'Aurea'
Golden bay
Golden leaves; a slightly hardier variety than the species when both are small plants.

L.n. 'Angustifolia'
Willow leaf bay
This narrow-leaved variety was promoted as less susceptible to wind damage – an aim not achieved.

L. nobilis

Stem
Solid, round, rich purple-brown, becoming woody and gray.

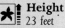 **Lifespan**
Evergreen tree. When mature, leaves may die in freezing winds

Height
23 feet

Levisticum officinale (Ligusticum levisticum)

Lovage Umbelliferae

Lovage is a handsome plant with a powerful flavor and numerous uses, both traditional and modern. Its leaves used to be laid in shoes to revive the weary traveler, and at inns it was served in a popular cordial, which was flavored with tansy and a variety of yarrow known as *Achillea ligustica* as well as lovage. A modern form is made by steeping fresh lovage seed in brandy, sweetening it with sugar and then drinking it to settle an upset stomach.

Lovage leaves add a strong savory flavor to dishes, so use cautiously at first.

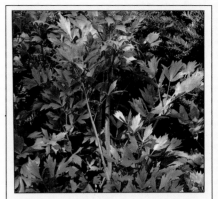

Seed
Brown, ridged, crescent shaped, oblong-sectioned and aromatic; about $\frac{1}{4}$ inch long.

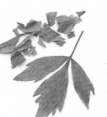

Dried leaves
These contain a strong flavor of yeast and celery; excellent infused as broth or for seasoning.

Dried root
These retain their aroma and are used medicinally.

Flower
Tiny, pale greenish-yellow clusters appear from mid- to late summer.

Leaf
Large, aromatic, toothed, deeply divided and glossy dark green on long stems; those leaves near top are smaller and stalkless.

Stem
Hollow, ridged, round, branching near top and greenish-red.

Lifespan
Hardy herbaceous perennial

Height
7 feet

Root
Thick, gray-brown, aromatic and branching with white flesh.

CULTIVATION

Site Full sun or partial shade.
Soil Rich, moist and well drained.
Propagating Sow fresh ripe seed in late summer. (Lovage self-seeds readily.) Take root cuttings with buds in spring or autumn.
Growing Thin or transplant to 2 feet apart. Tie straw around stems 2–3 weeks before harvesting for blanched tender vegetable. Not suitable for growing indoors.
Harvesting Pick leaves as needed, but retain young central leaves. Gather young blanched stems in spring. Dig second- and third-season roots before flowers open each year. Gather seed when ripe.
Preserving Freeze or dry leaves. Dry seeds and roots.

USES

Decorative
● *Leaf and stem* Arrange fresh leaves and stems in a clear tall vase.

Culinary
● *Seed* Add to liqueurs and cordials. Crush in bread and pastries. Sprinkle on salads, rice or mashed potatoes.
● *Leaf* Make lovage soup (see p. 166). Add fresh or dried leaves to stock, stews and cheese, and fresh young leaves to salads. Rub leaf on chicken and around salad bowl. Drink tea for its savory taste.
● *Stem and leaf stalk* Steam and serve with white sauce. Chop into stews and soup. Crystallize young stems. Eat raw shoots, 4 inches long, dressed with oil and vinegar.
● *Root* Peel; then cook or pickle.

Medicinal
● *Seed, leaf and root* Infuse any of these to reduce water retention, assist in removal of waste products, act as a deodorizer, and aid rheumatism. This infusion should not be taken during pregnancy or by those with kidney problems.

Marrubium vulgare

Horehound *Labiatae*

For thousands of years, horehound has been much valued as a cough remedy. Egyptian priests honored its medicinal properties and called it "seed of Horus," "bulls' blood" and "eye of the star." The Greek physician Hippocrates and other physicians down the ages have also held this herb in high esteem as a cure for many ills. It was also thought to break magical spells.

Horehound's botanical name comes from the Hebrew *marrob*, which translates as bitter juice. Its common name is derived from the Old English term for downy plant, *har hune*.

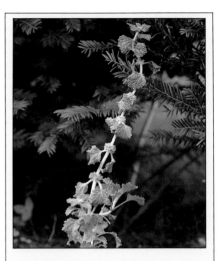

Seed
Shiny, dark brown, tear-shaped, $\frac{1}{12}$ inch long.

	Lifespan
	Hardy perennial
	Height
	18 inches

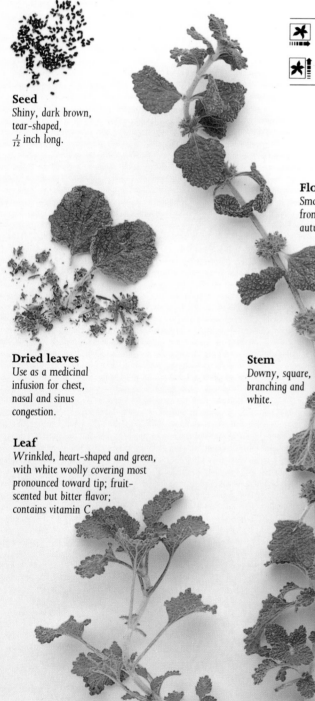

Flower
Small, white clusters borne from midsummer to early autumn from second year.

Dried leaves
Use as a medicinal infusion for chest, nasal and sinus congestion.

Stem
Downy, square, branching and white.

Leaf
Wrinkled, heart-shaped and green, with white woolly covering most pronounced toward tip; fruit-scented but bitter flavor; contains vitamin C.

CULTIVATION
Site Full sun. Protect from winds.
Soil Dryish and alkaline.
Propagating Divide horehound in midspring. Sow in late spring. Take stem cuttings in late summer.
Growing Thin or transplant to 1 foot apart. Protect from excessive winter wet. Prune in spring. Horehound can be cultivated indoors.
Harvesting Pick leaves and flowering tops at flowering time or as needed.
Preserving Dry leaves and flowering tops or make into syrup.

USES
Decorative
● *Flowers* Use dried in flower arrangements.

Household
● *Flower* Attracts bees to gardens.
● *Leaf* Infuse as a spray for cankerworm in trees. Infuse in fresh milk and set in a dish as a fly killer.

Medicinal
● *Leaf* At the first sign of a cold: finely chop nine small horehound leaves, mix with 1 tablespoon honey and eat slowly to ease sore throat or cough. Repeat several times if necessary. Suck horehound cough candy as an expectorant. To make cough candy: put 4 ounces fresh horehound leaves, $\frac{1}{2}$ teaspoon crushed aniseed and 3 crushed cardamom seeds in $2\frac{1}{2}$ cups water and simmer for 20 minutes. Strain through a fine filter. Over a low heat, dissolve 2 cups of white sugar and $1\frac{1}{2}$ cups of moist brown sugar in the liquid. Then boil over medium heat until the syrup hardens when drops are put in cold water. Pour into an oiled tray. Score when partially cooled. Store in waxed paper. Drink a cold infusion to ease digestion and heartburn, and to destroy intestinal worms.

Melilotus officinalis

Melilot/Sweet clover Leguminosae

The name melilot derives from *meli* meaning honey, and *lotos* meaning fodder or clover, hence its other name, sweet clover. A native of Europe, Asia and North America, it was once a popular strewing herb and fodder crop, until replaced by common clover, and was also a source of many successful medical remedies.

M. *alba*, with white flowers, originates from the Mediterranean and also decorates the highways of northern Alberta. There it is called Canadian sweet clover, and it is a valued honey plant. Near Gruyère, the Swiss pick a local blue form (M. *caerulea*) to flavor their cheese.

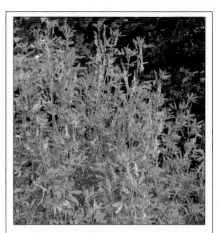

Seed
Small, brown, egg-shaped fruit pod, wrinkled and one-seeded.

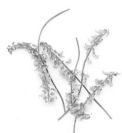

Dried flowers
Provide color and a little scent for potpourri; use in eye lotion.

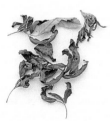

Dried leaves
Drying process develops coumarin — a long-lasting scent of new-mown hay — in the leaves.

Flower
Yellow, honey-scented, pealike flowers throughout summer and autumn.

Stem
Hollow, ridged, round, branching and green — occasionally red.

Leaf
Unevenly toothed and mid-green, with lighter underside. Faintly aromatic, leaves arranged in threes.

Lifespan
Hardy biennial. Behaves as an annual if sown in early spring

Height
M. officinalis 2–4 feet
M. alba 7 feet

CULTIVATION
Site Sun; tolerates light shade.
Soil Well drained.
Propagating Sow in spring or late summer. Self-seeds in light soils.
Growing Thin or transplant 18 inches apart. Not suitable indoors.
Harvesting Gather leaves and flowers anytime.
Preserving Dry leaves and flowers.

USES
Culinary
● **Leaf** Use dried leaves in a "cordial" and add small amounts to sausages, pork marinades and rabbit stuffings. Gives an original flavor to beer and cheese. Used in the Swiss green cheese Schabzieger and in Gruyère.

Household
● **Flower** Attracts bees to gardens.
● **Leaf** Scatter dried leaves among clothes to deter moths.

Cosmetic
● **Flower** Add to bathwater for a comforting bath. According to *The Fairfax Stillroom* (1651), to make a "Bath for Melancholy": take 3 handfuls each of mallows, pellitory-of-the-wall; one handful each of chamomile flowers and melilot flowers, and 1 ounce of celery seed. Boil in 10 gallons of water until reduced to $3\frac{1}{2}$ gallons, then add 4 cups of new milk and "go into it blood warm or something warmer."

Aromatic
● **Leaf** Add to potpourri.

Medicinal
● ***Whole plant*** Used dried as a mild antiseptic, in salves and to reduce the likelihood of thrombosis. Infuse for indigestion and headaches.
● **Flower** Use as a diluted infusion in a lotion or eyewash.
● **Leaf** Apply fresh leaves as a poultice for aching joints and cuts.

Mentha species

Mints Labiatae

In Greek mythology, Minthe was a nymph beloved by Pluto, who transformed her into this scented herb after his jealous wife took drastic action. Mint has been highly esteemed ever since, its value being epitomized by biblical references to the Pharisees collecting tithes in mint, dill and cumin. The Hebrews laid it on synagogue floors, and this idea was repeated centuries later in Italian churches, where the herb is called *Erba Santa Maria.*

Mint as a symbol of hospitality is mentioned by the Roman poet Ovid, who wrote of two peasants, Baucis and Philemon, who scoured their serving board with mint before feeding guests. Gerard enlarged on this theme in 1597: "they strew it in rooms and places of recreation, pleasure and repose, where feasts and banquets are made." The Romans also flavored wines and sauces with mint. However, when women who drank wine were threatened with death, secret drinkers would mask their breath by chewing a paste of mint and honey. In Japan, the refreshing, restorative scent of mint was so highly prized that the Japanese wore pomanders of its leaves.

Many mint varieties had been introduced into Europe by the ninth century. A monk writing during this time said that there were so many he would rather count the sparks of Vulcan's furnace. With more than 600 varieties, which continue to hybridize, the best way to select a good plant is by nose rather than by name.

Seed
Dark brown, roughly spherical and small.

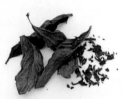

Dried leaves
These retain their flavor well for teas, cooking and medicinal uses.

Stem
Square, green and branching in the upper part.

Leaf
Oval, pointed, aromatic, green and wrinkled from deep veins.

**M. requienii
Corsican mint**
Tiny, peppermint-scented, bright green leaves and miniature flowers. Ht: 1 inch.

**M.s. 'Variegata'
Variegated applemint**
Cream-edged leaves with mild applemint flavor. Lasts longer into winter than other mints. Ht: 16 inches.

**M. spicata 'Moroccan'
Moroccan spearmint**
Closely set, toothed, bright green leaves with clean spearmint flavor. Ht: 2 feet.

**M. x gentilis 'Variegata'
Ginger mint**
Smooth gold-splashed leaf with a hint of spiciness. Prune to renew golden growth. Ht: 16 inches.

**M. raripila rubra
Red raripila spearmint**
Pointed, dark green leaves, with sweet spearmint flavor, purple stems and flowers borne in late summer. Ht: 2 feet.

**M. suaveolens
Applemint**
Hairy, apple-scented, bright green leaves. Ht: 2 feet.

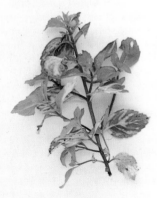

Lifespan
Hardy herbaceous perennial

Height
1 inch–3 feet; smaller species make good ground cover.

**M. spicata 'Crispii'
Curly mint**
Crinkled, deep green leaves, with savory apple scent. Ht: 16 inches.

OTHER SPECIES AND VARIETIES

Exact naming is difficult as mints interbreed so readily.

M. pul. 'Upright'
Upright pennyroyal
Smooth, bright green leaves, with strong peppermint scent.
Ht: 12 inches.

M. pulegium
Creeping pennyroyal
Bright green, peppermint-scented leaves, lax stems, which root where they touch earth.
Ht: 6 inches.

M. x aquatica 'Citrata'
Lemon mint
Smooth, lemon-scented, mid-green leaves.
Ht: 16 inches.

M. x villosa 'Alopecuroides'
Bowles' mint
Large, round, hairy, apple/spearmint-scented, mid-green leaves, pink flowers. Ht: 3 feet.

M. x p. 'Crispa'
Crinkle-leaved black peppermint
Vibrant green leaves with strong peppermint scent, purple stems. Ht: 2½ feet.

M. piperita 'Citrata'
Eau de cologne mint
Smooth, bergamot-scented, purple-tinged, dark green leaves, purple stems.
Ht: 18 inches.

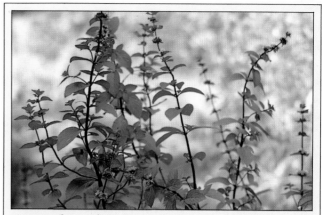

The mauve flowers of **M. spicata** appear in mid- to late summer.

CULTIVATION

Site Partial shade or sun.
Soil Moist, well-drained, alkaline soil, rich in nutrients.
Propagating Take root or stem cuttings, or divide mint, in spring and autumn. In summer, root stem cuttings in water. (Pennyroyal) Sow in spring.
Growing Thin or transplant, to 12 inches apart, into large pots or polythene bags to restrain invasive roots. Remove all flowering stems to avoid cross-pollination between species. If rust appears, dig up plant and burn. Mints can be grown indoors.
Harvesting Pick leaves just before flowering.
Preserving Dry, freeze or infuse leaves in oil or vinegar.

USES

Decorative
● *Leaf* Use in herb posies and invalid bouquets.

Culinary
● *Leaf* Infuse either individual or blended mints as a refreshing tea. (Spearmint and peppermint) Use for mint sauce, vinegar, syrups and with chocolate in rich desserts (see p. 165). Crystallize as a sweet for decoration. (Spearmint and applemint) Add fresh leaves to new potatoes, peas, fruit salads, drinks and punches. (Pennyroyal) Use sparingly in soups and stuffings.

Household
● *Whole plant* (Spearmint and peppermint) Grow near roses to deter aphids.
● *Leaf* Scatter fresh or dried leaves around food to deter mice. (Spearmints) Rub on a new beehive to attract bees. Use leaf oil to overpower tobacco smells. (Pennyroyal) Strew in cupboards and beds to deter ants and fleas.

Cosmetic
● *Leaf* (Spearmint) Decoct strongly to heal chapped hands. Add to bathwater for an invigorating bath. (Eau de cologne) Makes a refreshing bath.

Aromatic
● *Leaf* Use in potpourri and herb bags.

Medicinal
● *Leaf* (Spearmints) Inhale drops of essential oil, or sprinkle on a handkerchief, for relief from heavy colds. (Peppermints) Infuse as a tea to help digestion, colds and influenza. Sip cold tea for hiccups and flatulence. (Spearmint and peppermint) Macerate leaves in oil; then massage affected areas for migraines, facial neuralgia and rheumatic and muscular aches, especially in winter.

Note: *Do not take pennyroyal in large doses when pregnant or suffering from kidney problems. Use only under medical supervision.*

Melissa officinalis

Lemon balm *Labiatae*

Sacred to the temple of Diana, and used medicinally by the Greeks some 2,000 years ago, lemon balm was called "heart's delight" in southern Europe and the "elixir of life" by the Swiss physician Paracelsus. He believed the herb could completely revive a man, and this view was endorsed by the *London Dispensary*, in 1696: "Balm, given every morning, will renew youth, strengthen the brain and relieve languishing nature." Lemon balm was reputed to be among the regular morning teas imbibed in the thirteenth century by Llewelyn, Prince of Glamorgan, who lived to 108 years, while John Hussey, of Sydenham, England, lived to be 116 after 50 years of breakfasting on lemon balm tea with honey. Its virtue of dispelling melancholy has been praised by herbal writers for centuries, and it is still used today in aromatherapy to counter depression.

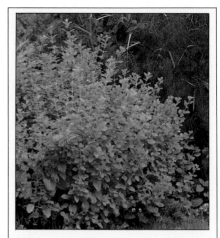

Seed
Shiny dark brown with white tip, tear-shaped, $\frac{1}{16}$ inch long.

Dried leaves
Drying lemon balm reduces its scent and medicinal properties.

**M.o. var. *variegata*
Variegated lemon balm**
Gold-splashed, lemon-scented leaves. Grow in light shade, as hot sun scorches leaves, creating pale spots. Ht: 1 foot.

Flower
Small, two-lipped, pale yellow blooms in clusters, maturing through white to pale blue, borne from summer to autumn.

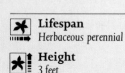

Lifespan
Herbaceous perennial

Height
3 feet

Stem
Hairy, square, branching and light green, with occasional purple markings.

Leaf
Lemon-scented, hairy, strongly veined, toothed, oval and light green. Leaves turn yellow and harsh-scented when grown in full sun and dry soil.

CULTIVATION
Site Full sun with midday shade.
Soil Grows in any moist soil.
Propagating Sow in spring, slow to germinate. Divide plant or take stem cuttings in spring or autumn.
Growing Thin or transplant to 2 feet apart. Small plants can be grown indoors.
Harvesting Pick leaves anytime, but handle gently to avoid bruising. Their flavor is best when flowers begin to open.
Preserving Dry leaves. Add fresh leaves to vinegar.

USES
Decorative
● *Leaf* Use in invalid posies.

Culinary
● *Leaf* Finely chop fresh leaves into salads, white sauces for fish, mayonnaise, sauerkraut, pickled herrings, poultry and pork. Add to fruit salads, jellies, custards, fruit drinks and wine cups. Infuse fresh leaves for melissa tea or float in Indian tea. Add to blended vinegars: try lemon balm with tarragon.

Household
● *Leaf* Plant around beehives and orchards to attract pollinating bees. Rub on beehives before introducing a new swarm. Add juice to furniture polish. Once a strewing herb.

Cosmetic
● *Leaf* Infuse as a facial steam and as a rinse for greasy hair. Add to bathwater. It is an essential ingredient in Carmelite water.

Aromatic
● *Leaf* Use in potpourri and pillows.

Medicinal
● *Leaf* Place fresh leaves directly onto insect bites and sores, or apply in a poultice. Infuse as a tea for relief from chronic bronchial catarrh, feverish colds, headaches, and to calm and uplift tension.

Monarda didyma

Bergamot/Bee balm Labiatae

This North American native became a popular garden and tisane plant in Europe after settlers sent back seed. The name *Monarda* honours the Spanish medical botanist Dr Nicholas Monardes of Seville, who wrote his herbal on the flora of America in 1569. He probably called this herb bergamot because its leaf scent resembles that of the small, bitter, Italian bergamot orange, *Citrus aurantium bergamia*, which produces the oil used in aromatherapy, perfumes and cosmetics. The Oswego Indians infused bergamot as a drink, and it became a popular tea substitute in New England after the Boston Tea Party, in 1773. Several Indian tribes used wild bergamot for colds and bronchial complaints, and, as it contains the powerful antiseptic thymol, it is worthy of further research.

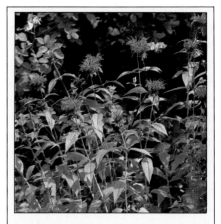

M.d. 'Blue Stocking'
Purple-blue flowers. Leaves are slightly less aromatic than the species.

Dried flowers
These retain their color well. Add to potpourri and teas.

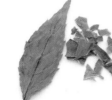

Dried leaves
Dry carefully and use for potpourri and teas.

Flower
Shaggy heads are a tight cluster of tubular scarlet blooms borne in late summer.

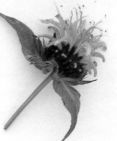

**M. fistulosa
Wild bergamot**
Lavender flowers (shown in bud).

Leaf
Toothed, oval, pointed, dark green with reddish veining, exuding eau de cologne scent strongest in young leaves.

M.d. 'Croftway Pink'
Soft pink flowers.

Stem
Hairy, hard, ridged, square, branching and tinged red at leaf joints.

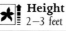 **Lifespan**
Hardy herbaceous perennial

Height
2–3 feet

CULTIVATION
Site Sun, or part shade in hot climate. Add a mulch in spring.
Soil Rich, light and moist.
Propagating Divide or take root cuttings in spring, stem cuttings in summer. (Species) Sow in spring.
Growing Thin or transplant to 18 inches apart. Divide every 3 years, discarding dead center. Bergamot is not suitable for growing indoors.
Harvesting Collect leaves in spring or in summer when flowers form. Pick flowers when open.
Preserving Dry leaves and flowers.

USES
Decorative
● *Flower* Use fresh and dried in flower arrangements.

Culinary
● *Flower* Scatter in salads.
● *Leaf* Infuse, or simmer for 10 minutes in an enamel saucepan for greater flavor, as a tea. Put fresh leaf into China tea for an Earl Grey flavor, into wine cups and into lemonade. Add sparingly to salads, stuffings, pork. Use for jams, jellies and bergamot milk: pour 1 cup of boiling milk over 1 tablespoon dried or 3 tablespoons shredded leaves, steep for 5–7 minutes, strain and serve.

Household
● *Flower* Attracts bumble bees (honey bees are unable to reach nectar unless holes have been made by other insects).

Cosmetic
● *Flowering top* (Wild bergamot) Boiled by Omaha and Ponca Indians to make a hair oil.

Aromatic
● *Flower and leaf* Use in potpourri.

Medicinal
● *Leaf* Infuse as a tea to relieve nausea, flatulence, menstrual pain and insomnia. Try steam inhalation for bronchial catarrh and sore throats.

Myrrhis odorata

Sweet cicely/Myrrh Umbelliferae

The attractive, fernlike leaves of sweet cicely are among the first to appear in spring and the last to depart in autumn. The soft green leaves have a myrrhlike scent with overtones of moss and woodland and a hint of aniseed, the botanic name of this plant being from the Greek word for perfume.

An extra bonus of sweet cicely is the cluster of large, upstanding green seeds or, more properly, fruits, which appear in early summer. They have a delicious nutty flavor and characteristic scent and, besides being excellent when eaten raw, they also provide an aromatic furniture polish.

A similar North American plant, *Osmorhiza longistylis*, flowers in early summer and has a sweet, aniseed-flavored root.

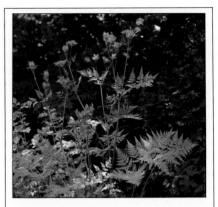

CULTIVATION

Site Light shade. Tolerates sun.
Soil Rich in humus.
Propagating Sow outdoors in autumn; seed requires several months of cold winter temperatures before germination.
Growing Transplant 2 feet apart in spring.
Harvesting Pick young leaves any time. Collect unripe seed when green; ripe seed when dark brown. Dig up roots in autumn.
Preserving Dry or pickle unripe seed. Clean and peel root, then infuse in wine or brandy.

USES

Culinary
● *Seed* Toss unripe seeds, which have a sweet flavor and nutty texture, into fruit salads. Chop into ice cream. Use ripe seed whole in cooked dishes such as apple pie; otherwise use crushed. Used to flavor chartreuse liqueur.
● *Leaf* Chop finely and stir into salad dressing and omelettes. Add to soups, stews and to boiling water when cooking cabbage. Cook with tart fruits (rhubarb, gooseberries, currants) to reduce acidity, thereby decreasing amount of sugar required. Add to cream for a sweeter and less fatty taste.
● *Root* Chop, peel and serve raw with salad dressing. Cook as a root vegetable and serve with butter, or cool and chop into salads.

Household
● *Seed* Crush as a furniture polish.

Medicinal
● *Whole plant* Considered to be a "wholesome" tonic (especially the root in brandy), mild antiseptic and digestive aid.
● *Leaf* A valuable "sweetener," especially for diabetics.
● *Root* When infused, enigmatically listed in old herbals as a valuable tonic for girls aged 15 to 18. Boiled root was prescribed to strengthen the elderly.

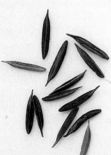

Ripe seed
Dark brown, glossy, ridged, ¾ inch long.

Dried leaves
These retain a little scent; occasionally used medicinally, also to decorate paper and candles.

Flower
Small white flowers appear in late spring. One of the earliest nectarous flowers for bees.

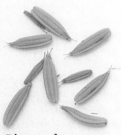

Unripe seed
Green, ridged, ¾ inch long appear late spring. Eat raw.

Leaf
Up to 18 inches long, downy beneath, green above. White markings may appear as season progresses.

Stem
Hollow, furrowed, downy surface; branching.

Root
Thick brown taproot, occasionally branching, with white, aromatic flesh.

Lifespan
Hardy herbaceous perennial

Height
3 feet

Myrtus communis

Myrtle Myrtaceae

In Greek legend, Myrrha was a favorite priestess of Venus, who transformed her into this fragrant evergreen to preserve her from too ardent a suitor. Venus wore a myrtle wreath when Paris awarded her the Golden Apple for beauty, and this herb was planted around all temples dedicated to her. Representing Venus and love, myrtle is often woven into bridal wreaths, and the Romans displayed it lavishly at feasts, weddings and celebrations. An Arabian story tells of Adam, banished from paradise, bringing a sprig of myrtle from the bower where he declared his love to Eve, and Shakespeare planned that Venus and Adonis should meet under myrtle shade. The apothecary John Parkinson wrote, "we nourish Myrtles with great care for their beautiful aspect, sweet scent and rarity."

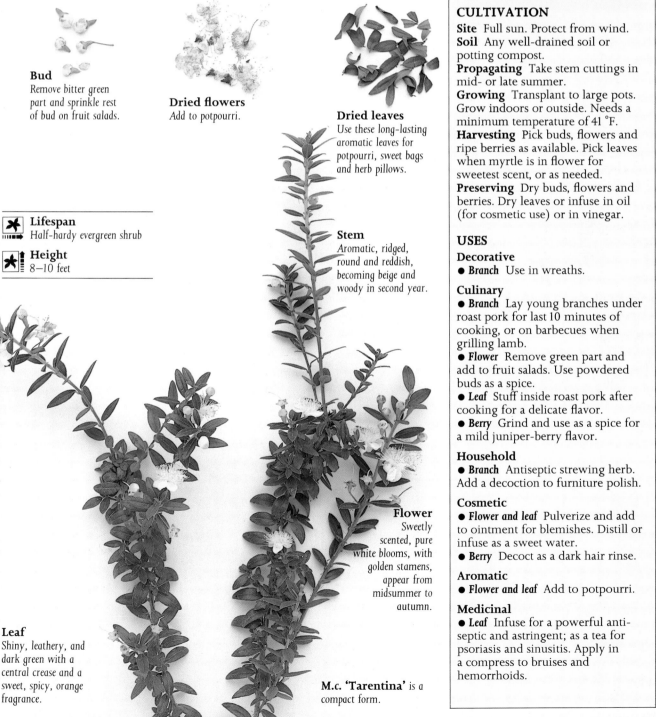

Bud
Remove bitter green part and sprinkle rest of bud on fruit salads.

Dried flowers
Add to potpourri.

Dried leaves
Use these long-lasting aromatic leaves for potpourri, sweet bags and herb pillows.

Stem
Aromatic, ridged, round and reddish, becoming beige and woody in second year.

✻ Lifespan
Half-hardy evergreen shrub

✻ Height
8–10 feet

Flower
Sweetly scented, pure white blooms, with golden stamens, appear from midsummer to autumn.

Leaf
Shiny, leathery, and dark green with a central crease and a sweet, spicy, orange fragrance.

M.c. 'Tarentina' *is a compact form.*

CULTIVATION
Site Full sun. Protect from wind.
Soil Any well-drained soil or potting compost.
Propagating Take stem cuttings in mid- or late summer.
Growing Transplant to large pots. Grow indoors or outside. Needs a minimum temperature of 41 °F.
Harvesting Pick buds, flowers and ripe berries as available. Pick leaves when myrtle is in flower for sweetest scent, or as needed.
Preserving Dry buds, flowers and berries. Dry leaves or infuse in oil (for cosmetic use) or in vinegar.

USES
Decorative
● **Branch** Use in wreaths.

Culinary
● **Branch** Lay young branches under roast pork for last 10 minutes of cooking, or on barbecues when grilling lamb.
● **Flower** Remove green part and add to fruit salads. Use powdered buds as a spice.
● **Leaf** Stuff inside roast pork after cooking for a delicate flavor.
● **Berry** Grind and use as a spice for a mild juniper-berry flavor.

Household
● **Branch** Antiseptic strewing herb. Add a decoction to furniture polish.

Cosmetic
● **Flower and leaf** Pulverize and add to ointment for blemishes. Distill or infuse as a sweet water.
● **Berry** Decoct as a dark hair rinse.

Aromatic
● **Flower and leaf** Add to potpourri.

Medicinal
● **Leaf** Infuse for a powerful antiseptic and astringent; as a tea for psoriasis and sinusitis. Apply in a compress to bruises and hemorrhoids.

Nepeta cataria

Catnip/Catmint Labiatae

The name *Nepeta* may derive from the Roman town Nepeti, where catnip was cultivated when it was more highly valued than today. It had a reputation as a seasoning and medicinal herb, and in less favorable times the mildly hallucinogenic dried leaves were smoked to relieve the pressures of life.

Set in a border, catnip can be a pretty plant, with its whorls of lavender or white flowers attracting the bees, if it is not damaged by cats. These animals will lie in the center of the plant, rubbing the leaves in a state of sheer bliss, thus giving catnip its common name. The smaller catmint, N. mussinii, receives less attention from cats, and its compact form, which produces masses of lavender-blue flowers, is traditionally planted in front of lavender and roses.

Seed
Small, rich brown, oval, flattish, with a white fleck on one end. Seeds are viable for 5 years.

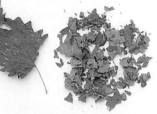

Dried leaves
Develop a sharp, balsamlike taste; use for tea and medicinal infusions.

Stem
Tall, hairy, ridged, square and branching; has pungent scent.

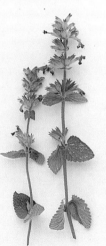

N. mussinii Catmint
An attractive edging plant with mildly fragrant 6 inch spikes of lavender-blue flowers from late spring to early autumn. Ht: 12–18 inches.

Leaf
Coarsely toothed, heart-shaped and gray-green with downy underside. Leaves grow in pairs opposite each other and have a penetrating, mintlike scent that is loved by cats.

 Lifespan
Hardy herbaceous perennial

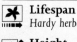 **Height**
18 inches–3 feet

A bed of flowering catmint.

CULTIVATION
Site Sun or light shade.
Soil Well drained.
Propagating Sow or divide whole plant in spring. Take softwood cuttings in late spring.
Growing Thin or transplant to 12 inches apart. Cut back in autumn. The scent released by any bruised leaf or root will attract cats, who then molest the plant, so plants grown from seed in situ are less likely to be damaged than transplanted plants, which may need protection. N. mussinii grows indoors.
Harvesting Gather leaves when young and flowering tops.
Preserving Dry whole plant.

USES
Decorative
● *Whole plant* (N. mussinii) Makes a good garden edging plant.

Culinary
● *Leaf* Rub on meat to flavor. Drunk as tea before China tea was introduced to the West.
● *Shoot* Use in salads, when young.

Household
● *Whole plant* Attracts bees.
● *Leaf* Dry and stuff into cloth "mice" as toys for cats. Catnip scent repels rats. Plant near vegetables to deter flea beetles.

Medicinal
● *Leaf and flowering top* Contain vitamin C. Infuse to relieve colds and fevers (as catnip induces sleep and perspiration but does not increase body temperature); for restlessness and colic in children, for headaches and upset stomachs, as a mild sedative. Apply infusion externally to soothe scalp irritations. Mash leaves and flowering tops for a poultice for external bruises.

Ocimum basilicum

Basil *Labiatae*

This important culinary herb, with its warm spicy flavor, sends cooks into poetic raptures. A native of Africa and Asia, basil is held in reverence as a plant imbued with divine essence, and therefore the Indians chose this herb upon which to swear their oaths in court. Basil was found growing around Christ's tomb after the resurrection, so some Greek Orthodox churches use it to prepare the holy water, and pots of basil are set below church altars.

There are many varieties of basil, including shrubby basil, which is a tropical species. In Haiti, it belongs to the pagan love goddess Erzulie, as a powerful protector, and in rural Mexico it is sometimes carried in pockets to magnetize money and to return a lover's roving eye.

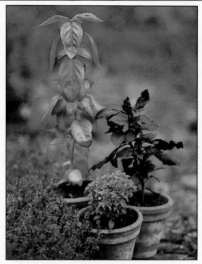

A selection of pot-grown basils.

CULTIVATION

Site Warm sun. Protect from wind, frost and scorching, midday sun.
Soil Well drained and moist.
Propagating Sow thinly in heated location. After danger of frost has passed, sow in pots or in position.
Growing Avoid overwatering seedlings as they are prone to "damping off." Thin to 8 inches; avoid transplanting. Always water at midday, not in the evening. Syringe leaves in hot weather. Basil is excellent pot-grown indoors.
Harvesting Pick leaves when young. Gather tops as flowers open.
Preserving Freeze leaves (first paint both sides with olive oil) or dry them. Store whole leaves in olive oil with salt or dry-pack them with salt. Infuse leaves in oil or vinegar.

USES
Culinary
● *Leaf* Pound with oil or tear with fingers rather than chop. Add at last minute to cooked dishes. Sprinkle over salads and sliced tomatoes. Basil's rich pungent flavor complements garlic. Used in pesto sauce and many Mediterranean dishes, and to flavor blended vinegars. See p. 164 for further ideas.

Household
● *Whole plant* Place pots on window sills to deter flies.

Cosmetic
● *Flowering top and leaf* Add a fresh infusion for an invigorating bath.

Medicinal
● *Leaf* Steep a few leaves in wine for several hours as a tonic. Infuse as a tea to aid digestion. Basil has many uses in aromatherapy. Put a drop of essential oil on a sleeve and inhale to allay mental fatigue.

Seed
Dark brown, faceted, tear-shaped, $\frac{1}{16}$ inch long.

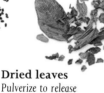

Dried leaves
Pulverize to release the clove scent and use in potpourri and scented beads.

O.b. 'Purpurascens'
Dark opal basil
Crinkled purple leaves with good medium flavor, pale pink flowers.

Flower
Small, scented, whitish blooms, in circular clusters of six, appear in late summer.

O.b. 'Citriodorum'
Lemon basil
Lemony scented, green leaves, white flowers.
Ht: 12 inches.

O.b. 'Minimum'
Bush, or Greek, basil
Compact. Tiny green leaves with good medium flavor. Hardiest variety in poor conditions.
Ht: 8 inches.

Leaf
Large, toothed, oval, pointed and bright green, with a warm yet fresh, strong, clovelike scent.

Stem
Hairy, finely ridged, square, branching and light green to reddish at base.

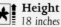

Lifespan
Tender annual

Height
18 inches

Oenothera biennis

Evening primrose Onagraceae

A plant for a moonlit garden: the clear yellow flowers of evening primrose unclasp their hooked cover at twilight and open their blossom to the moon, welcoming the night with their delicate sweet fragrance and mysterious emissions of phosphorescent light. As the season progresses, the flowers often stay open all day as well.

Though probably grown in nineteenth-century monastery gardens, the evening primrose was overlooked by the Austrian monk Gregor Mendel when choosing plants for his famous experiments on inheritance. However, it is now grown by geneticists to demonstrate the principles of heredity. Medical research is also currently exploring ways in which the seeds, which contain the rare gamma-linoleic acid, may alleviate premenstrual tension, menopausal discomfort, psoriasis, reduce thrombosis and control multiple sclerosis and other degenerative diseases. The increasing uses of evening primrose seed may well signal a time when whole fields billow with these glorious yellow flowers.

Lifespan
Hardy biennial

Height
3–6 feet

Seed
Beige, round, oily; contains gamma-linoleic acid and unknown anticoagulant compounds of interest to medical researchers.

Flower
Fragrant clear yellow flowers, 3 inches across, open from early summer to midautumn.

Root
Thick and conical, with yellow outside and white inside.

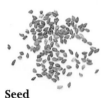

Stem
Sturdy, rough, hairy and reddish.

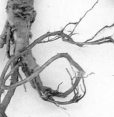

Leaf
Long, oval, pointed and mid-green, arranged in rosettes the first year; along the stem in the second.

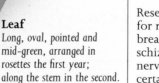

CULTIVATION
Site Sunny and open.
Soil Well drained.
Propagating Sow spring to early summer. Self-seeds in light soil.
Growing Transplant to 12 inches apart by autumn. Not suitable indoors.
Harvesting Collect seed when ripe. Gather leaves and stem "bark" when flowering stems have grown. Dig up roots in second year.
Preserving Dry seeds and leaves.

USES
Decorative
● *Whole plant* Long flowering season. Excellent in any garden.

Culinary
● *Leaf and stem* Once a popular food with North American Indians.
● *Root* Boil root, which tastes like sweet parsnip. Pickle and toss in salads or use as an aperitif.

Cosmetic
● *Leaf and stem* Infuse to make an astringent facial steam. Add to hand cream as a softening agent.

Medicinal
● *Seed* Take evening primrose oil capsules for premenstrual tension, menopausal discomfort and psoriasis. Gamma-linoleic acid lowers levels of cholesterol and blood pressure. Seems to reduce the risk of thrombosis, and to relieve symptoms of multiple sclerosis and other degenerative diseases.
● *Leaf and stem* Infuse peeled "bark" and leaves to soothe cough spasms.

Research continues into treatments for rheumatoid arthritis, benign breast tumors, hyperactivity, schizophrenia, alcoholism, anorexia nervosa, Parkinson's disease, and certain forms of infertility.

Onopordum acanthium

Cotton thistle *Compositae*

Readers of A. A. Milne's *Winnie the Pooh* will know how fond donkeys are of thistles, and the botanic name of this herb derives from the Greek *onos*, meaning "an ass," and *pedron*, meaning "I disperse wind." This perhaps provides a clue as to why the character Eeyore led such a solitary and sorrowful existence.

O. *acanthium* is thought to be the true Scotch thistle, the emblem of Scotland. This symbol was firmly fixed by 1503, when the poet Dunbar wrote "The Thrissill and the Rose" on the union of the Scottish James IV and the English Princess Margaret. The Order of the Thistle, which ordained Scottish knighthoods, was instituted by King James V in 1540.

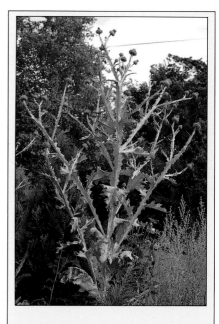

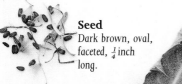

Seed
Dark brown, oval, faceted, $\frac{1}{4}$ inch long.

Dried leaves
These were once used medicinally. Down used to be collected for stuffing pillows.

Flower
Magenta-purple, tufted blooms, 2 inches across, borne in second summer.

First year plant
Clusters of silvery leaves appear in first season; tall flowering stems then grow in second season.

Stem
Spiny, winged stem of triangular section, covered with fine silvery down.

Root
Dark brown taproot, with beige side roots and white astringent flesh.

Leaf
Long, narrow, toothed with prickles, green with white down.

 Lifespan
Hardy biennial

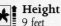 **Height**
9 feet

CULTIVATION
Site Full sun or light shade.
Soil Tolerates any soil, but requires rich loam to reach maximum height.
Propagating Sow in late spring in situ or in pots to be transplanted in autumn. May self-seed in warm climates. Cotton thistle can be started in early spring under glass.
Growing Thin or transplant to $2\frac{1}{2}$ feet apart. Not suitable for indoor growth.
Harvesting Pick flowers, leaves and stems as required. Collect seed and dig up roots in autumn of the plant's second season.
Preserving Dry leaves.

USES
Decorative
● *Whole plant* Makes a striking garden feature.
● *Flower* Popular in decorations.

Culinary
● *Seed* In the past, Cotton thistle seeds were used to produce an oil for cooking and lamps.
● *Flower* Prepare and cook large disk containing the florets in the same way as artichokes: remove petals and tough outer bracts and boil or steam until tender.
● *Stem* Blanch and peel young stems. Eat raw with oil and vinegar, or steam and serve like asparagus.

Medicinal
● *Leaf* Juice was said to relieve cancer and skin ulcers. Gerard's *Herbal* of 1597 declared it a remedy for "those with their bodies drawn backwards" (crick in the neck), based on the authority of the Roman writer Pliny.
● *Root* Decoction may diminish mucous discharges.

Origanum species

Marjorams & Oregano Labiatae

The Greeks have given us the legends and the name of this ancient culinary herb: *oros ganos*, joy-of-the-mountain. Those who have visited Greece, where oregano (wild marjoram) covers the hillsides and scents the summer air, would probably endorse the name. The sweet spicy scent of sweet marjoram was reputedly created by Aphrodite as a symbol of happiness. Bridal couples were crowned with garlands of marjoram, and plants were placed on tombs to give peace to departed spirits. Aristotle reported that tortoises who swallowed a snake would immediately eat oregano to prevent death, so it was taken as an antidote to poisoning. The Greeks enjoyed its scent after a bath, when marjoram oil was massaged into their foreheads and hair. Earlier still, in ancient Egypt, oregano's power to heal, disinfect and preserve was well known and has been treasured ever since.

Sweet marjoram was introduced into Europe in the Middle Ages and was in demand by ladies "to put in nosegays, sweet bags and sweet washing waters." Its leaves were also rubbed over heavy oak furniture and floors to give a fragrant polish. In thundery weather, dairymaids would place marjoram by pails of fresh milk in the curious belief that this plant would preserve its sweetness. This task might well have been followed by marjoram tea – advised by the herbalist Gerard for those who "are given to overmuch sighing."

Seed
Dark brown, tear-shaped and tiny.

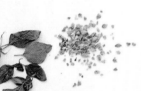

Dried leaves
These retain their flavor well and can be used in cooking.

Leaf
Oval, pointed; mid- to dark-green.

O. vulgare
Oregano
Slightly sprawling habit, dark green peppery-flavored leaves, (containing the powerful antiseptic thymol), white or pink flowers. Ht: 2 feet.

Stem
Erect to lax, hairy, round and green mottled with red.

Roots
Horizontal stems root wherever they touch the soil.

O. majorana
Sweet/Knotted marjoram
Tender, sweet spicy-flavored pale green leaves and white or purplish flowers producing seed clusters like "knots."

O. onites
Pot/French marjoram
Mid-green savory-flavored leaves and white or pink flowers.

Lifespan
Hardy herbaceous or shrubby perennial

Height
6 inches–2 feet

OTHER SPECIES AND VARIETIES

O.v. 'Variegatum' Gold variegated marjoram
Mild savory-flavored green leaves, splashed with gold in full sun, pale pink to white flowers.

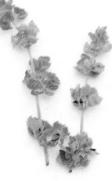

O.o. 'Crinkle Leaf'
Curled, savory-flavored, golden leaves that scorch in full sun, seldom flowers. Compact form.

O.v. 'Compact pink flowered'
Pungent, savory-flavored, dark green leaves. Compact, dark pink flower heads.

O. heracleoticum Winter marjoram
Tender. Sweet spicy aromatic leaves, pink flowers. Ht: 9 inches.

O.v. 'Aureum' Golden marjoram
Mild, savory-flavored golden leaves that scorch in full sun.

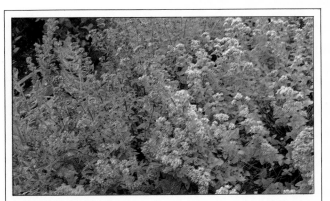

A bed of marjorams in flower.

CULTIVATION
Site Full sun. (Gold leaf forms) Need midday shade.
Soil Well drained, dryish, alkaline, nutrient rich. Unlike most other herbs from the same family, marjorams have a stronger flavor when grown in rich soil.
Propagating Sow in spring (germination can be slow). (Hardy perennials) Divide in spring or autumn. Take root or stem cuttings from late spring to midsummer.
Growing Thin out or transplant to 12–18 inches apart. Cut back marjoram plants by two-thirds before they die down for winter. If site is not too windy, leave seed heads for bird food. Marjorams can be grown indoors.
Harvesting Pick young leaves anytime. If leaves are to be used for preserving, gather just before flowers open.
Preserving Freeze or dry leaves. Macerate in oil or vinegar. Dry flowering tops.

USES
Culinary
● **Leaf** (Sweet marjoram) Infuse as an aromatic tea. Chop finely for salads and butter sauces for fish. Add to meat dishes in last few minutes of cooking. (Pot marjoram, oregano) Blend with chili and garlic. Add to pizza, tomatoes, egg and cheese dishes. Stuff fresh haddock with marjoram and breadcrumbs. Rub into roasting meat. Often included in bouquet garni (see also p. 165).
● **Stem** Give food a faint marjoram flavor by laying stems on barbecue embers.

Household
● **Flower** Grow to attract bees and butterflies.
● **Leaf** (Sweet marjoram) Add pulverized leaves or a strong decoction to furniture polish (see p. 195).

Cosmetic
● **Leaf** (Oregano) Infuse for a relaxing bath. Infuse strongly as a hair conditioner.

Aromatic
● **Leaf** (Sweet marjoram) Use in potpourri and pillows.

Medicinal
● **Flowering top** (Sweet marjoram) Infuse as a tea for colds, headaches, simple gastrointestinal and nervous disorders. Add a decoction or essential oil to bathwater, ointments or compress for relief from rheumatic pains and tension. Sprinkle a few drops of essential oil on a pillow to promote sleep. (Oregano) Infuse as a tea for coughs, stomach and gallbladder disorders, nervous headaches and irritability, general exhaustion and menstrual pains. Drink as a sedative to prevent sea-sickness. Apply externally as an antiseptic poultice for swellings, rheumatism and stiff necks.
● **Leaf** (Oregano) Chew, or rub on a drop of essential oil for temporary relief of toothache.

Papaver species

Poppies *Papaveraceae*

Around 3000 B.C., the Sumerians revered poppies as cult plants. The species gives us flowers described as the handmaidens of cornfields, voluptuous garden plants, an oil, edible seed and opium.

The laboratory analysis of the opium poppy is historically the transition from the magical and religious use of plants to scientific use. It also highlights the dangers of reducing plants to their chemical components. The opium poppy gives us morphine and codeine, our most important painkillers, and heroin, which is also addictive and results in much human misery. Its growth is strictly controlled in many countries.

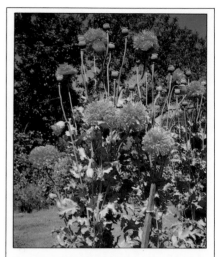

Ornamental double-form poppy.

Flower
White, pink, purple or dull red flowers appear in late summer. There is also a double form (below).

P. somniferum
Opium poppy

Seed
Minute blue-gray and kidney shaped (called maw seed). Indian or white flower seed is cream and smaller; flavors are similar.

Seed head
Bulbous, flat-capped, hairless capsule, becoming woody.

P. rhoeas
Field poppy/Corn poppy
Long, slender stem with solitary, dark-centered red flower. Ripe seed capsule has ring of pores near top.

Leaf
Smooth, deeply lobed, unsymmetrical and pale gray-green. Upper leaves clasp the stem.

Stem
Tall, slightly hairy, rigid and occasionally branching.

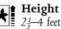

Lifespan
Hardy annual

Height
$2\frac{1}{2}$–4 feet

CULTIVATION
Site Full sun.
Soil Well drained and cultivated.
Propagating Sow in spring or autumn in flowering site, just pressing seed into soil. Field poppy requires a cold spell to trigger germination. Self-seeds freely.
Growing Thin to 12 inches. Not suitable for indoor cultivation.
Harvesting Collect seed when capsule is ripe.
Preserving Dry seed heads; then shake to extract seeds.

USES
Decorative
● *Whole plant* (Field poppy) Make a "poppy doll": bend back petals and tie around stem with grass; for arms, push dried stalk through capsule "head."
● *Seed* Use dried seed heads for winter arrangements.

Culinary
● *Seed* Sprinkle on bread, cake and biscuits for a pleasant nutty flavor. Add to curry powder for texture, flavor and as a thickener. Gives a culinary oil from first cold pressing.

Household
● *Seed* Feed to birds. An artist's oil is made from the second pressing.
● *Flower* (Field poppy) Petals used to color medicines and wines.

Medicinal
● *Seed* (Opium poppy) Latex from unripe capsule used originally to relieve pain, diarrhea, and some coughs, but is now main source of morphine, which has not yet been synthesized.

Note: *All parts of opium poppy except ripe seed are dangerous and should be used only by trained medical staff.*

Pelargonium species

Scented geraniums Geraniaceae

Most pelargoniums originate from the Cape of Good Hope in Africa, and although they were introduced to Britain in 1632, they remained relatively unknown until 1847, when the French perfume industry realized their aromatic potential. From the leaf of the rose-scented geranium, P. *graveolens*, the French distilled an oil with a delightful light rose perfume and a fresh green note. It is popular in cosmetics and important in aromatherapy. Unfortunately, it is an easy oil to adulterate, so purchase it from a reputable supplier.

In winter, the Victorians brought pot-grown pelargoniums indoors, and positioned them so that their long skirts would brush against the plants, thus scenting a room. In summer, they moved the pots outdoors and put them along paths for a similar effect.

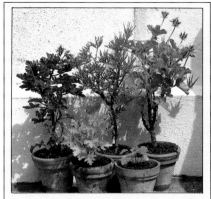

A collection of potted pelargoniums.

CULTIVATION

Site Sunny, well-ventilated position.
Soil Well-drained potting compost.
Propagating Sow in early spring. Take tip cuttings in spring (from over-wintered plants) or in late summer. May root well in sand.
Growing Grow pelargoniums in pots so they can be moved indoors in winter. Thin or transplant to individual pots. Pinch out growing tips when plants reach 6 inches. Cut back one-third of growth before bringing indoors.
Harvesting Pick leaves just before flowers open.
Preserving Dry leaves.

USES

Culinary
● **Flower** Toss in salads.
● **Leaf** Chop finely, or infuse in liquid, then discard leaves, and use to flavor sauces, custards, jellies, buns, water ices, butters, jams, sugar, syrups and vinegars. Crystallize to decorate cakes. Lay leaves under baked apples or cakes to impart flavor (see p. 186). Infuse as a tea or add to a wine cup. (Rose-peppermint scented) Add to liver pâté. (Piney-nutmeg scented) Cook in watercress soup and Welsh rarebit. (Apple scented) Bake with fish in cider.

Cosmetic
● **Leaf** Add essential oil to perfume and face creams (to balance sebum of oily and dry or inflamed skin). Infuse as a mild astringent to clean and help circulation of pale, sluggish complexions. Add to bathwater.

Aromatic
● **Leaf** Use in potpourri and pillows.

Medicinal
● **Leaf** Essential oil used in aromatherapy massages for premenstrual tension and fluid retention, dermatitis, eczema, herpes and dry skins. Add to massage oil for tonic to the nervous system.

Dried leaves
These retain their scent well, as do leaves that die on the plant.

P. *graveolens* 'Variegatum'
Rose-peppermint scent

P. *quercifolium*
"Oak" leaves smell of incense

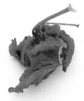

P. *crispum* 'Prince of Orange'
Orange scent

P. *radens*
Rose-lemon scent

P. × *fragrans*
Piney-nutmeg scent

Flower
Fragrant, pink or white blooms appear in summer to autumn.

Seedhead
Stork's bill-shaped, containing small black seed.

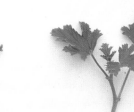

P. *odoratissimum*
Apple scent

P. *capitatum*
Rose scent

Stem
Hairy, round and green, becoming woody.

Leaf
Rose-scented, hairy, toothed, mid-green, with five to seven lobes.

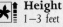 **Lifespan**
Tender evergreen perennial

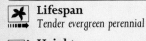 **Height**
1–3 feet

Petroselinum crispum

Parsley Umbelliferae

Held in high esteem by the Greeks, parsley was used to crown victors at the Isthmian Games and to decorate tombs, being linked with Archemorus, the herald of death. The Greeks also planted parsley and rue along the edges of herb beds, thereby instigating the expression "being at the parsley and rue," meaning to be at the start of an enterprise. Although the Greeks used parsley medicinally, and Homer recorded that warriors fed parsley to their horses, it appears that the Romans were the first to use it as a food. They consumed parsley in quantity and made garlands for banquet guests to discourage intoxication and to counter strong odors.

There are many excellent parsley varieties, including Hamburg parsley (*P.c.* 'Tuberosum'). This has flat leaves and a large, edible, well-flavored root. All parsleys are rich in vitamins, minerals and antiseptic chlorophyll, making it a beneficial as well as attractive garnishing herb. Set out a dish of the leaves each day and enjoy a flavor described as the "summation of all things green."

Seed
Small, gray-brown and sickle-shaped with cream ridges; contains apiole, which can be toxic.

Leaf
Finely cut, curled, with toothed margins and bright green, with fresh taste; rich in vitamins A, B and C, salts of iron, calcium, magnesium and chlorophyll.

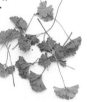

Dried leaves
These retain most flavor when dried quickly. Use in cooking and boil with stem for a yellow-green dye.

**P. crispum
Curled parsley**

P.c. 'Neapolitanum' Italian, or French, parsley
Flat, cut, dark green leaves with stronger, coarser flavor than the species, and edible, succulent stems. Ht: 2 feet.

Stem
Solid, ridged, semi-circular, branching and mid-green; more strongly flavored than leaves.

Root
Thin, brownish-yellow, smooth taproot with tiny hairlike roots; contains strongest parsley flavor.

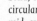 **Lifespan**
Hardy biennial

 Height
15 inches

CULTIVATION
Site Full sun or light shade.
Soil Rich, moist and deeply dug.
Propagating Sow from spring to late summer. For fast germination: soak seed overnight in warm water, pour boiling water in drill before sowing or grow in seed tray and maintain 70 °F. Self-seeds.
Growing Thin or transplant to 9 inches apart. Protect in cold weather. Grows well indoors.
Harvesting Pick leaves during first year. Collect seeds when ripe. Dig up roots in autumn of second year.
Preserving Dry or freeze leaves. Dry or blanch and freeze roots.

USES
Culinary
● *Leaf* Add raw to salads. Finely chop and sprinkle over sandwiches, egg dishes, vegetable soups, fish, and boiled potatoes. Add to mayonnaise and many classic sauces. When cooked, parsley enhances other flavors, but add towards end of cooking time (see p. 165). Use in bouquet garni.
● *Root* Use in bouquet garni. Add to soups and stews. (Hamburg parsley) Boil as a root vegetable. Grate raw into salads.

Household
● *Whole plant* Grow by roses to improve their health and scent.

Cosmetic
● *Leaf* Infuse as a hair tonic and conditioner. Add to facial steam and lotion for dry skin and to minimize freckles. Use infusion as a soothing eyebath.

Medicinal
● *Leaf* Chew raw to freshen the breath and promote healthy skin. Infuse for a digestive tonic. Use in a poultice as an antiseptic dressing for sprains, wounds and insect bites.
● *Root* Decoct for kidney troubles and as a mild laxative. Apply juice to reduce swellings.

Pimpinella anisum

Anise/Aniseed Umbelliferae

This graceful feathery annual has been cultivated for centuries. Around 1500 B.C., the Egyptians grew their native anise in quantity to supply food, drink and medicine from its leaves and seed. The fields of Tuscany were planted with anise by the Romans, who developed a special spiced cake, *mustaceum*, as a finishing dish for feasts. It was baked with anise, cumin and other digestive herbs and established a tradition thought to be the precursor of spiced wedding cakes. Charlemagne's edict of the ninth century, that every herb growing in St. Gall's monastery should be planted on all his royal estates, spread anise throughout Europe. It became so valued in England that its import was taxed. Early colonists carried the seed to North America, where Shakers grew it in their medicinal herb crops.

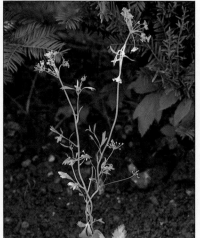

Flower
Small, starlike, white blooms, in clusters, appear in late summer.

Seed
Aromatic, light gray-brown, ridged, elongated, pointed egg-shape; requires a sunny summer to ripen fully.

Stem
Ridged, round, branching and mid-green.

Leaf
Aromatic, toothed, round, lobed and mid-green lower leaves; finely divided and feathery upper leaves.

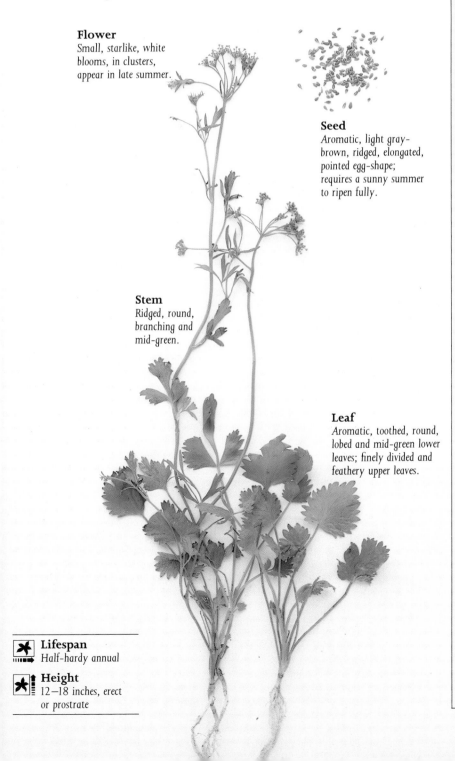

Lifespan
Half-hardy annual

Height
12–18 inches, erect or prostrate

CULTIVATION
Site Sunny and sheltered.
Soil Well drained and alkaline.
Propagating Sow in situ in late spring. Seed loses viability after second year.
Growing Thin to 8 inches apart; do not transplant, so keep well weeded. Can be grown indoors.
Harvesting Pick lower leaves as required. Collect flowers as they open. For seed, cut plant at ground level when fruit begins to turn gray-green at the tips. Gather stems and dig up roots in autumn.
Preserving Dry seed by suspending plant until ripe (see p. 270).

USES
Culinary
● **Seed** Use whole or crushed in breads, cakes, apple pies, apple sauces, creams and confectionery. Add to cream cheese, pickles, curries and water for boiling shellfish. Chew slightly roasted seed after a meal as a breath sweetener and digestive. It flavors many liqueurs.
● **Flower** Mix into fruit salads.
● **Leaf** Add to fruit salads with figs, dates and chestnuts. Use to garnish.
● **Stem and root** Mix into soups and stews for a hint of licorice.

Household
● **Seed** Set as a bait in mouse traps.

Cosmetic
● **Seed** Add ground to a face pack. Seed oil is used in perfumes, tooth-pastes, soaps and mouthwashes.

Aromatic
● **Seed** Use crushed in potpourri.

Medicinal
● **Seed** Infuse as a comforting antiseptic tea for colds, coughs and bronchial problems; to soothe colic in babies, relieve nausea, and as a gland stimulant for nursing mothers to increase their milk supply.

Herbal trees

Although rarely considered for their herbal attributes, trees provide sap, bark, leaves, blossoms, berries and nuts – many of which have potent herbal properties. They have always supplied people's basic needs – fuel, food, building material and furniture – and given us herbal gifts such as dyes, medicines, salad and liqueur ingredients, household articles and aromatic items. Each month has its useful trees; the ancient Druids created a 13-month lunar calendar with a valued tree for each month, featuring oak for the summer solstice. Reaching great heights and extending deep into the earth, trees also give us spiritual sustenance as an almost universal symbol of wisdom and strength. They can provide an inspirational framework for a large herb garden.

Prunus dulcis
Sweet almond (*above*)
Yields rich almond oil, used in cosmetics and aromatherapy. (See p. 274.)

Sambucus nigra
Elder (*left*)
Flowers and fruit yield food, drinks, medicines, cosmetics, insect repellent and dyes. (See p. 115.)

Ginkgo biloba
Maidenhair tree (*above*)
Seeds and leaves are used medicinally in China. (See p. 273.)

Ilex aquifolium
English holly (*right*)
The tonic leaves have been used medicinally. Berries are toxic. (See p. 273.)

Betula pendula
Silver birch (*right*)
Birch leaves are antiseptic; all parts of the tree are useful. (See p. 112.)

Crataegus monogyna
Hawthorn (*left*)
The ripe fruits are an excellent tonic for the heart and circulatory system. (See p. 112.)

Picea abies
Norway spruce (*above*)
Yields a medicinal pitch and resin. Leaf tips used to make beer. (See p. 114.)

Tilia cordata
Linden (*right*)
Linden-blossom tea is a popular remedy for nervous tension. (See p. 115.)

Quercus robur
English oak (*above*) Oak bark yields dye and tannin. Highly valued for centuries. (See p. 274.)

Juglans regia
Walnut (*above*)
Provides edible nuts and has other useful properties. (See p. 113.)

Cytisus scoparius
Broom (*below*)
Attractive flowering tree with many useful properties, including a dye and fibrous bark. (See p. 113.)

Populus balsamifera '**Aurora**'
Balsam poplar (*left*)
"Balm of Gilead" scented buds obtained from the species and this variegated form. (See p. 274.)

Juniperus communis
Juniper (*above*)
Berries are used as flavoring and are antiseptic. (See p. 114.)

111

Herbal trees

Betula pendula
Silver birch *Betulaceae*

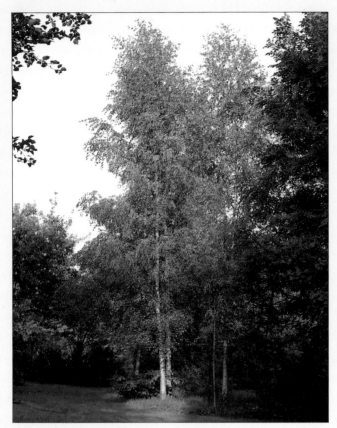

An elegant and graceful tree, with its silvery bark and mid-green oval leaves, the silver birch has a lovely fragrance after rain. It can grow to a height of 20–60 feet with a spread of 8–12 feet and bears male and female catkins in spring. In ancient times its softish wood was used in roof- and boat-building, and its bark served as a writing material as well as a medication.

CULTIVATION
Sow seeds in boxes in early spring. When large enough, prick out into nursery rows outdoors. After two to three years, plant out during autumn or spring in permanent positions. Thriving in any site and soil type, silver birch needs plenty of space to allow room for its wide-spreading surface roots.

USES
Birch twigs make strong, effective brooms, and are traditionally used in a sauna. Wine and vinegar can be made from the sap, and beer from the bark. Birch tea, made from the leaves, used to be recommended for rheumatism and gout. Oil extracted from the bark is used for dressing leather and in medicated soaps for skin conditions such as eczema.

Crataegus monogyna
Hawthorn *Rosaceae*

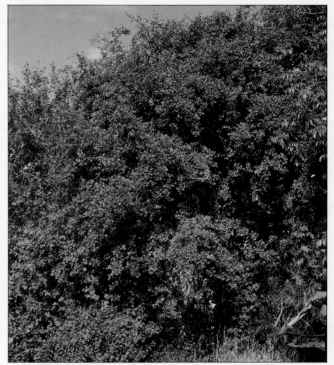

A tough, thorny perennial, the hawthorn grows very rapidly once established. It will thrive in semi-shade, but is happiest in an open, sunny position where it can reach a height of 30 feet with a spread of 15–20 feet. Its dark-green leaves are lobed and toothed and, in late spring, it bears clusters of lovely, sweetly scented white flowers, followed by bright-red berries from late summer well into the autumn. Tradition links the tree with Christianity. Christ wore a crown of thorns and, according to legend, in A.D. 60 when Joseph of Arimathea went to Britain to deliver the Holy Grail, he struck his staff into the ground at Glastonbury, where it took root, flowering twice a year, once in spring and once at Christmas.

CULTIVATION
Sow ripe seeds outdoors in late winter/early spring, or plant young shrubs from autumn until early spring. Protect with tree sleeves. For a hedge, plant shrubs at 12–16 inch intervals and trim between midsummer and spring.

USES
Hawthorn makes a good, thick hedge or an attractive specimen tree for a lawn. When burned, it gives off a great deal of heat. Today the flowers and especially the berries are used in cardiac tonics. A liqueur can be made from the berries mixed with brandy.

Cytisus scoparius
Broom   Leguminosae

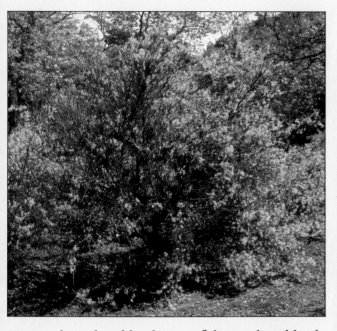

Honored as a heraldic device of the medieval lords
of Brittany and the Plantagenet rulers of England,
common broom is a deciduous perennial shrub
that could once be found extensively growing
wild. With a height and spread of 8 feet, it
has long, erect branches which remain bright
green even in winter. In late spring and early
summer the branches are covered with a mass of
yellow, fragrant flowers, followed by black seed
pods. The flowers, rich in pollen, attract bees, and
hybrids are available in a variety of colors from
white to red.

CULTIVATION
Although very adaptable, broom prefers full sun and a
well-drained, slightly acid soil. Sow seeds as soon as
they are ripe, and transplant the seedlings to their
permanent position in autumn. Broom can also be
increased by layering. Prune annually after flowering
to prevent the plant becoming leggy.

USES
A colorful and useful addition to the garden, broom
will bind the soil on a steep bank and provide shelter
for other shrubs until they become established. It
derives its common name from the fact that its tough
and flexible branches were made into brooms. The
tannin in its bark was once employed to tan leather and
the seeds have been used as a substitute for coffee.
Before hops were introduced to brewing, the young
green tops added bitterness to beer, and broom buds
were held to be a delicacy, often pickled to resemble
capers. Known for its medical properties in Anglo-
Saxon times, broom was thought to cure kidney and
bladder complaints. Today it is an ingredient of a
number of pharmaceutical drugs, including diuretics.
Slightly narcotic, and dangerous in large doses, broom
is considered unsafe and not suitable for domestic use.

Juglans regia
Walnut   Juglandaceae

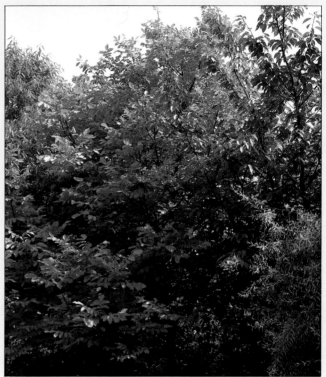

This handsome, deciduous tree, with its massive
trunk and large, spreading branches, can reach a
height of 100 feet. It bears both male and female
flowers in late spring: the insignificant tiny green
female flowers in small clusters and the yellowish-
green male flowers in catkins. The glossy, bright-
green oval leaves have a strong aroma. Walnut
trees are cultivated commercially for their timber
as well as for their nuts.

CULTIVATION
Sow seeds in nursery beds in mid- to late autumn and
leave for two or three years before transplanting during
the autumn or spring. Choose an open site with fertile,
well-drained soil, where the tree will be protected
from spring frosts. Trees raised from seed will produce
edible nuts after about 15 years.

USES
Green, unripe walnuts can be pickled in vinegar,
preserved in syrup or made into a liqueur. Mature nuts
are added to cake mixtures, stuffings and sauces. They
are an essential ingredient of some salads and a variety
of salad oil. The boiled green husks of the nuts give a
yellow dye, and a brown hair dye can be obtained
from the leaves and outer shells. An infusion of the
dried leaves can help skin complaints such as eczema
and herpes, while an infusion of the powdered bark is
said to act as a laxative.

Herbal trees

Juniperus communis

Juniper Cupressaceae

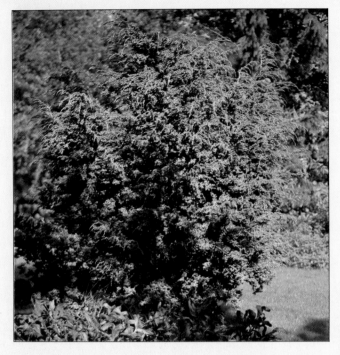

This low, prickly bush or tree, between 4 and 10 feet high, is a slow-growing coniferous evergreen. It has silvery-green spiny needles and, from late spring to early summer, bears small yellow flowers. The juniper is cultivated for its berries, which take up to three years to ripen, when they change from green to silvery-purple. The slightly resinous, sweetly flavored berries are borne only by the female bush, and can be found in various stages of ripeness on the same plant. Their flavor is stronger the farther south the plant is grown. Many ornamental varieties are available.

CULTIVATION
Suitable for an exposed, sunny site, the juniper will tolerate an alkaline soil. Sow seeds taken from ripe berries in cold frames in early autumn. Grow the seedlings on in nursery rows outdoors for one or two years before planting in permanent positions. Both male and female plants are necessary for berry production. To be sure of the plant's gender, it is best to cultivate from semi-hardwood cuttings taken late summer to early autumn.

USES
As well as giving gin its characteristic flavor, juniper berries are used to flavor other spirits and beer. Crushed berries are added to marinades for game and stuffings for poultry (see p. 164). An infusion of the berries is thought to have diuretic properties and to be good for cystitis. It also soothes aching muscles. Juniper berries should not be taken during pregnancy or by people with kidney problems.

Note: *Repeated use can cause kidney damage.*

Picea abies

Norway spruce Pinaceae

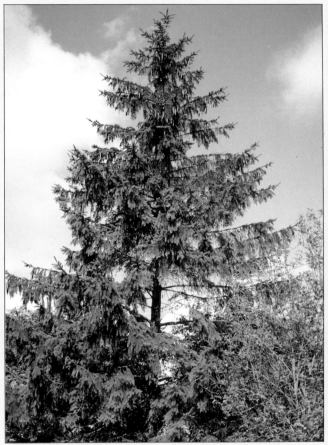

Familiar to millions of people as the traditional Christmas tree, the Norway spruce can reach a height of 150 feet (40–60 feet is average), with a spread of 20–30 feet. Its evergreen, needlelike leaves appear on the upper side of its branches only. When the tree is about 40 years old, it begins to produce 6 inch-long cylindrical cones, which hang downward. Like many conifers, it is grown commercially for its light but strong timber.

CULTIVATION
Sow seeds in pots in early spring. Move the seedlings to nursery beds the following spring. Plant in their permanent positions in the autumn or spring two or three years later. Choose a sheltered site, where the soil is moist and acid.

USES
Oil of turpentine, rosin and oil of tar are all obtained from the resin of spruce and other members of the pine family. Its leaves and twigs fermented with yeast and sugar produce spruce beer.

Sambucus nigra
Elder *Caprifoliaceae*

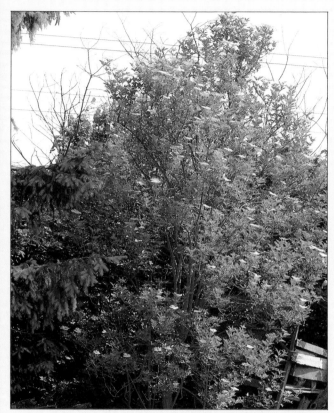

A perennial, deciduous large shrub or small tree, with oval, serrated leaves, the elder has a height and spread of about 15 feet. Its spreading branches bear large, flat heads of small, star-shaped, creamy-white flowers in late spring and early summer. These are followed, in early autumn, by drooping bunches of purplish-black, juicy berries. A common wild plant, it is part of the folklore of several countries, where ancient legends link it with magic.

CULTIVATION
Sow ripe berries 1 inch deep in a pot outdoors. Plant seedlings out in a semi-shaded position when large enough. Or plant 1 foot long hardwood cuttings in a nursery bed in mid- to late autumn and plant out the following autumn. Cut back hard in winter. Elders tolerate most soils; *S. canadensis* is a more hardy species.

USES
This important and valuable tree, once called "the medicine chest of the country people," has innumerable uses. An infusion of the sweet-scented flowers can be used to treat colds. Elderflower water is good for the complexion and the eyes. The flowers are also used in an ointment to treat burns, while an ointment made from the leaves is suitable for bruises and sprains. The berries are rich in vitamin C and are often the main ingredient in jellies and cordials. For centuries, wine has been made from both the berries and the flowers (see p. 193).

Tilia cordata
Linden *Tiliaceae*

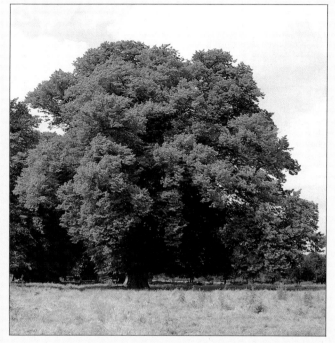

The small-leaved linden (above) is a fast-growing, hardy, deciduous tree, reaching a height of 35 feet. Its heart-shaped leaves are a glossy dark-green with serrated edges. The clusters of yellowish, heavily scented flowers, which appear in midsummer, have a sweet nectar that attracts bees. The leaves often harbor aphids which produce "honeydew," a sticky substance which also attracts bees but eventually drips off as an unpleasant residue.

CULTIVATION
Sow seeds in a cold frame in early spring. Plant out in nursery beds in midautumn. After growing on for at least four years, transplant to permanent positions, in full sun or semi-shade, in well-drained soil.

USES
Linden tea is made from the dried flowers and is very popular in European countries, where it is drunk as a digestive and calming tonic. The flowers are also used to flavor sweets and liqueurs. Linden blossom is used in beauty preparations to soothe the skin. Although not particularly durable, the white, close-grained wood of the linden is the most suitable for intricate carving. Note that very old flowers should be avoided when making preparations as they may produce symptoms of mild intoxication.

Poterium sanguisorba (Sanguisorba minor)

Salad burnet Rosaceae

The dainty decorative leaves of this refreshing herb belie its hardiness – its leaves often survive a mild winter. Should they fail to do so, they are then among the earliest leaves to appear in spring. Salad burnet, which the early Pilgrims carried to New England, was thought by Gerard to "make the hart merry and glad, as also being put in wine, to which it yeeldeth a certaine grace in the drinking." The young leaves have a pleasant if somewhat sharp cucumber flavor. The green flowering globes expand amid tiny red dots with the unfulfilled promise of an explosion of color. This pretty plant was recommended by Francis Bacon to be set in alleys with wild thyme and water mint, "to perfume the air most delightfully, being trodden on and crushed."

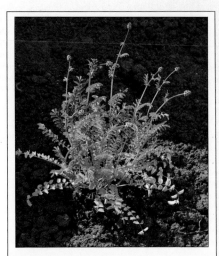

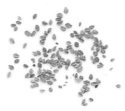

Seed
$\frac{1}{8}$ inch long. Beige, ridged, oval shaped.

Flower
Tiny green blooms, with red points packed into a $\frac{1}{2}$ inch sphere, appear in early to midsummer. They contain no nectar and have to be wind-pollinated.

Leaf
Rosettes of hardy, lacy, graceful foliage, composed of finely toothed leaflets, survive mild winters.

Lifespan
Hardy herbaceous perennial

Height
8–30 inches

Stem
Grooved, with branching flowering stems.

CULTIVATION
Site Sun or light shade.
Soil Prefers limy soil.
Propagating Sow seeds in spring or autumn. If allowed to flower, salad burnet will self-seed.
Growing Plant seedlings 12 inches apart, when large enough to handle. Cut flowering stems and old leaves regularly to produce plenty of tender young leaves.
Harvesting Pick young tender leaves whenever required.
Preserving Dry leaves.

USES
Decorative
● *Whole plant* Plant as edging for formal herb garden designs.

Culinary
● *Leaf* Introduce this nutty and slightly sharp cucumber flavor into garnishes, salads, herb butters and soft cheeses, or sprinkle on vegetables. Add at beginning of cooking to casseroles and creamy soups. Combine with other herbs, particularly rosemary and tarragon. Serve in a sauce with white fish: add 2 tablespoons each of chopped burnet and tarragon or mint to 4 ounces melted butter, simmer for 10 minutes. Use to flavor vinegar, salad dressing and to give a cooling effect to summer drinks and punch.

Household
● *Leaf* Press dried leaves into sides of slightly melted candles.

Cosmetic
● *Leaf* Infuse to make a facial wash for sunburn and for troubled skin.

Medicinal
● *Whole plant* Try as an infusion to relieve hemorrhoids or diarrhea.
● *Leaf* Sprinkle fresh leaves, which contain vitamin C, on food to aid digestion. Use as a tonic and mildly diuretic tea.

Primula veris   *Primula vulgaris*

Cowslip & Primrose Primulaceae

These two flowers of spring never fail to gladden the heart. Favorite of favorites, the primrose is the first to appear. Although picked for jams and cosmetics, its real attraction is the soft yellow simplicity of its perfect flower. Its leaves are enjoyed by silkworms.

The cheerful, nodding cowslip, the "Keys of St Peter," has a unique milky scent likened to a cow's breath or to that of a new baby. In some areas, it has almost been picked to extinction, mainly to make seductive cowslip wine, but also for the childish delight of sucking the sweet nectar from the flowers. It can be found wild here in some areas, having escaped from cultivation. Primroses tend to be found only in gardens.

Primrose.

Flower
Pale yellow heart-shaped petals with deeper yellow centers. One flower per stalk; multiples are hybrids.

Leaf
Crinkled, oblong and yellow-green.

Primula vulgaris Primrose

Seed
Dark brown, faceted, $\frac{1}{16}$ inch long.

Dried flowers
These make a mild, sedative tea.

Root
Tan aromatic rootstalk with small, pale yellow roots.

Dried leaves
Used occasionally as a medicinal tea.

Primula veris Cowslip

Flower
Golden petals, each with an orange dot at the base, appear in spring.

Seed
Dark brown, faceted, $\frac{1}{16}$ inch long.

Dried flowers
Retain their color well for dried decorations and potpourri.

Stem
Sturdy, solid, round stalk supports 1 to 30 flowers.

Leaf
Bluer green than primrose, slightly crinkled and rosette-forming.

Dried leaves
Used medicinally.

Lifespan
Hardy herbaceous perennial

Height
Cowslip 5–9 inches
Primrose 3–6 inches

CULTIVATION
Site Semishade or sun.
Soil Cowslip favors limy soil; primrose prefers moist soil.
Propagating Divide large plants in autumn. Seed picked in early autumn, when still slightly succulent, will germinate quickly; ripe, dry seed needs cold then warm temperatures to break its dormancy. Sow in autumn and cover with glass.
Growing Plant out in the following autumn, 6 inches apart. Primrose, unlike cowslip, is not suitable for indoor cultivation.
Harvesting Pick leaves and flowers as they open. Harvest roots in autumn.
Preserving Crystallize flowers. Dry leaves and roots.

USES
Decorative
● **Flower** Include in spring posies.

Culinary
● **Flower** (Cowslip) Use for jam and wine, or pickle. (Primrose) Eat raw in salads. Crystallize for decoration. Once used in jams and an ancient dessert with rice, almonds, honey, saffron and ground flowers.
● **Leaf** (Cowslip) Use in salads and for meat stuffing. (Primrose) Boil as a vegetable.

Cosmetic
● **Flower** Soak in distilled water to make lotion for spots and wrinkles.

Aromatic
● **Flower and root** Use dried flowers and powdered roots in potpourri.

Medicinal
● **Whole plant** (Primrose) Infuse fresh plant to make a cough remedy and mildly sedative tea.
● **Flower** Try fresh or dried in tea as a sedative and for headaches.
● **Leaf** (Cowslip) May heal wounds in a salve. (Primrose) Use for a medicinal tea.
● **Root** (Primrose) Infuse as a tea for nervous headaches.

Rosmarinus officinalis

Rosemary Labiatae

Rosemary, "dew of the sea," holds a special place in the affections of many as the essence of a summer herb garden. It has been used by cooks and apothecaries from earliest times. With a reputation for strengthening the memory, it became the emblem of fidelity for lovers; some brides have even worn rosemary wreaths "richly gilded and tied with silken ribands of all colors." The Spanish revere rosemary as the bush that sheltered the Virgin Mary on her flight to Egypt. As she spread her cloak over the herb, the white flowers turned blue.

In times past, resinous rosemary was burned in sick chambers to purify the air and branches were strewn in law courts as a protection from "jail fever" (typhus). During the Plague of 1665, it was carried in the handles of walking sticks and in pouches to be sniffed when traveling through suspicious areas. In some Mediterranean villages, linen is spread over rosemary to dry, so the sun will extract its moth-repellent aroma.

Rosemary also makes a good garden hedge. In Shakespeare's time, it was used for topiary and clipped to a sphere or cone shape.

Apart from common rosemary, there are several named varieties, including a vigorous new upright form, 'Sawyer's Selection,' with large, mauve-blue flowers, which can reach 8 feet within three years. There is a variable gold-tipped form, and ancient texts mention a silver variegated form.

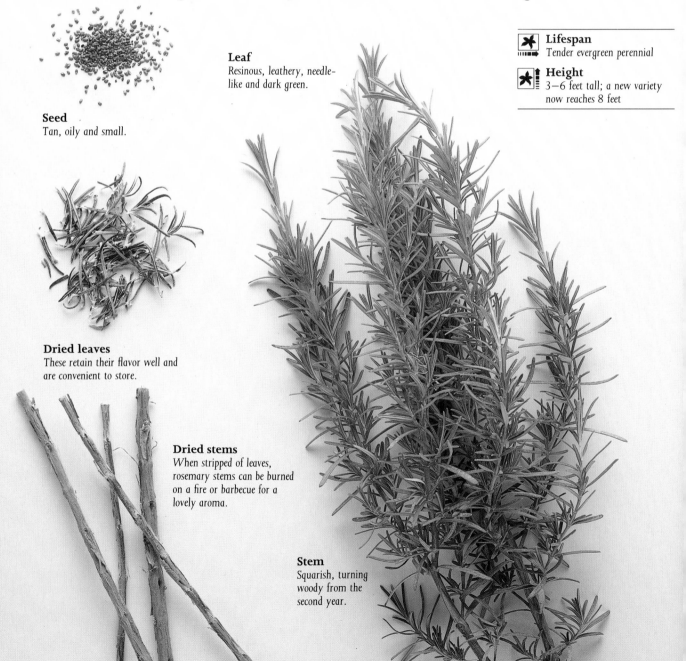

Seed
Tan, oily and small.

Leaf
Resinous, leathery, needle-like and dark green.

Lifespan
Tender evergreen perennial

Height
3–6 feet tall; a new variety now reaches 8 feet

Dried leaves
These retain their flavor well and are convenient to store.

Dried stems
When stripped of leaves, rosemary stems can be burned on a fire or barbecue for a lovely aroma.

Stem
Squarish, turning woody from the second year.

118

OTHER VARIETIES

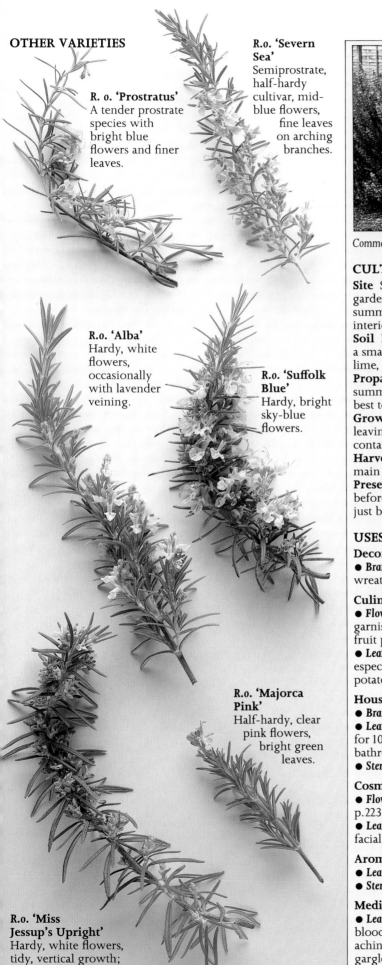

R. o. 'Prostratus'
A tender prostrate species with bright blue flowers and finer leaves.

R.o. 'Severn Sea'
Semiprostrate, half-hardy cultivar, mid-blue flowers, fine leaves on arching branches.

R.o. 'Alba'
Hardy, white flowers, occasionally with lavender veining.

R.o. 'Suffolk Blue'
Hardy, bright sky-blue flowers.

R.o. 'Majorca Pink'
Half-hardy, clear pink flowers, bright green leaves.

R.o. 'Miss Jessup's Upright'
Hardy, white flowers, tidy, vertical growth; useful for hedging.

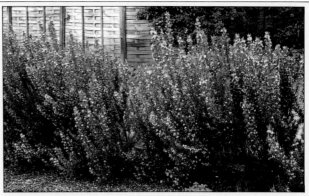

Common rosemary has pale blue orchidlike flowers in early summer.

CULTIVATION

Site Sunny. Protect from cold winds. In cold or exposed gardens, grow in a large pot; sink it in outdoor soil in summer, but return it to the greenhouse or a sunny interior in winter.

Soil Needs excellent drainage. On limy soil, rosemary is a smaller but more fragrant plant. To provide additional lime, apply eggshells or potash.

Propagating Sow under heat in spring or outdoors in summer. Germination is erratic; needs at least 70 °F. It is best to propagate by cuttings or layering.

Growing Transplant when large enough to handle, leaving 2–3 feet spaces between plants. Rosemary can be container-grown indoors in a sunny position.

Harvesting Pick small amounts all year round. Gather main leaf crop before flowering.

Preserving Dry sprigs and branches. Strip off leaves before storing. To release the aroma, crush leaves only just before use.

USES

Decorative
● **Branch** Provides a fragrant "skeleton" when woven into wreaths and garlands.

Culinary
● **Flower** Toss fresh rosemary into salads. Crystallize for a garnish. Pound with sugar, mix with cream, and add to a fruit purée.
● **Leaf** Add sparingly to a wide range of meat dishes, especially lamb and pork. Use rosemary to flavor baked potatoes and to make an herb butter for vegetables.

Household
● **Branch** Place fresh boughs in a room to cool the air.
● **Leaf** Boil a handful of rosemary in 2 cups of water for 10 minutes to yield an antiseptic solution for washing bathroom fixtures.
● **Stem** Shape into barbecue skewers.

Cosmetic
● **Flower** Use the essential oil in "Hungary water" (see p.223).
● **Leaf** Stimulates blood circulation in a bath. Use as a facial steam. Makes a rinse for dark hair.

Aromatic
● **Leaf** Use in potpourri. Lay sprigs among linens.
● **Stem** Scatter on a barbecue to discourage insects.

Medicinal
● **Leaf** Stimulates circulation and eases pain by increasing blood supply where applied. Aids fat digestion. Good for aching joints and rheumatic pains. Use as an antiseptic gargle and mouthwash.

Rosa species

Roses Rosaceae

For sheer fragrance and beauty, the rose reigns supreme. Its cultivation spread from Persia and China, bringing inspiration to artists,
warriors and lovers in every land. Cleopatra seduced Antony knee
deep in roses, and Roman banquets were garlanded with petals. In
1187, on entering Jerusalem, the Muslim conqueror Saladin even had
the Omar mosque washed in rosewater to purify it.

This "gift of the angels" was also popular for its gentle healing
powers. Rose essence is among the safest healing substances known,
and the delicate flavor of rosewater is excellent for cooking. Rose
wine dates from ancient Persia, and the candy known as Turkish
delight is made with rosewater. Rose petals were historically valued
for jam, vinegar, pies and as a garnish. Once again, all the myriad
uses for the rose are being rediscovered and enjoyed.

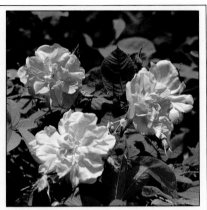
Damask roses in bloom.

CULTIVATION
Site Sunny, or light shade, and
open; not too windy.
Soil Well-drained loam.
Propagating Take cuttings in
autumn. Plant seed for species.
Growing Thin or transplant from
autumn to spring. Deadhead in
summer. Prune lightly in spring.
Do not grow indoors.
Harvesting Pick buds when
formed, petals when first open, hips
when ripe or, for wine, after the
first frost when softened.
Preserving Dry petals and buds.
Crystallize petals. Dry hips.

USES
Decorative
● **Flower** Use in arrangements.

Culinary
● **Flower** Use scented petals with
bitter white heel removed. Sprinkle
in salads, apple or cherry pie. Make
syrup, vinegar, sorbets and sweets
(see p. 183). Crystallize as a garnish.
Flavor sweets and drinks with
rosewater. Pickle rosebuds. Flavor
pork with Chinese rose liqueur.
● **Hip** Remove irritant hairs first.
Use in teas, wine, syrup and jams.
Purée, sweeten and add lemon juice
for a lamb sauce.

Cosmetic
● **Flower** Use rosewater as an antiseptic tonic to soothe skin, especially
dry, inflamed, mature and sensitive
skins. Use rose oil as perfume.

Aromatic
● **Flower** Add petals to potpourri.

Medicinal
● **Flower** Use blended oil in massage
to aid circulation, cleanse the blood
and tone capillaries. Soothes tension.
Splash eyes with rosewater for
conjunctivitis.
● **Leaf** Infuse for a tonic and
astringent tea.
● **Hip** Contains vitamins B, E, K;
high in C. Take as tea or syrup.

Dried hips
*Hips from the wild (dog)
rose are especially rich in
vitamin C.*

Leaf
*Elliptical with finely
serrated edges, five to
seven mid-green
leaflets on a stalk.*

**R. gallica 'Versicolor'
Rosamundi** Attractive
striped petals.

Stem
*Green and
densely
covered with
small thorns.*

**R. damascena
Damask rose**

Flower
*Rose-pink, highly
scented, semidouble
flowers borne in summer.
Source of rose oil and
rosewater.*

Dried petals and buds
*Pick petals once flowers
open as a main ingredient
in potpourri and sweet bags.*

**R.g.
'Officinalis'
Apothecary rose/
Red rose of
Lancaster**

**R. canina
Wild rose** Strong,
arching, prickly stems,
mid-green leaflets, pink or
white fragrant flowers and
bright red hips.

**R. eglanteria
(R. rubiginosa)
Sweetbrier/Eglantine**
Small, pink, fragrant,
single flowers with
apple-scented leaflets,
densely prickled,
arching stems and
bright red hips.

Fragrant old roses
Charles de Mills rose and petals
of 'Maiden's Blush,' 'Mme Isaac
Pereire,' 'Alba
Maxima,' 'Old
Blush.'

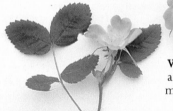

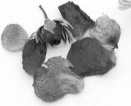

Lifespan
Hardy shrub

Height
4–8 feet

Rumex acetosa

Sorrel *Polygonaceae*

Prolific flowering stalks of sorrel, rising above grass on an acid soil, can cause a hay meadow to assume a reddish tint at harvest time. On a hot summer day, haymakers would frequently eat the succulent leaves to quench their thirst. Most sorrel leaves have an intriguing sharp acidic flavor, which is used to advantage in many dishes. However, buckler leaf sorrel (*R. scutatus*) boasts a milder lemony zest but still with an interesting sharpness. It is preferred by the French for sorrel soup and is known by many as French sorrel. Confusingly, both species have been called French sorrel and garden sorrel.

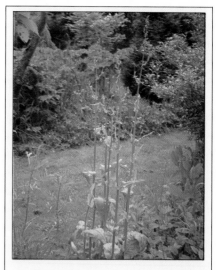

Seed
Small, rich brown, shiny, pointed and ridged with three curved facets.

Flower
Whorled reddish-green spikes borne during summer. Remove to ensure continued supply of succulent young leaves.

Leaf
Lance-shaped with broad base, containing potassium and vitamins A, B1 and C.

Stem
Juicy, ridged and reddish.

R. scutatus
Buckler leaf (French) sorrel
Silvery patches on light green leaves, which have sharp flavor; a "more grateful acidity" than broad leaf sorrel.

R. acetosa
Broad leaf (Garden) sorrel
Fresh sap-green leaves that are almost tasteless in early spring: acidity develops as season progresses.

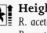 **Lifespan**
Hardy perennial

 Height
R. acetosa 2−4 feet
R. scutatus 6−18 inches

CULTIVATION

Site (*R. acetosa*) Sun or light shade; (*R. scutatus*) Full sun; sheltered spot.
Soil (*R. acetosa*) Moist, rich with iron; (*R. scutatus*) Well drained.
Propagating Sow seed in spring; germination takes 7−10 days. Divide roots in autumn.
Growing Thin seedlings or transplant to 12 inches apart. Water to keep leaves juicy; protect from snails. Divide and replant every 5 years. Grow indoors in pots.
Harvesting Gather leaves when young for culinary use. For a winter supply, cover sorrel with cloches.
Preserving Dried sorrel has little flavor. Best frozen in cooked dishes.

USES

Culinary
● **Leaf** Eat raw young leaves (especially *R. scutatus*) in salads (reducing vinegar or lemon in dressing) and in sorrel soup. Cook like spinach, changing the cooking water once to reduce acidity. Use to season vegetable soups, omelettes, lamb and beef dishes, and in sauces for fish, poultry and pork.

To make a green sauce, wash a handful each of sorrel and lettuce leaves with half a handful of watercress. Cook in a little water with a whole onion until tender. Remove onion. Mix 1 tablespoon olive oil with 1 tablespoon wine vinegar, pepper and salt. Stir into sorrel mixture until creamy.

Household
● **Leaf** Use juice to bleach rust, mold and ink stains from linen, wicker and silver.

Medicinal
● **Leaf** Infuse as a tea to treat kidney and liver ailments. Apply to mouth ulcers, boils and infected wounds.

Note: *Large doses may damage kidneys.*

Ruta graveolens

Garden rue *Rutaceae*

Leonardo da Vinci and Michelangelo both claimed that, owing to rue's metaphysical powers, their eyesight and creative inner vision had been improved. Branches of rue were used to sprinkle holy water before high mass, and it was an important strewing herb and antiplague plant. Robbers who stripped plague victims protected themselves with "Vinegar of the four thieves," rue being an ingredient, and it was also a main component of *mithridate*, a Greek all-purpose poison antidote. Rue is shown on the heraldic Order of the Thistle and inspired the design of the suit of clubs in playing cards.

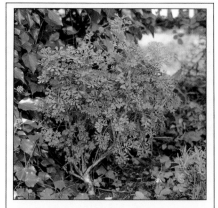

R.g. 'Jackman's Blue' *has compact, metallic blue leaves.*

Seed
Black and crescent-shaped; used in Roman cooking in the first century A.D.

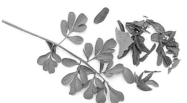

Dried leaves
These contain a powerful germ killer and insecticide; crush and sprinkle as insect repellent.

Flower
Frilled, slipper-shaped, greenish-yellow petals on flowers borne in late summer.

R.g. 'Variegata'
Bright cream splashes on leaf tips. Prune in spring to encourage new variegated foliage. May revert to green.

Leaf
Small, rounded, lobed and blue-green, dotted with oil glands.

Root
Cream-colored, branching and fibrous; thought to resemble the arrangement of blood vessels in the human eye.

Stem
Round and chalky blue-green, becoming woody in second year. Sap may cause a rash.

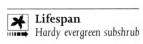

Lifespan
Hardy evergreen subshrub

Height
2 feet

CULTIVATION
Site Full sun. Tolerates light shade.
Soil Well drained and alkaline; poor to moderate fertility for hardiest plants.
Propagating Divide in spring. Take stem cuttings in late summer. (Species only) Sow in spring, slow to germinate.
Growing Thin or transplant to 18 inches apart. Prune in late spring. In severe winters, give protection. Rue can be grown indoors.
Harvesting Pick young leaves just before flowers open. Collect seeds.
Preserving Dry leaves and seed.

USES
Decorative
● *Whole plant* (R.g. 'Jackman's Blue') Use as low hedge in knot gardens.
● *Leaf* Include in small posies and nosegays.

Culinary
● *Seed* Infuse with lovage and mint as a marinade for partridge.
● *Leaf* Rue leaf tastes bitter but very small amounts give unusual muskiness to cream cheese, egg and fish dishes. Mix with damsons and wine for a delicious meat sauce.

Cosmetic
● *Leaf* Infuse to bathe tired eyes.

Medicinal
● *Leaf* Infused as a tea that acts as a menstruation stimulant, appetizer, perspiration inducer and bile stimulant. Added to compresses for wounds and skin ulcers. Drunk as a tonic for extra iron and mineral salts. Used by herbalists for hysteria, epilepsy and abnormal blood pressure. Fresh leaves used in a homeopathic tincture for rheumatism, arthritis and neuralgia.

Note: *Rue should be taken only under strict medical supervision and never during pregnancy. It may irritate some skins.*

Santolina chamaecyparissus (S. incana)

Santolina Compositae

Although it has long been known as lavender cotton, santolina is not a lavender but a member of the daisy family. The whole plant is highly aromatic and has been used to sweeten the air in Mediterranean regions for centuries. It is valued as an insect repellent and was much used medicinally in medieval times. Santolina was probably brought into Britain in the sixteenth century by French Huguenot gardeners, who were skilled in creating the popular knot gardens. It is neater than the thrift, germander, marjoram and thyme previously planted in such gardens. With three color forms available, it is still a popular plant for edging and hedging.

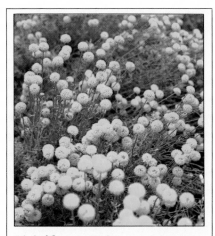

A bed of flowering **S. chamaecyparissus**.

CULTIVATION

Site Full sun.
Soil Well drained, preferably sandy. If soil is too rich, santolina growth is soft and less silvery.
Propagating Take 2–3 inch stem cuttings in spring or from mid-summer to autumn (give protection in frosty weather).
Growing Transplant to 18 inches– 2 feet apart or to 12–15 inches apart for hedging. Clip to shape in spring or summer; never in autumn in frosty climates. Deadhead in autumn. If temperatures drop below 5 °F, protect with a sleeve of two layers of chicken wire filled with straw, spruce or salt hay, 5 inches thick. Santolina can be grown indoors.
Harvesting Pick flowering stems in late summer. Gather leaves anytime.
Preserving Dry flowering stems and leaves.

USES

Decorative
● **Whole plant** Use for hedges, edging and knot gardens. Create patterns with the three color forms.
● **Flower** Dry for decorations.

Household
● **Branch** To deter moths and other insects, lay in drawers and under carpets, hang in closets and distribute among books.

Aromatic
● **Leaf** Add to potpourri.

Medicinal
● **Flower and leaf** A decoction was thought to kill intestinal worms and to give mild stimulation to menstrual flow. An infusion was taken to cleanse kidneys and to help jaundice. Wash with a decoction to heal ringworm and scab.
● **Leaf** Mix in herbal tobacco with chamomile and coltsfoot.

Note: Do not take internally.

S. rosmarinifolia
Yellow flowers and small, rosemarylike, willow-green leaves, which have a less pungent, sweeter scent than S.c.

Flower
Bright yellow button flowers, one on each stalk, borne from mid- to late summer.

Leaf
Pungent, finely divided, silver-gray, evergreen foliage forming low mounds.

S. virens (S. viridis)
Bright yellow button flowers and thread-like pungent, vivid green leaves.

Santolina chamaecyparissus

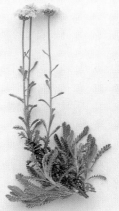

S.c. 'Lemon Queen'
Cream button flowers (the only cultivar that doesn't have yellow flowers!) and willow-green foliage with slightly fresher scent.

Stem
Soft, round and white felted; greenish-brown and woody in second season.

S. neapolitana
Bright yellow button flowers and silver-gray leaves which are longer, more feathery and slightly fruitier scented than S.c.
Ht: 2½ feet.

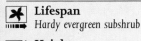

Lifespan
Hardy evergreen subshrub

Height
1–2 feet

Salvia officinalis

Sage Labiatae

"The desire of sage is to render man immortal," instructs a late medieval treatise. Indeed, the sage plant has been praised highly throughout history and on many continents for its powers of longevity. "How can a man grow old who has sage in his garden?" is the substance of an ancient proverb much quoted in China and Persia and parts of Europe. It was so valued by the Chinese in the seventeenth century that Dutch merchants found the Chinese would trade three chests of China tea for one of sage leaves.

The name *salvia*, from the Latin *salvere*, to be in good health, to cure, to save, reflects its benevolent reputation. To the Romans it was a sacred herb gathered with ceremony. The appointed person would make sacrifices of bread and wine, wear a white tunic and approach with feet bare and well washed. Roman instructions advised against using iron tools, a sensible edict as iron salts are incompatible with sage.

This powerful healing plant is also a strong culinary herb, often best used on its own. As one chef wrote: "In the grand opera of cooking, sage represents an easily offended and capricious prima donna. It likes to have the stage almost to itself." However, it is valuable as an aid to digesting fatty foods, both savory and sweet.

To complete its commendation, sage is also a beautiful aromatic shrub, popular with bees yet often undervalued as a flowering garden plant.

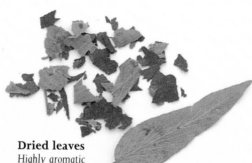

Dried leaves
Highly aromatic
and pungent.

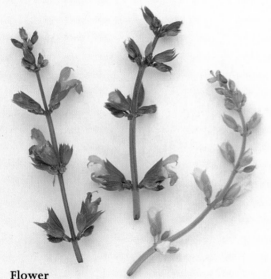

Flower
Deep throated, two-lipped, generally mauve-blue. The white and pink forms are less common.

Leaf
Set in pairs, gray-green, often with yellow blotches on old leaves. Thick, downy and "pebbly" with pronounced veining on underside.

Seed
Dark brown, ovoid and tiny; form in fruits at the base of each flower.

Stem
Square, green with fine hairs; woody from the second year.

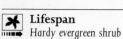

Lifespan
Hardy evergreen shrub

Height
1–2½ feet

OTHER VARIETIES

S. lavandulifolia
Spanish sage/
Narrow leaf sage
Slight balsamic
flavor; good for
teas.

S.o. 'Tricolor'
Half hardy.
Leaves green
splashed pink,
white margins.
Mild flavor.

S.o. 'Purpurea
variegata'
Variegated
purple sage
Strong flavor, good
for medicinal tea.

S.o.
'Prostratus'
Prostrate sage
Most balsamic
flavor. Keeps
blue leaf color
all summer.

S.o. 'Icterina'
Gold variegated
sage Milder
flavor than
common sage.

S.o. 'Purpurea'
Purple (or red)
sage
Strongly
flavored leaf. Use
in tea for sore
throats.

S. sclarea
Clary sage
Biennial. Large wrinkled
leaf, long-lasting lilac flowers.

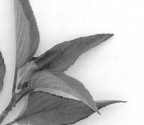

S. elegans (S. rutilans)
Pineapple sage
Half hardy. Scarlet
flowers late summer.
Pineapple-flavored
leaves.

S.o. 'Broad leaf'
Broad leaf sage
Seldom flowers in
cooler climates. Good
culinary and medicinal form.

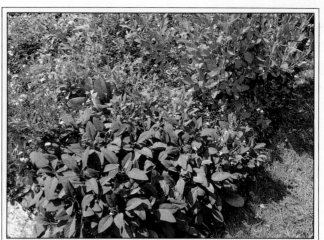

A bed of sages, purple sage in the foreground.

CULTIVATION

Site Full sun.
Soil Light, dry, alkaline and well drained.
Propagating Grow common sage from seed. All forms
take easily from cuttings; rooting time is about four
weeks in summer.
Growing Cut back after flowering; replace woody plants
every four to five years. Plant out 18–24 inches apart.
Prune frequently to keep bushy. Yellowing leaves can
mean roots need more space. Small green caterpillar eats
leaves; remove by hand, or prune and burn leaves.
Suitable indoors with sun.
Harvesting Pick leaves just before flowers appear.
Preserving Dry leaves slowly to preserve best flavor and
avoid mustiness.

USES

Decorative
● *Leaf* Attractive in wreaths and nosegays.

Culinary
● *Flower* Scatter in salads. Infuse for a light, balsamic tea.
● *Leaf* Mix with onion for poultry stuffing. Cook with
rich, fatty meats: pork, duck, sausage. Combine with
other strong flavors: wrap around tender liver and sauté
in butter; blend into cheeses. Dip and fry whole leaves in
batter (see p. 177) or young leaves in cream, and eat with
sugar and orange. Make sage vinegar and sage butter.

Household
● *Leaf* Put dried leaves among linen to discourage insects.
Burn on embers or boil in water to disinfect a room. Sage
smoke deodorizes animal and cooking smells.

Cosmetic
● *Leaf* Use in facial steams and astringent cleansing
lotion, and as a rinse to condition and darken gray hair.
Rub on teeth to whiten. Use in a mouthwash.

Medicinal
● *Seed* Clary sage seed infused in water may be used to
remove foreign matter from eyes painlessly.
● *Leaf* Aids digestion and is antiseptic, antifungal and
contains estrogen. Helps to combat diarrhea. A sage
sandwich or sage tea after a meal benefits digestion. Sage
tea and sage wine are nerve and blood tonics. Tea reduces
sweating, soothes coughs and colds and may be used to
treat irregular menstruation and menopause. Clary sage
beer was once famous for its intoxicating properties.

Note: *Sage should not be taken in large doses for a long period.*

Saponaria officinalis

Soapwort *Caryophyllaceae*

Soapwort is worth searching for, as it is a lovely garden herb. It yields a soapy sap that is excellent for laundering and revitalizing precious fabrics, and is now used in museums for this purpose. It also exudes the most delicious raspberry-sorbet scent with a hint of clove, thus revealing its family connection with pinks. This sweet fragrance will fill the air on hot summer evenings.

In the Middle East, soapwort has been used both as a cleaning agent and as a medicinal herb for skin problems such as eczema, acne and those caused by venereal diseases. For these qualities, as well as for its believed ability to help eliminate toxins, especially from the liver, and soothe poison ivy rashes, soapwort was grown on the nineteenth-century herb farms of the American Shakers.

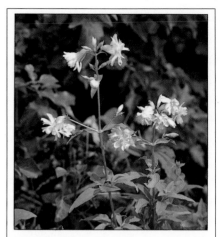

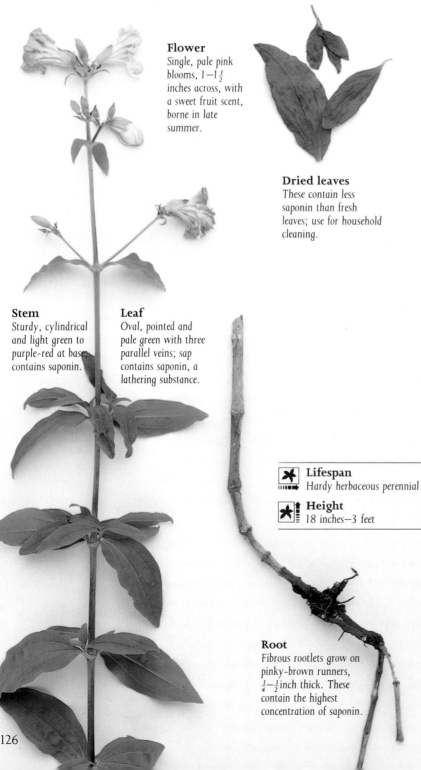

Flower
Single, pale pink blooms, 1–1½ inches across, with a sweet fruit scent, borne in late summer.

Dried leaves
These contain less saponin than fresh leaves; use for household cleaning.

Stem
Sturdy, cylindrical and light green to purple-red at base; contains saponin.

Leaf
Oval, pointed and pale green with three parallel veins; sap contains saponin, a lathering substance.

✳ Lifespan
Hardy herbaceous perennial

✳ Height
18 inches–3 feet

Root
Fibrous rootlets grow on pinky-brown runners, ¼–½ inch thick. These contain the highest concentration of saponin.

CULTIVATION
Site Full sun or light shade.
Soil Fertile and moist.
Propagating Sow in spring. Divide plants or take pieces of underground runners in late autumn to early spring. Self-seeds.
Growing Thin or transplant to 2 feet apart. Use twiggy sticks to support stems. Cut back after flowering to induce second blooms. Scent strength varies according to where soapwort is planted. Do not grow near fish ponds as its root excretions can poison fish. Not suitable for indoor cultivation.
Harvesting Pick flowers, leaves, stems and roots in autumn or as required.
Preserving Dry flowers and leaves. Slice roots and and dry in the sun.

USES
Culinary
● **Flower** Garnish green and fruit salads. Sometimes used in brewing to produce a "head" on beer.

Household
● **Leaf, stem and root** Just cover in rain- or soft water (not chemically treated tap water) and boil for 30 minutes; then use soapy liquid to wash and miraculously revive delicate old fabrics. The Romans used soapwort as a water softener.

Cosmetic
● **Leaf, stem and root** Boil in soft water, strain and use to wash hair and sensitive skins (see p. 225).

Aromatic
● **Flower** Perfume a room with bouquets of soapwort. Use dried in potpourri, although only a little scent is retained.

Medicinal
● **Root** Decoct and use as a wash for acne and psoriasis.

Note: *Soapwort root is poisonous and should not be taken internally.*

Satureja montana (Satureia montana)

Winter savory Labiatae

Savory, with its peppery spiciness, is one of the oldest flavoring herbs and has long been considered an antiseptic herb beneficial to the whole digestive tract. It is also a stimulant and was in demand as an aphrodisiac – a possible reason why it was named *Satureia*, meaning satyr. Virgil, in a poem of country life, described savory as highly aromatic and valuable when planted near beehives. The Romans added savory to sauces and to vinegars which they used liberally as a flavoring. They also introduced savory into northern Europe, where it became a valued disinfectant strewing herb. Later, it was among the herbs listed by John Josselyn in *New-England's Rarities Discovered* (1672) as being taken to North America by early settlers.

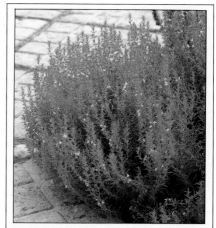

Tiny, pink to white flowers appear on winter savory in summer.

CULTIVATION
Site Full sun.
Soil Well drained and alkaline. (Summer savory) Rich loam.
Propagating Sow in early autumn or late spring. Press lightly into soil. Divide plant in spring or autumn. Take stem cuttings in summer. (Summer savory) Sow in spring.
Growing Thin or transplant to 18 inches apart. Prune in late spring. Winter savory may need some protection in winter. Can be grown indoors. (Summer savory) Thin or transplant to 9 inches apart. Prune to prevent woody growth.
Harvesting Pick leaves just as flower buds are formed. Collect flowering tops in late summer.
Preserving Dry leaves. Infuse to make savory vinegar and savory oil.

USES
Decorative
● *Whole plant* A useful edging plant.

Culinary
● *Leaf* Cook with beans. Make into savory jelly using grape juice. Used commercially to flavor salami. Peppery winter savory is good for salt-free diets (see also p. 165).

Household
● *Branch and leaf* Throw on fires as an aromatic disinfectant.
● *Flower* Provides nectar for bees.

Cosmetic
● *Flowering top* Use as an astringent and antiseptic in facial steams or baths for oily skin.

Medicinal
● *Flowering top* Infuse as a tea to stimulate appetite, ease indigestion and flatulence; also use as an antiseptic gargle. Steep in wine as a tonic, especially good after fevers.
● *Leaf* Crush and apply to insect bites or wasp stings for pain relief.

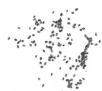

Seed
Shiny, mid-brown, elongated sphere, halved lengthways, with tiny tip.

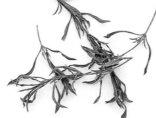

Dried flowering tops
These contain an antiseptic that aids digestion and is used medicinally. Crumble leaves for cooking.

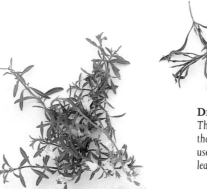

S. montana repanda
Creeping winter savory
Rock-garden carpet of strongly flavored deep green leaves sprinkled with tiny white flowers in late summer. Ht: 3 inches.

Leaf
Small, narrow, pointed and dark green, gland-dotted and aromatic with a distinctive central vein that creates a fold.

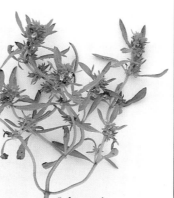

S. hortensis
Summer savory
Annual. Sparser, slightly larger and more rounded leaves than winter savory, and pale lilac to white flowers in late summer. Ht: 18 inches.

Stem
Hairy, square, branching and green, turning reddish-brown; woody in second season.

Root
Dark brown, dense and fibrous.

Lifespan
Hardy evergreen subshrub

Height
15 inches

127

Sempervivum tectorum

Houseleek *Crassulaceae*

According to legend, as a gift from Jupiter for protection from lightning, thunder, fire and witchcraft, houseleek has always been considered a form of home fire insurance. Its wild origins are unknown: even in the fourth century B.C., the Greek botanist Theophrastus recorded its presence on walls and roof tiles. The Romans planted courtyard urns of houseleek, and Charlemagne ordered one plant to be grown on every roof. This spread the houseleek throughout Europe, and eventually to the New World.

In the language of flowers, houseleek symbolizes vivacity and industry. It is also one of the oldest first-aid herbs, with similar but reduced healing properties to aloe vera. Houseleek's advantage is that it will survive several degrees of winter frost.

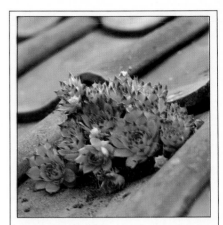

Offset
Houseleek produces small rosettes which develop roots and become separate plants. Occasionally, in midsummer, a spray of 1 inch rose-purple flowers will appear on an erect round stem covered with scale-like leaves. The rosette that produced the flower stem then dies.

Leaf
Fleshy and mid-green, forming rosettes 2–6 inches wide, with spiny-pointed maroon tips.

Runner
Smooth red rootstalk which extends some of the offsets outward.

Root
Fibrous; clings to surfaces, especially to roofs.

Split leaf
Contains a succulent mucilage which has healing and soothing qualities.

 Lifespan
Hardy evergreen perennial succulent

Height
2–3 inches; flowering stem 8 inches

CULTIVATION
Site Sunny; traditionally positioned on porches or roofs.
Soil Dry, well drained and thin; suitable for rock gardens.
Propagating In spring, take offsets and leaf cuttings (cut a leaf at the base with an eye from the stem); sow seed in spring.
Growing Thin or transplant to 9 inches apart. Will grow indoors.
Harvesting Gather the thickest leaves for use.
Preserving Extract and freeze juice (no tests appear to have measured its properties after being frozen).

USES
Culinary
● *Leaf* The Dutch add it to salads.

Cosmetic
● *Leaf* Soak fresh leaves in a bath or facial steam to heal and nourish the skin. Apply juice (from sliced fresh leaf) or a decoction to warts and other skin blemishes.

Medicinal
● *Leaf* Relieves small injuries; either slice open fresh leaves to reveal their succulent interior and apply directly to skin, or pulp and use in a poultice or dressing. Apply to minor burns, wasp and nettle stings, cuts, ulcers, insect bites, itching, burning skin and warts. To soften skin around corns, bind on leaves for a few hours, soak foot in hot water, then attempt to remove corn. Repeat procedure as necessary.

Infuse as a tea for septic throats, bronchitis and mouth ailments.

Sium sisarum

Skirret *Umbelliferae*

This Chinese pot herb, grown for its aromatic edible root, was brought to Rome by early traders and became so valued by the Emperor Tiberius that he accepted skirret as tribute. In the sixteenth century, skirret was introduced to northern Europe as "the most delicious of root vegetables." As a perennial that multiplies quickly, it was an invaluable crop for peasants. Writing in 1699, John Evelyn praised skirret as "Exceedingly nourishing, wholesome and delicate; of all the root-kind, not subject to be windy. This excellent root . . . is very acceptable to all palates."

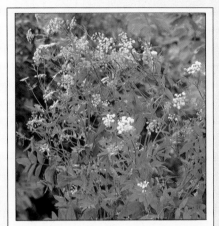

Flowers
Small clusters of tiny, fragrant, white, five-petaled flowers, open toward evening in mid- to late summer.

Seed
Brown, ridged, crescent-shaped, $\frac{1}{8}$ inch long?

Leaf
One to five pairs of narrow, pointed, finely toothed, mid-green leaflets and one terminal leaflet; older leaflets are more rounded. Some turn red in autumn.

Stem
Sturdy, hollow, ridged, round, branching and light green; red toward the base.

Lifespan
Hardy herbaceous perennial

Height
2–4 feet in first two seasons; mature plants can reach 6 feet

Root
Hairlike roots and numerous light brown, oblong tubers, 4–5 inches long, with white flesh and pleasant aromatic smell and taste.

CULTIVATION
Site Full sun or light shade.
Soil Rich, well-drained, alkaline loam; but tolerates most soils.
Propagating In spring, sow seed or divide crown (stem base), leaving about three tubers to each piece. Plant each piece 3 inches deep, 12 inches apart.
Growing Thin or transplant seedlings to 12 inches apart. Keep moist in summer, and feed with liquid comfrey fertilizer (see p. 131) or dilute liquid manure. Not suitable for indoor cultivation.
Harvesting Gather young shoots in spring. Dig roots as required or lift in autumn; sever from base of stem.
Preserving Store tuberous roots in sand until required, or lightly scrub, blanch for 1 minute, cool and freeze.

USES
Decorative
● *Whole plant* Boasts elegant foliage for back of herb or flower border.

Culinary
● **Shoot** Lightly steam or stir-fry young shoots.
● **Root** Lightly scrub, steam or boil and serve with butter and seasoning or with white sauce; or purée cooked root and serve with butter and nutmeg. Add sliced to meatballs and new potatoes for traditional German fare. Cook whole roots in stews, vegetable pies and Chinese stir-fried dishes. Pickle whole root and serve with salads or cold meats.

Medicinal
● **Shoot** Fresh young shoots said by Culpeper to be a "wholesome food, of a cleansing nature, and easy digestion, provoking urine."
● **Root** Boil and eat skirret root for, according to Culpeper, "opening and cleansing, to promote urine and to free the bladder of slimy phlegm; helps the jaundice and liver disorders." May also help relieve chest complaints.

Smyrnium olusatrum

Alexanders Umbelliferae

This aromatic plant resembles both lovage and angelica, which
occasionally leads to mistaken identity, but its bright green glossy
leaf has rounded tips and lacks the deep indentations of the other
two. However, it is called black lovage by some. The medieval Latin
name for this herb was *Petroselinum alexandrinum*, the parsley of
Alexandria, illustrating its Mediterranean heritage, and it was one of
many useful plants introduced by the Romans to northern Europe.

Although alexanders was listed as an official medicinal plant for
two centuries, its historical importance was more as a culinary herb:
its leaves, root tops, stems and flower buds all feature in medieval
recipes. The dried leaves were among the herbs taken on long sea
voyages to prevent scurvy.

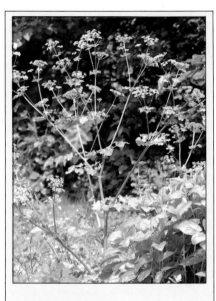

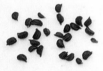

Seed
Two $\frac{1}{4}$ inch long, almost
half-globular seeds, ridged,
black and aromatic, form in
each fruit.

Flower
Greenish-yellow flowers,
full of nectar, borne in
early to midsummer.

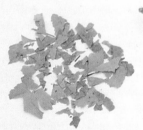

Dried leaves
These retain slight flavor and can
be used in cooking or medicinally.

Leaf
Glossy, serrated, and
bright green. Lower leaves
can reach 12 inches in
length.

 Lifespan
Biennial; sometimes perennial,
but not reliably hardy

Height
3–5 feet

Stem
Solid and furrowed.

Root
Thick at the top,
branching to three or
four main roots.

CULTIVATION

Site Sun or part shade. Grows wild
near some seacoasts.
Soil Grows readily in any soil.
Propagating In late summer or the
following spring, sow ripe seed
outdoors where it is to flower.
Alexanders will self-seed readily.
Growing Thin out seedlings until
2–2½ feet apart. In spring of second
year, cover over with soil or straw
for three or four weeks to blanch
for a sweeter flavor. Alexanders
is not a suitable plant for indoor
growth.
Harvesting Gather leaves in
summer, and stems when young or
blanched. Dig up roots in late
summer of second year.
Preserving Dry only leaves
gathered before flowering time.

USES

Decorative
● *Seed* Use dried seed heads for
winter arrangements.

Culinary
● *Seed* Grind and use like pepper.
● *Flower* Toss buds in salads and
flowers in savory fritters.
● *Leaf* Eat raw young leaves in
salads or use as flavoring in stew.
Serve with fish. Include in a "Lenten
potage" with watercress and nettles.
● *Stem* Stew, steam or braise young
stems, which taste like asparagus;
serve with a white sauce.
● *Root* Boil upper part, which tastes
like parsnips. Crystallize as a sweet.

Aromatic
● *Seed* Grind coarsely and add to a
potpourri.

Medicinal
● *Root* May be used in a decoction
to improve jaded appetites.

Symphytum officinale

Comfrey *Boraginaceae*

Among plants, comfrey's claim to be a miracle worker must be preeminent. The list of beneficial substances in its leaves sounds impressive and includes calcium, potassium, phosphorus, vitamins A, C and B12 – but not in sufficient amounts to meet our daily requirements, especially as comfrey should only be taken internally in moderation. As it has more protein in its leaf structure than any other known member of the vegetable kingdom, it is cultivated in many countries for fodder. From two to five crops a year can be produced, depending on climate. Comfrey also sends down a 10-foot or longer taproot, to raise moisture and valuable minerals to the upper soil levels. The leaf and roots contain allantoin, a protein that encourages cell division, and the plant is credited with some remarkable cures, from stubborn leg ulcers to broken bones.

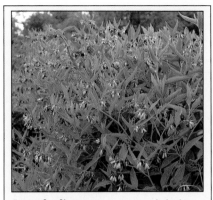

S. x uplandicum, a rust-resistant hybrid.

CULTIVATION
Site Full sun. Position carefully as comfrey is difficult to eradicate.
Soil Rich in nitrogen; neutral pH.
Propagating Take root offsets (root section with growing tip) any time except midwinter.
Growing Transplant and set 2 feet apart. For a higher nutritional yield, give each plant a bucketful of crude manure in spring and late summer.
Harvesting Pick leaves in summer. Dig up roots in autumn or winter.
Preserving Clean roots. Chop finely and dry. Dry leaves, or make into a skin-healing "oil" (see below).

USES
Culinary
● **Leaf** Chop young leaves into salads. Cook as spinach or in fritters.
● **Stem** Blanch; cook like asparagus.

Household
● **Leaf** Soak in water for four weeks to make perfect fertilizer for tomato and potato plants, owing to high potash content. Pick leaves, allow to wilt for at least 48 hours, then apply as a mulch. Boil fresh leaves for a golden-brown fabric dye.

Cosmetic
● **Leaf and root** Infuse and add to baths and lotions to soften the skin.

Medicinal
● **Leaf** Make an "oil" to use externally on skin irritations. Pick clean dry leaves and cut into 1 inch squares. Pack into a clean dark jar. Apply a screw-top lid, label and date. Store for two years; do not open. This results in a viscous amber liquid with some sediment. Decant "oil" into a smaller container. Use on eczema and other skin inflammations. Put fresh leaves in a poultice for rough skin, aching joints, sores, burns, cuts, sprains and to reduce swelling around fractures.

Note: *Some authorities say comfrey should not be taken internally.*

Flower
Blue-mauve bells in drooping clusters open along the spiral flower stem from late spring.

Leaf
Oval base, tapering to a point; rough, thick-ribbed and dark green.

Other species
Clockwise from the top:
S. grandiflorum *creamy red flowers; good ground cover.*
S. officinale *white and pink flowers.* **S. asperum** *bright blue flowers.*

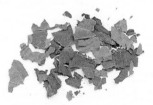

Dried leaves
Infuse for a medicinal tea.

Stem
Squarish, rough, hairy and branching near top.

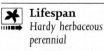

Lifespan
Hardy herbaceous perennial

Height
3–4 feet

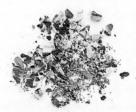

Dried root
Useful medicinally.

Root
Brown-black, thick, tapering and penetrating.

Salad herbs

As our culinary habits become more adventurous, herbs are being reintroduced, particularly in salads, giving us a range of flavors, colors and textures not experienced since the sixteenth century, when a salad might contain over 50 different leaves, buds, seeds, flowers, blanched stems and pickled roots.

Use leaves with a mild flavor such as lettuce, blanched endive, summer purslane or chickweed, to make up the bulk of the salad. Sharp-flavored leaves such as sorrel or nasturtium, and those with great pungency, such as basil should be shredded and used in small amounts as an accent. Flowers give special appeal, but consider their color when mixing ingredients so that they harmonize. Add other culinary herbs in small amounts: coriander, lemon balm, parsley, chervil, fennel stalks, leaves and bulb, thyme, lovage, tarragon, and seeds of sunflower or sprouted fenugreek.

Allium schoenoprasum
Chive flowers (below)
Sprinkle the flower petals of common chives in salads for a mild onion flavor. Try the white starry flowers of Chinese chives for a mild garlic flavor. (See p. 40.)

Lactuca sativa 'Lollo'
Lettuce (left)
Succulent crunchy leaf in green and red forms; a decorative presentation leaf for pâté or around a salad bowl. (See p. 135.)

Lactuca sativa 'Salad bowl'
Red salad bowl lettuce (right)
A "heartless" form, and a useful plant, as you pick only the number of leaves required. (See p. 135.)

Echium vulgare
Viper's bugloss (right)
Small blue, or sometimes pink, flowers with sweet nectar and a very mild taste. (See p. 275.)

Tropaeolum majus 'Variegata'
Variegated nasturtium (right)
Leaves add a sharp peppery zest to salads and sandwiches. Flowers and buds contribute a milder flavor. (See p. 137.)

Stellaria media
Chickweed (below)
Worth nurturing for its tender leaves, available most of the year. (See p. 278.)

Rosa species
Rose petals (above)
Use the petals of any scented rose. Remove the bitter white heel at the base. (See p. 120.)

Brassica juncea 'Mizuna'
Mizuna mustard greens (right)
An attractive cut leaf and tasty stalk with a fresh mild flavor; can be available most of the year from successive sowings.

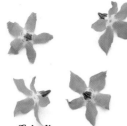

Portulaca oleracea
Summer purslane
(right)
The perfect salad
herb: its crunchy leaves
have a succulent, nutty
flavor. (See p. 137.)

Calendula officinalis
Calendula petals (right)
The glamour herb
for salads; a mild
flavor, and visually
stunning when
varnished with
salad oil.
(See p. 61.)

Borago officinalis
Borage flowers (above)
Beautiful starry blue flowers.
To pick, grasp the black
stamens and gently wiggle
the flower away from the
green backing. (See p. 53.)

Alliara petiolata
Jack-by-the-hedge (above)
A wild plant with a hint
of garlic. Choose tender young
unblemished leaves and chop
finely. (See p. 134.)

Geranium pratense
Meadow cranesbill
(above)
Mild flavored blue
or crimson-veined blue
flowers most of the summer.

Bellis perennis
Lawn daisy (above)
Both the flowers and young leaves
can be used in salads. Separate
the petals, or use small
flowers whole.
(See p. 275.)

Montia perfoliata
Winter purslane
(right)
Available almost
all year round. Second
stage leaves are shown;
early leaves are narrow.
(See p. 136.)

Lepidium sativum
Garden cress (right)
The hot-flavored
leaf is usually seen
in its seedling
stage as
"mustard and
cress." Allowed
to grow on; it is a
pretty salad crop.
(See p. 136.)

Atriplex hortensis
Orach (right)
Pick tender young
purple or gold leaves
for a colorful medium-mild flavored
addition to salads. (See p. 134.)

Eruca vesicaria
Arugula (above)
Young leaves have a hot spicy flavor;
older leaves become bitter. The flowers
can also be tossed in salads. (See p. 135.)

Viola x
Wittrockiana
Garden pansy
(right)
A colorful
addition to the
salad bowl.

Cichorium endivia
Endive (right)
Easy-to-grow salad leaf,
with a bitter flavor
unless blanched or
picked young.

Brassica napus
Rape cabbage
(right)
Young leaves have a
mustardy-cabbage flavor.
Best grown as a seedling crop.

Salad herbs

Alliaria petiolata (Sisymbrium alliaria)
Jack-by-the-hedge Cruciferae

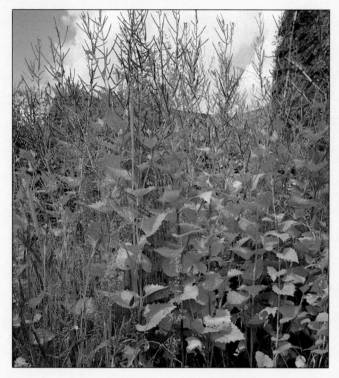

An early-flowering perennial or biennial found growing wild in hedgerows. It reaches a height of between 2 and 3 feet and is topped by a cluster of small white flowers. The broad, somewhat heart-shaped, heavily indented leaves give off a strong smell of garlic when crushed. For this reason, the plant is also known as garlic mustard.

CULTIVATION
Rarely cultivated, the leaves of the wild plant were gathered by country people as and when they were needed. For garden cultivation, seeds can be obtained from a specialist in wild-plant seeds.

USES
The leaves make a tasty accompaniment for meat or cheese in a sandwich or, when finely chopped, add flavor to a salad. They can be eaten fried or boiled in sauces, although they lose flavor slightly when cooked. The juice of the leaves is said to be diuretic.

Atriplex hortensis
Garden orach Chenopodiaceae

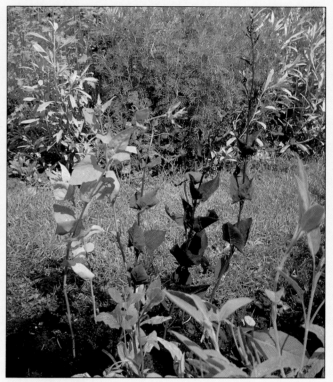

This tall, erect hardy annual, also known as mountain spinach, was once commonly grown in the vegetable garden as a substitute for spinach. It grows to over 5 feet high. The large leaves are indented and the whole plant resembles a large dock. Gold and purple varieties are available as well as green. A row of orach plants can be grown to form a temporary hedge.

CULTIVATION
Sow seeds in rows 2 feet apart in rich soil in late spring or early summer. Water freely to encourage quick growth. Pinch out the flower heads of all but a few plants, which will then seed themselves.

USES
No longer used medicinally, garden orach was once known to every housewife for its healing properties. It was prescribed for sore throats, gout and jaundice. Although considered inferior to spinach, it is now grown a great deal in France, where it is used in soups. The different forms, particularly the purple variety, make it a decorative salad ingredient. Young leaves can be eaten raw, older leaves should be cooked.

Eruca vesicaria (E. sativa)
Arugula Cruciferae

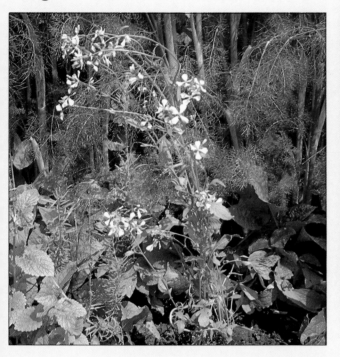

An easy-to-grow salad herb that can be found running wild on wasteland. The cultivated variety grows to a height of 2–3 feet, with small creamy-yellow flowers that appear in late spring and early summer. The pointed, lance-shaped leaves are deeply indented near the base of the plant and have a characteristic smell when bruised and a peppery flavor.

CULTIVATION
Sow rows of seed in rich, moist soil in a lightly shaded position from early spring to early summer. Grow quickly for tender leaves, which are ready to pick within six to eight weeks of sowing and should be gathered before flowering.

USES
Once used medicinally in a cough syrup, arugula is now grown only as an edible herb. The Ancient Romans prized the flavor of its leaves and seeds. Added to a green salad, the leaves impart a pungent, spicy flavor, which is milder the earlier the leaves are picked. They can also be used in sauces or steamed as a vegetable. The flowers can be used to garnish a salad and in flower language, arugula means deceit.

Lactuca sativa
Lettuce Compositae

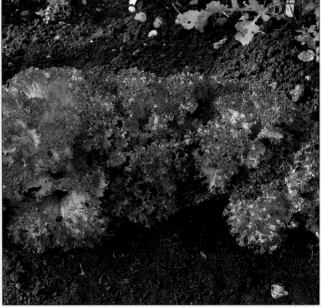

The best-known and most universally used of all the salad herbs, lettuce is now available in a variety of shapes, textures and colors as well as in all seasons. One of the most attractive and reliable is the 'Lollo' (above). With its pretty, frilled, red leaves, this rosette type is almost completely pest- and disease-resistant. Other attractive forms are the red 'Salad bowl' and the cut-and-come-again varieties such as 'Saladisi.'

CULTIVATION
Lettuce needs a light, well-drained, fertile soil, which retains moisture. For a steady supply, sow seed little and often in an open site while the weather is cool. Thin as early as possible to 10 inches apart.

USES
The Ancient Greeks and Romans were aware of its soporific and health-giving properties. In Greek mythology Aphrodite is said to have laid the dead Adonis on a bed of lettuce leaves. The juice is used in a cooling lotion for sunburn. Mainly eaten raw in green or mixed salads, lettuce can also be braised or made into soup.

Salad herbs

Lepidium sativum
Garden cress Cruciferae

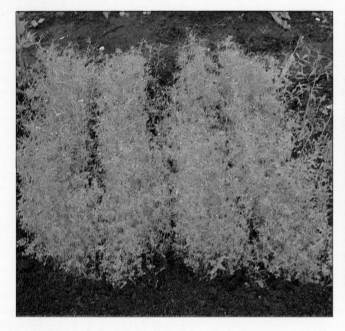

Sown on a dish indoors, this is the cress of
"mustard and cress." Outdoors it can reach a
height of 18 inches and bears small white flowers,
typical of the crucifer family, in early
summer. It is cultivated for its narrow, lance-
shaped leaves, which have a biting, peppery taste.

CULTIVATION
Sow frequently in light, well-drained soil anytime from
early spring to early autumn. Water freely and gather
the young leaves before they have time to toughen in
hot weather.

USES
Another favorite with the Ancient Romans, this useful
cut-and-come-again crop adds piquancy to salads,
garnishes and sauces. As a very young plant it gives a
tang to mustard and cress, but the leaves develop a
hotter flavor as the plant matures. Although it does
contain a natural antibiotic, garden cress is not used
medicinally.

Montia perfoliata (Claytonia perfoliata)
Winter purslane Portulacaceae

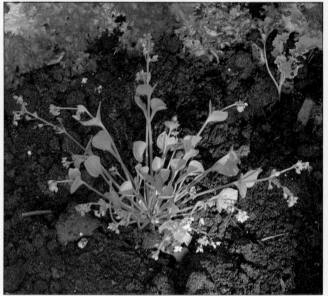

Also known as miner's lettuce in some areas, this
hardy annual deserves more attention as a salad
herb. It can provide several winter crops and is
useful as a substitute when the soil is too poor for
spinach. During spring it grows extremely rapidly,
producing small white flowers on long stalks. The
early leaves are narrow, while later leaves, just as
succulent to eat, are rounded and become
wrapped around the stem.

CULTIVATION
For winter use, sow very thinly in rows in late
summer. Any soil is suitable, but the plants need cold-
frame protection in a severe winter. When they run to
seed and die in midsummer, leave a few to seed
themselves, then transplant seedlings that autumn, or
the following spring for a summer crop.

USES
A cut-and-come-again crop that is indispensable for
providing cool and juicy bulk in winter and early-
spring salads. The stalks, leaves and flowers are all
edible, and the leaves can also be cooked like spinach.

Portulaca oleracea
Summer purslane   *Portulacaceae*

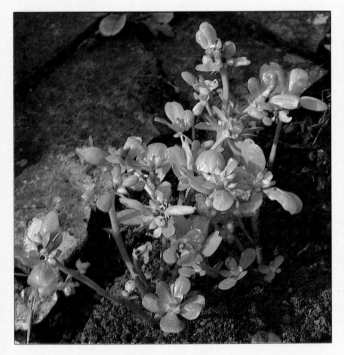

Cultivated for hundreds of years in India and the Middle East, summer purslane was very popular in Europe during the sixteenth century. There are several varieties of this half-hardy annual, which grows to a height of 6 inches with rounded, fleshy, green or, in some forms, golden leaves and reddish stems. In midsummer it bears short-lived small yellow flowers.

CULTIVATION
Sow each month during summer for a continuous supply. Choose a sheltered, sunny site with light, well-drained soil and sow in rows 1 foot apart with 6 inch spaces between plants. Water well and harvest after six to eight weeks.

USES
The golden-leaved variety can make a very attractive display in a more formal herb garden. The plant was once thought to afford protection from evil spirits. It is high in vitamin C and, eaten raw, has diuretic properties. The thick leaves and stems can be pickled in vinegar, but the plant is usually eaten cooked in the East. With sorrel, it is one of the traditional ingredients in the French dish *soupe bonne femme*. An excellent crunchy salad plant, its cooling leaves blend well with hotter-flavored salad herbs.

Tropaeolum majus
Nasturtium   *Tropaeolaceae*

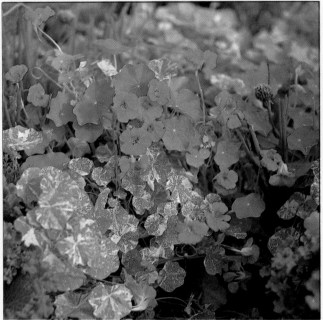

There are many varieties of this colorful annual: climbers, semi-trailers, spreading and compact dwarfs. It has round, flat leaves with yellowy-green veins and red, yellow or orange, trumpet-like flowers which appear from midsummer to midautumn.

CULTIVATION
Nasturtiums thrive in full sun or partial shade. Sow the seeds singly 8 inches apart in late spring in any free-draining soil. In general, the poorer the soil, the more flowers you can expect.

USES
Both the leaves and flower buds have a cress-like flavor and add bite to salads and sandwiches. The young seeds have a stronger flavor and are sometimes used chopped as a substitute for horseradish in sauce tartare. Pickled in vinegar, they resemble capers. Used whole, the flowers can make a stunning garnish. The leaves have a high vitamin-C content and are thought to relieve cold symptoms. The nasturtium seems to attract hoverflies, which will attack aphids on nearby plants, making it a useful companion plant.

Tagetes patula

French Marigold Compositae

Tagetes offers a unique asset to gardeners: it can deter eelworm (nematodes). Its root secretions will deaden the detector mechanism of eelworms so that they don't "wake up" to the presence of their host plant. In Holland recent experiments have confirmed that eelworm among roses can be controlled by interplanting with French marigold. Tulip and potato growers also find it invaluable, and the foliage scent deters insects from tomato plants.

African marigold (T. *erecta*) has similar properties to French marigold, but most effective of all is the Inca marigold (T. *minuta*), which can grow to a height of 10 feet. For hundreds of years, South American Indians have grown potatoes on the same land and prevented eelworm attack by interplanting with this "sacred weed."

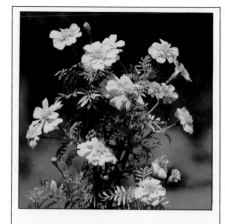

Flower
Pungent-scented, vibrant dark orange, crimson or yellow flowers, double or single, borne from early summer to first frost.

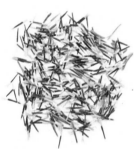

Seed
Like miniature paintbrush: cream-tipped, shiny, flat, dark "handle," $\frac{3}{8}$ inch long, with cream "bristles."

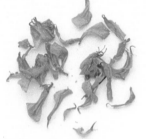

Dried petals
These retain their rich color for potpourri or for implanting in homemade papers.

Leaf
Finely divided and mid-green; bruised foliage emits pungent scent.

Stem
Sturdy, hollow (near base), round and green with pungent scent.

Root
Fine and beige.

 Lifespan
Half-hardy annual

Height
T. patula 12 inches

CULTIVATION
Site Sunny and open.
Soil Well cultivated; prefers moderately rich loam but tolerates dry and poor soil.
Propagating Sow under glass in early spring.
Growing (T. *patula*) Transplant to 12 inches apart in late spring. Deadheading improves growth. Can be grown indoors. (T. *minuta*) Start under glass, when 6 inches tall, transplant 12 inches apart.
Harvesting Gather open flowers.
Preserving Separate petals and dry.

USES
Decorative
● **Flower** Cut flowers are long lasting. Dry for potpourri.

Household
● **Whole plant** Emits scent that deters white fly from tomato plants.
● **Flower** Boil for a yellow dye with alum mordant for wool and silk.
● **Root** Exudes secretions which repel eelworm (nematodes). Grow T. *patula* and T. *erecta* as protection against most noncyst-forming eelworms. The most damaging cyst-forming eelworms are clustered 90–500 in a chemical-proof cyst. They have a mechanism to detect potatoes which triggers their release. New research indicates that secretions of T. *minuta* deaden this detector (it does not eliminate the eelworm). T. *minuta* root secretions also kill certain weeds in a circle round it (the "Tagetes Effect"). It is strongest against ground elder (*Aegopodium podagraria*), quite strong against bindweed (*Calystegia sepium*) and less strong against couch grass (*Agropyron repens*).

Aromatic
● **Leaf** (T. *tenuifolia* var. pumila "Tangerine Gem") Plant for its orange scent. (T. *tenuifolia*) Cultivate for its fresh lemon verbena scent. Dry for potpourri.

Tanacetum parthenium (*Chrysanthemum parthenium*)

Feverfew Compositae

Some medicinal properties of this ancient herb have been known by herbalists, including Culpeper, for centuries. These were its ability to aid "melancholy and aches and pains in the head." However, feverfew's ability to soothe headaches was not given much attention until recently and, after detailed scientific analysis of the plant, several new healing substances have been discovered and patented. For example, in trials to prevent or reduce migraine, 70 percent of patients experienced some improvement after eating a number of feverfew leaves every day, while the best drug on the market currently has a 50 percent cure rate. Feverfew's success in combating migraines may be due to its accumulative effect in slowly reducing the smooth muscle spasms, which are implicated in many forms of migraine.

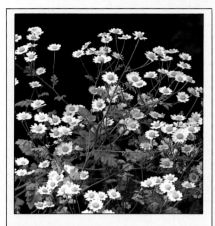

Seed
Small, beige-brown, narrow and flat.

Dried flowers
Add to potpourri for petal color; also used medicinally in infusions, disinfectants, and as a mild sedative.

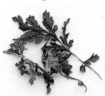

Dried leaves
Exude penetrating aroma, so store away from other herbs.

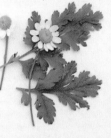

Flower
Small loose clusters of single white flowers with flat yellow centers borne from midsummer. (Their flat centers distinguish them from chamomile flowers, which have conical ones.)

Leaf
Aromatic, divided and mid to yellow-green.

Stem
Slightly downy, ridged, round, branching and green.

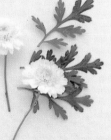

Double-flowered form
White flowers resemble button chrysanthemums; very finely cut leaves. Lasts well in flower arrangements.

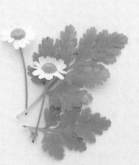

T.p. 'Aureum' Golden feverfew
Single white flowers and aromatic golden-green leaves; makes an attractive edging plant, especially in winter. Ht: 12 inches.

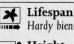

Lifespan
Hardy biennial/perennial

Height
2 feet

CULTIVATION
Site Prefers sunny position.
Soil Dry and well drained.
Propagating Sow in spring or autumn. (Feverfew self-seeds profusely.) Take stem cuttings in summer. Divide roots in autumn.
Growing Thin or transplant to 12 inches apart. Feverfew can be grown indoors in cool air.
Harvesting Pick leaves and flowers anytime.
Preserving Dry leaves and flowers.

USES
Decorative
● *Whole plant* Cultivate golden feverfew for year-round color.
● *Flower* Adds color to potpourri.

Culinary
● *Leaf* Add small amounts to food to "cut" the grease; bitter flavored.

Household
● *Leaf* Decoct or infuse for a mild disinfectant. Use dried in sachets to deter moths.

Cosmetic
● *Leaf* Used by Gervase Markham in the 17th century in the first commercial skin lotion reputed to remove freckles and blemishes.

Medicinal
● *Leaf* Eat three to five fresh leaves between slices of bread every day to reduce migraines. In trials, 70 percent of patients experienced reduced migraines, and 43 percent felt other beneficial side effects, including more restful sleep and relief from arthritis; while only 18 percent had unpleasant side effects. Research has not tested gold or double-flowered forms, but experience suggests they act similarly. Infuse as a mouth rinse after tooth extraction and as a mild laxative. Once used for fever, melancholy and vertigo.
● *Leaf and flower* Infuse as a mild sedative, a tonic to the appetite, and to relieve muscle spasms.

Tanacetum vulgare (Chrysanthemum vulgare)

Tansy *Compositae*

Tansy was believed to arrest decay, and its name derives from the Greek *athanasia*, meaning immortality. In some ancient cultures, its strong antiseptic properties were used to preserve the dead and, according to classical legend, a drink made from tansy was given to the beautiful young man Ganymede to make him immortal, so that he could serve as Zeus's cup-bearer.

In the 1,100-year-old monastery plan of St Gall in Switzerland, tansy is shown in the physic garden. This monastery garden was Charlemagne's favorite, and he ordered that all its herbs should be grown on his imperial estates. Tansy was also popularly used as an insecticide, disinfectant and strewing herb, and, at Easter, was made into "Tansy," a rich custardy pudding. John Evelyn, in 1699, wrote that the new leaves, stir-fried and eaten hot with orange juice and sugar, made a most agreeable dish.

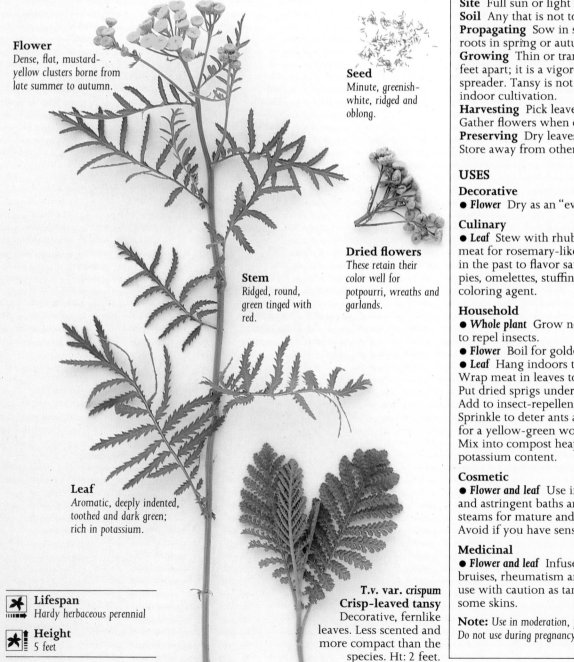

Flower
Dense, flat, mustard-yellow clusters borne from late summer to autumn.

Seed
Minute, greenish-white, ridged and oblong.

Stem
Ridged, round, green tinged with red.

Dried flowers
These retain their color well for potpourri, wreaths and garlands.

Leaf
Aromatic, deeply indented, toothed and dark green; rich in potassium.

**T.v. var. crispum
Crisp-leaved tansy**
Decorative, fernlike leaves. Less scented and more compact than the species. Ht: 2 feet.

Lifespan
Hardy herbaceous perennial

Height
5 feet

CULTIVATION
Site Full sun or light shade.
Soil Any that is not too wet.
Propagating Sow in spring. Divide roots in spring or autumn.
Growing Thin or transplant to 2–3 feet apart; it is a vigorous spreader. Tansy is not suitable for indoor cultivation.
Harvesting Pick leaves as required. Gather flowers when open.
Preserving Dry leaves and flowers. Store away from other herbs.

USES
Decorative
● **Flower** Dry as an "everlasting."

Culinary
● **Leaf** Stew with rhubarb. Rub on meat for rosemary-like flavor. Used in the past to flavor sausages, meat pies, omelettes, stuffings, and as a coloring agent.

Household
● **Whole plant** Grow near fruit trees to repel insects.
● **Flower** Boil for golden yellow dye.
● **Leaf** Hang indoors to deter flies. Wrap meat in leaves to preserve. Put dried sprigs under carpets. Add to insect-repellent sachets. Sprinkle to deter ants and mice. Boil for a yellow-green woolen dye. Mix into compost heap for its potassium content.

Cosmetic
● **Flower and leaf** Use in stimulating and astringent baths and facial steams for mature and sallow skins. Avoid if you have sensitive skin.

Medicinal
● **Flower and leaf** Infuse as a wash for bruises, rheumatism and sprains, but use with caution as tansy can irritate some skins.

Note: *Use in moderation, potentially toxic. Do not use during pregnancy.*

Trigonella foenum-graecum

Fenugreek *Leguminosae*

Fenugreek is one of the herbs whose medicinal use and commercial cultivation is at present on the increase. Its seed contains not only mucilage but also diosgenin, which is important in the synthesis of oral contraceptives and sex hormone treatments. Its leaves contain coumarin, which gives them a sweet hay scent when dried, so they are sometimes used to mask inferior hay. *Foenum-graecum*, in fact, is the Latin for Greek hay and it is a well-known fodder crop.

Archaeological evidence suggests that the Egyptians valued fenugreek for eating, healing and embalming. The Greeks and Romans, too, enjoyed the seed as food and medicine. On the Indian subcontinent, its spicy seed has long been included in curry powder and its leafy shoots have been curried as a vegetable.

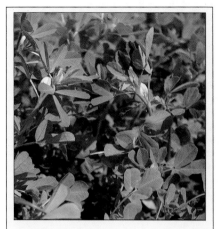

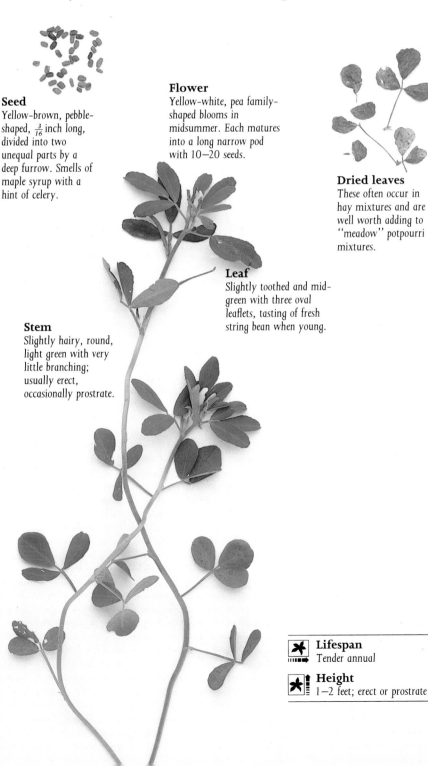

Seed
Yellow-brown, pebble-shaped, $\frac{3}{16}$ inch long, divided into two unequal parts by a deep furrow. Smells of maple syrup with a hint of celery.

Flower
Yellow-white, pea family-shaped blooms in midsummer. Each matures into a long narrow pod with 10–20 seeds.

Dried leaves
These often occur in hay mixtures and are well worth adding to "meadow" potpourri mixtures.

Leaf
Slightly toothed and mid-green with three oval leaflets, tasting of fresh string bean when young.

Stem
Slightly hairy, round, light green with very little branching; usually erect, occasionally prostrate.

Lifespan
Tender annual

Height
1–2 feet; erect or prostrate

CULTIVATION
Site Full sun.
Soil Fertile, well drained, alkaline.
Propagating Sow thickly in rows 9 inches apart in spring for main crop, and throughout summer for young salad leaves.
Growing Thin to 4 inches apart; difficult to transplant. Small plants can be grown indoors.
Harvesting Pick young leaves as needed. Cut whole plant in autumn. Pick seed when ripe.
Preserving Dry leaves and seed.

USES
Culinary
● *Seed* Used as a spice in curries and chutneys. Roast gently to develop flavor before grinding (overheating turns seed red and bitter). Sprout and use as a winter salad herb (ready in 4–6 days). As sprouts grow, curry flavor recedes.
● *Leaf* Toss sprouted seed leaves into salads. When fenugreek is 8 inches tall, eat raw or boil or curry as a vegetable.

Household
● *Seed* Boil for a yellow dye.

Cosmetic
● *Seed* Contains up to 30 percent mucilage, protein, lecithin, vitamins and other valued conditioners. Infuse for a complexion wash. Powder and mix with oil for chapped lips, or use as a scalp massage for glossy hair. Try soaking seed until gummy and add to hand lotion recipes as an enriching, softening and thickening agent.

Medicinal
● *Seed* Grind coarsely, infuse and drink as a tonic tea to stimulate digestion and milk flow, ease coughing, flatulence and diarrhea. Make a mushy poultice of crushed seed and hot milk for inflammation, ulcers, swollen glands, sciatica and bruises. Fenugreek is said to be effective in treating fevers.

Thymus species

Thymes Labiatae

Thyme has inspired poetic praise from Virgil to Kipling, who wrote of "wind-bit thyme that smells of dawn in Paradise." Its fragrance is particularly strong on the warm, sunny hillsides of Mediterranean lands. To the Greeks, thyme denoted graceful elegance: "to smell of thyme" was an expression of stylish praise. After bathing, the Greeks would include oil of thyme in their massage.

Thymus may derive from the Greek word thymon, meaning "courage," and many traditions relate to this virtue. Roman soldiers, for example, bathed in thyme water to give themselves vigor. In the Middle Ages, European ladies embroidered a sprig of thyme on tokens for their knights-errant. A soup recipe of 1663 recorded the use of thyme and beer to overcome shyness, while Scottish highlanders drank tea made of wild thyme for strength and courage, and to prevent nightmares.

The powerful antiseptic and preservative properties of thyme were well-known to the Egyptians, who used it for embalming. It is still an ingredient of embalming fluid, and it will also preserve anatomical and herbarium specimens, and protect paper from mold. Sprigs were included in judges' posies and clasped by nobility to protect themselves from disease and odor. Thyme is the first herb listed in the Holy Herb Charm recited by those with "herb cunning" in the Middle Ages, and it is featured in a charming recipe from 1600 "to enable one to see the Fairies."

THYME-SCENTED THYMES

T. pulegioides
Broad leaf thyme
Bushy shrub with mauve-pink flowers and strongly flavored leaves, which are larger and rounder than common thyme's. Ht: 15 inches.

T.v. 'Silver Posie'
Shrub with pale pink to lilac flowers and green leaves edged in silver. Ht: 15 inches.

T. 'Aureus'
Golden creeping thyme
Rose-purple flowers with golden leaves, which fade with insufficient sun. Ht: 4 inches.

Lifespan
Evergreen shrub

Height
3–15 inches; creeping varieties make good ground cover

T. richardii (T. nitidus)
Neat shrub with pale lilac flowers and narrow, bright green leaves. Ht: 6 inches. (Similar T. carnosus has white flowers.)

Flower
Pale lilac blooms borne from early to midsummer.

Seed
Tiny, spherical, brown and shiny.

Dried leaves
These have stronger flavor than fresh winter leaves.

T. pseudolanuginosus (T. lanuginosus)
Woolly thyme
Creeper with pale pink flower and very hairy, gray leaves. Ht: 3 inches

Leaf
Aromatic, pointed oval and mid-green, covered in fine hairs.

Stem
Square, green-brown, becoming woody in second season.

T. vulgaris
Common thyme

Root
Fine and grayish-brown, forming dense mat.

T. serpyllum 'Minus'
Creeper with pink flowers and tiny mid-green leaves. Ht: 2 inches.

T.p.a. 'Snowdrift' ('Albus')
Creeper with white flowers and small, faintly scented, bright green leaves. Ht: 3 inches.

T.p.a. 'Coccineus'
Creeper with crimson flowers and small, faintly scented, green leaves. Ht: 3 inches.

T. praecox arcticus (T. serpyllum)
English wild thyme
Very hardy creeper with mauve flowers and mildly scented leaves. Ht: 3 inches.

T. doerfleri
Creeper with mauve flowers and gray leaves, narrower and in closer clusters than woolly thyme's. Ht: 3 inches.

OTHER SCENTED THYMES

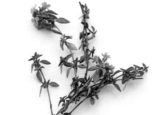

**T. caespititius
(T. azoricus)**
Creeper with pink
flowers and narrow,
pine-scented, green
leaves. Ht: 2 inches.

T. herba-barona
Prostrate subshrub with rose
flowers, arching branches and
caraway-scented, dark green
leaves. Ht: 4 inches.

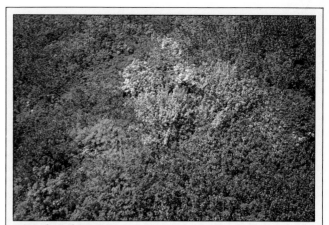

A bed of colorful thymes.

CULTIVATION
Site Full sun.
Soil Light and well drained, preferably alkaline.
Propagating Take 2–3 inch stem cuttings with a "heel"
anytime except winter. Divide roots or layer stems in
spring or autumn. (Species only) Sow in spring.
Growing Thin or transplant to 9–15 inches apart. In
summer, prune frequently. In very cold areas, protect
thyme in winter. Can be grown indoors.
Harvesting Pick leaves in summer. They are best while
thyme is in bloom.
Preserving Dry leaves. Make thyme vinegar and oil.

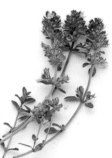

T. 'Fragrantissimus'
Shrub with pale lilac
flowers and sweet
fruity, blue-gray
leaves.
Ht: 15 inches.

**T. pallasianus
(T. odoratissimus)**
Shrub with pale
pink flowers, long
lax branches and
citrusy leaves.
Ht: 8 inches.

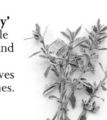

T. 'Doone Valley'
Creeper with pale
purple flowers and
lemon-scented,
bright green leaves
with gold splashes.
Ht: 3 inches.

**T.
'Aureus'
Golden lemon
creeping thyme**
Creeper with
pink flowers
and golden-
lemon leaves.
Ht: 3 inches.

**T. × citriodorus
'Silver Lemon Queen'**
Shrub with pale pink
flowers and lemony,
silver-splashed leaves.
Ht: 12 inches.

T. 'Lemon Curd'
Creeper with pink
flowers, long wiry
branches and narrow, sweet
lemon-scented, green leaves.
Ht: 2 inches.

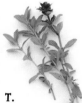

T. 'Citriodorus'
Creeper with pink
flowers and large,
strongly lemon-
scented, green
leaves. Ht: 6 inches.

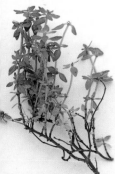

T. × citriodorus
Shrub with pale lilac
flowers and lemon-
scented, bright green
leaves. Ht: 12 inches.

USES
Decorative
● *Whole plant* Grow shrubs for low hedging and creepers
for aromatic carpets.
● *Flower and leaf* Include in summer posies.

Culinary
● *Leaf* (Common thyme) Mix with parsley and bay in
bouquet garni. Add to stocks, marinades, stuffings, sauces
and soups, using cautiously as thyme is extra pungent
when fresh. Aids digestion of fatty foods. Suits food
cooked slowly in wine – particularly poultry, shellfish
and game. Flavors benedictine liqueur. (Lemon-scented
thymes) Add to chicken, fish, hot vegetables, fruit salads
and jams. (T. herba-barona) Use to flavor beef.

Household
● *Flower* Thyme is loved by bees. Its honey is esteemed.
● *Leaf* Make a strong decoction for a household
disinfectant. Mix essential oil with alcohol, then spray on
paper and herbarium specimens for mold protection.

Cosmetic
● *Leaf* Make a decoction to stimulate circulation; use in
baths, facial steams and ointments for spots. Infuse with
rosemary as a hair rinse to deter dandruff. Use essential
oil as an antiseptic in toothpastes and mouthwashes.

Aromatic
● *Leaf* Use in potpourri. ·

Medicinal
● *Leaf* (English wild thyme) This has the strongest
medicinal qualities, although any thyme can be used.
Infuse as a tea for a digestive tonic and for hangovers.
Sweeten infusion with honey for convulsive coughs,
colds and sore throats. Apply infused thyme oil as a
massage for headaches. Use essential oil in an antiseptic
air spray. May also relieve insomnia, poor capillary
circulation, muscular pain, and stimulate production of
white blood corpuscles to resist infection.

Valeriana officinalis

Valerian *Valerianaceae*

This ancient medicinal herb, whose name derives from the Latin *valere* "to be in health," has long been valued around the world. Nordic, Persian and Chinese herbalists used the root, while the similar *V. sylvatica* was found in the medicine bag of Canadian Indian warriors as a wound antiseptic. Fresh valerian root smells like ancient leather but, when dried, it is nearer to stale perspiration. Its old name, *V. phu*, could be the origin of our expression for an undesirable scent. Nevertheless, valerian is still used to add a musky tone to perfume. Cats and rats are attracted to the smell, and the Pied Piper of Hamelin is said to have carried the root to lure the rats, his music being a decoy. Valerian returned to prominence in the First and Second World Wars for treating shell shock and nervous stress.

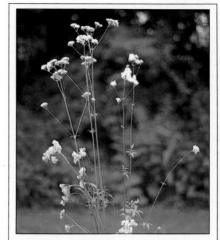

Flower
Tiny, peculiarly scented, pale lilac-pink clusters appear in midsummer.

Seed
Light brown, flat, tear-shaped, $\frac{1}{10}$ inch long.

Leaf
Narrow, toothed, dark green leaflets; exudes a sharp scent like horseradish.

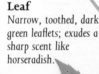

Young plant
Readily broken, shiny light green stems; leaves not yet divided into leaflets.

Stem
Round and green with *deep grooves*, which distinguish it from other valerians.

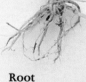

Root
Short rhizome with pale fibrous roots and offshoots from second season onward. Smells unpleasant.

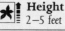

Lifespan
Hardy herbaceous perennial

Height
2–5 feet

CULTIVATION

Site Full sun or light shade. Prefers cool roots and warm foliage.
Soil Prefers rich, moist loam.
Propagating Sow in spring, pressing seed into soil but do not cover for germination. Divide roots in spring or autumn.
Growing Transplant or thin to 2 feet apart. Can be grown as an indoor plant.
Harvesting Dig complete root in second season in late autumn. Remove pale fibrous roots, leaving edible rhizome.
Preserving Slice rhizomatous root to dry.

USES

Decorative
● *Whole plant* Grow in the border.

Culinary
● *Root* Add to soups and stews.

Household
● *Whole plant* Boosts growth of nearby vegetables by stimulating phosphorus and earthworm activity. Infuse root and spray on ground to attract earthworms.
● *Leaf* Add mineral-rich leaves to raw compost.
● *Root* Attracts cats, vermin and earthworms. Used in rat traps.

Cosmetic
● *Root* Use decoction as a facial wash, for a soothing bath, and in lotion for acne or skin rashes.

Medicinal
● *Root* Acts as a depressant on central nervous system. Decoct root or, more effective, crush 1 teaspoon dried root and soak in cold water for 12–24 hours. Drink as a sedative for mild insomnia, sudden emotional distress, headaches, intestinal cramps and nervous exhaustion.

Note: *After 2–3 weeks, stop taking valerian for a few days. Then restart if needed.*

Verbascum thapsus

Mullein Scrophulariaceae

A magical herb of antiquity, mullein was given to Ulysses to protect him from the sorcery of Circe, who changed his crew into pigs. This tall and imposing plant has attracted over 30 common names, including Aaron's rod, candlewick plant, hag's taper, cow lungwort and velvet dock. The soft fine hairs on verbascum's leaves and stems make superb tinder. They also protect the herb from moisture loss, creeping insects and grazing animals, as the down irritates their mucous membranes. This skillfully constructed plant drops rain from its small leaves onto larger leaves and down to the roots.

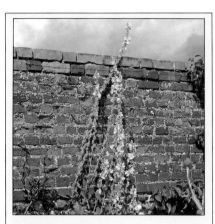

Seed
Tiny, brown, faceted and mildly toxic; many to a capsule.

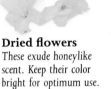

Dried flowers
These exude honeylike scent. Keep their color bright for optimum use.

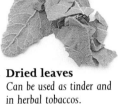

Dried leaves
Can be used as tinder and in herbal tobaccos.

Stem
Sturdy, downy, round and fibrous, enclosing white pith.

Leaf
Large, woolly and rosette-forming in first year, growing up stem in second year.

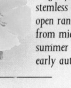

Flower
Bright yellow stemless blooms open randomly from mid-summer to early autumn.

Lifespan
Hardy biennial

Height
7 feet

CULTIVATION
Site Sunny and sheltered.
Soil Well drained; chalky or poor.
Propagating Sow in spring or summer. Self-seeds in light soils.
Growing Thin or transplant to 2 feet apart. Stake verbascum in exposed sites or on rich moist soil. Not suitable for indoor cultivation.
Harvesting Collect flowers as they open, and leaves in their first season.
Preserving Remove green parts from flowers; then dry gently, without artificial heat, as its healing power is connected with the yellow coloring matter. Dry leaves.

USES
Decorative
● **Flowering top** Use in arrangements. Dry to add color to potpourri.

Culinary
● **Flower** Use to flavor liqueurs.

Household
● **Flower** Verbascum pollen and nectar attract bees to gardens.
● **Leaf** Can be placed in shoes when soles become thin. The Romans wrapped figs in leaves to prevent them going bad. Use down stripped from leaves for tinder.
● **Stem** Dry and dip in suet or tallow for long-lasting iridescent torch.

Cosmetic
● **Flower** Use in a cream or facial steam to soften and soothe skin. Make a strong infusion to brighten fair hair.

Medicinal
● **Flower** Steep in hot water until water is yellow, then drink to relieve persistent coughs, respiratory mucus and hoarseness.
● **Leaf** Used in homeopathic products for migraine and earache. Infuse as a tea for coughs and strain through fine muslin to remove hairs or pollen, which can cause unpleasant itching in the mouth.

Note: *Take in small doses, as all verbascum parts, except the flower, are mildly toxic.*

Verbena officinalis

Vervain *Verbenaceae*

It is curious that such an unassuming plant as vervain should have become sacred to so many cultures. In Egypt, for example, vervain was believed to have originated from the tears of Isis, and Greek priests wore its root with their vestments. Being sacred to Venus, vervain was used in love potions. The Chinese names for this herb, "dragon-teeth grass" and "iron vervain," suggest hidden powers.

Vervain was the Roman word for altar plants used for spiritual purification, and the Druids, too, washed their altars with a flower infusion and used vervain in their lustral water for visions. It was a herb of prophecy for the magi, the mystic sages of Persia. To the Anglo-Saxons vervain was a powerful protector and part of the Holy Salve against demons of disease.

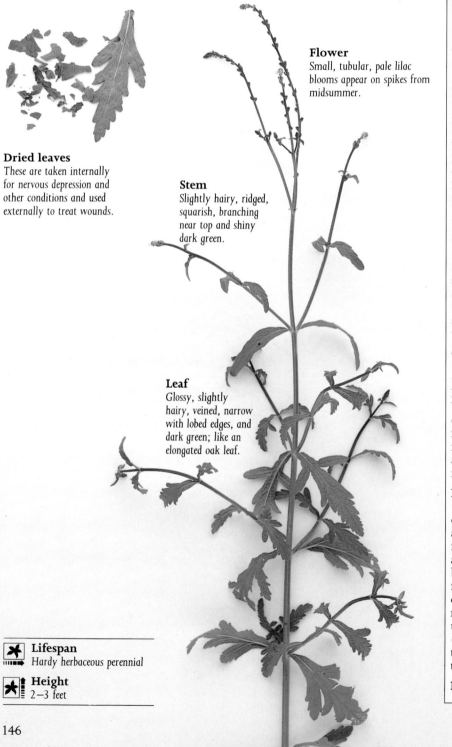

Flower
Small, tubular, pale lilac blooms appear on spikes from midsummer.

Dried leaves
These are taken internally for nervous depression and other conditions and used externally to treat wounds.

Stem
Slightly hairy, ridged, squarish, branching near top and shiny dark green.

Leaf
Glossy, slightly hairy, veined, narrow with lobed edges, and dark green; like an elongated oak leaf.

Lifespan
Hardy herbaceous perennial

Height
2–3 feet

CULTIVATION
Site Sun or light shade.
Soil Fertile, well-drained loam.
Propagating Sow in spring at 65–70 °F. Germination is erratic and may take 3–4 weeks.
Growing Thin or transplant to 12 inches apart. Can be grown indoors.
Harvesting Pick leaves as required. Cut whole plant when in bloom.
Preserving Dry leaves or whole plant if required.

USES
Culinary
● **Leaf** Because of its reputation as an effective love potion, vervain was sometimes included in dishes and added to homemade liqueurs. Note that vervain does not have a lemon scent and should not be confused with lemon verbena.

Cosmetic
● **Leaf** Infuse as an eye compress for tired eyes and inflamed eyelids. Decoct as an eye bath. The Victorians considered vervain an excellent hair tonic, especially when mixed with rosemary: massage infusion into the scalp and use it as a rinse. It was used in one of the first commercial hair tonics.

Medicinal
● **Whole plant** Infused as a tea for a digestive and for a sedative nightcap after nervous exhaustion, for detox-ification and for promotion of urine; as an anticoagulant; or as a wash for bruising and to cool feverish foreheads. Chinese herbalists use a decoction to treat suppressed menstruation, liver problems and urinary tract infections.
● **Leaf** Infuse as a gargle for sore throats. A poultice of dried leaves treats wounds.

Note: *Use with caution.*

Viola odorata

Sweet violet *Violaceae*

A delightful herald of spring, this modest spreading plant is the most highly scented violet. It has long been cultivated for its perfume and color and is added to cosmetics, drinks, sweets and syrups. Its seductive scent suggested strong emotions, and so sweet violet became a plant of Venus and Aphrodite, woven with other plants of love into the final scene of the famous Unicorn Tapestries, now held in the Cloisters museum in New York City.

The Greeks chose sweet violet as their symbol of fertility, while the Romans enjoyed sweet violet wine; for Napoleon, it was the emblem of the imperial party. It was said to be among the most popular scents in Victorian England, and the last Empress Dowager of China imported bottles of "Violetta Regia" from Berlin. Revered writers from Homer to Shakespeare and the old herbalists all speak with great affection of this charming flower. Its virtues were considered to be cool, moist and soothing.

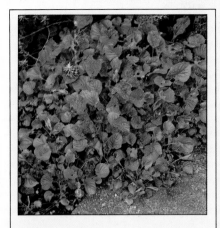

CULTIVATION
Site Semishade. Benefits from sun either early or late in the day.
Soil Rich and moist.
Propagating Easy to propagate from runners. Seed germination is erratic as many early flowers miss pollination.
Growing Transplant in early spring, leaving 4–5-inch spaces between plants. Sweet violets are not suitable as indoor plants.
Harvesting Pick leaves in early spring. Gather flowers when newly opened, and roots in autumn.
Preserving Dry leaves, flowers and roots. Crystallize flowers.

USES
Decorative
● **Flower** Add to a spring posy.

Culinary
● **Flower** Use crystallized to decorate cakes, puddings and ice cream. Eat raw in salads or make into syrup: to 2 ounces fresh flowers add 3 fluid ounces boiling water. Cover and infuse for 24 hours. Strain. Add $\frac{1}{2}$ cup sugar and heat to dissolve. (The color is retained by not allowing it to boil.) Cool and bottle.

Cosmetic
● **Flower** Make a decoction for an eyebath or mouthwash.
● **Leaf** Add to a facial steam.

Aromatic
● **Flower** Use in potpourri, floral waters and perfumes.

Medicinal
● **Flower** Take fresh or dried in an infusion or syrup as a mild laxative; also helpful for coughs and bronchitis, and soothing for nerves, headaches and insomnia.
● **Leaf** A decoction or infusion with dried leaves may alleviate catarrh and bronchitis. Try fresh leaves in a poultice for bruising.
● **Root** A decoction or infusion of dried root is said to alleviate catarrh and bronchitis.

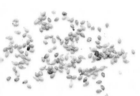

Seed
Light tan, hard, round and small.

Flower
Scented violet or white blooms from late winter to midspring. Provides nectar for early butterflies.

Dried leaves
Culpeper claimed that an infusion "doth purge the body of choleric humours."

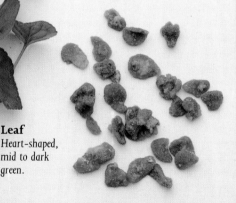

Leaf
Heart-shaped, mid to dark green.

Crystallized petals
A delicious sweetmeat alone or as decoration for cakes.

Runners
Horizontal runners root every 3–5 inches.

Root
Yellowy brown, knobbly rootstalk with hairlike roots.

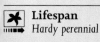
Lifespan
Hardy perennial

Height
4–6 inches; good ground cover

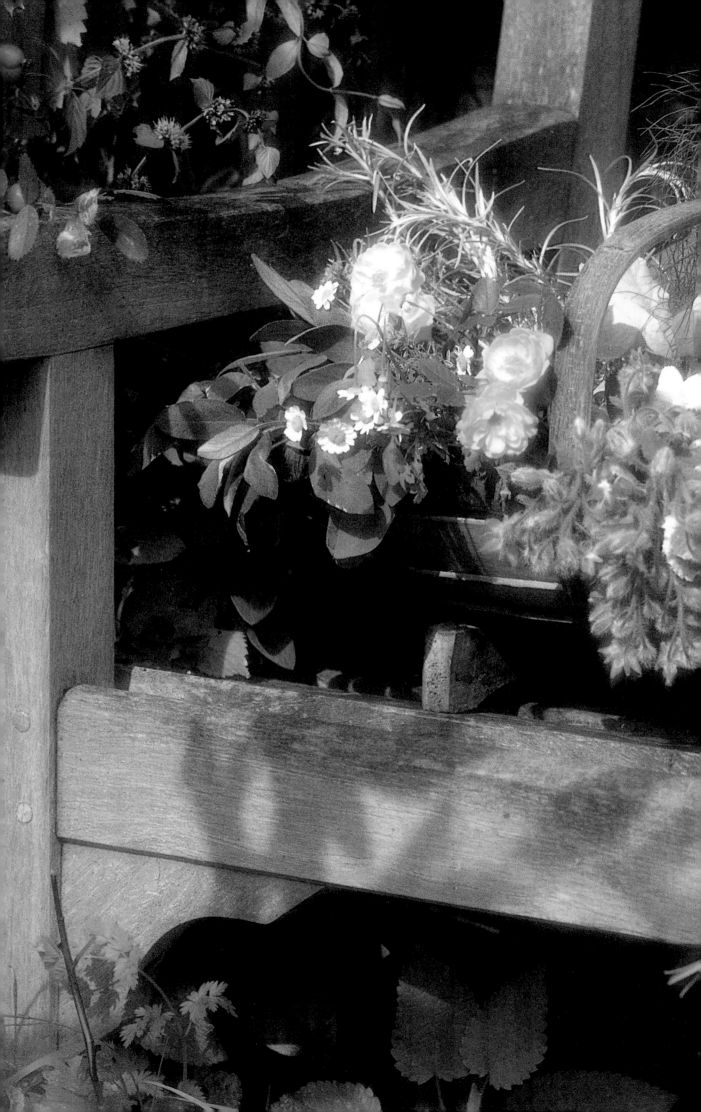

USING HERBS

For centuries, herbs were regarded as
essential to daily life. They played a significant
role in everyone's diet, were made into
household products and cosmetics, and provided
the main source of medical treatments. As manmade
and chemical products were introduced and
brought to the fore, the use of herbs fell into a
decline. However, since some of such "unnatural"
products have become the subjects of controversy,
herbs are enjoying a revival. They are cheap,
easy to grow and use, do not endanger the
environment and are generally much less
harmful than many of the synthetic ingredients
found in commercial foods, household
products and medicines.

The following chapters reveal a wealth of
practical, herbal knowledge, and provide an
inspiring source of ideas for the many ways
in which you can appreciate herbs. Arrange them
indoors to scent and decorate your home.
Taste their full flavors in mouthwatering recipes.
Use them as cleaning and coloring agents. Add
them to cosmetic preparations to soften the skin,
bring luster to your hair, brighten your eyes
and whiten your teeth. Enjoy their aromatic oils
in therapeutic massage treatments and reap the
benefit of their healing properties in a wide
range of simple home remedies.

A selection of colorful and aromatic herbs cut ready for use.

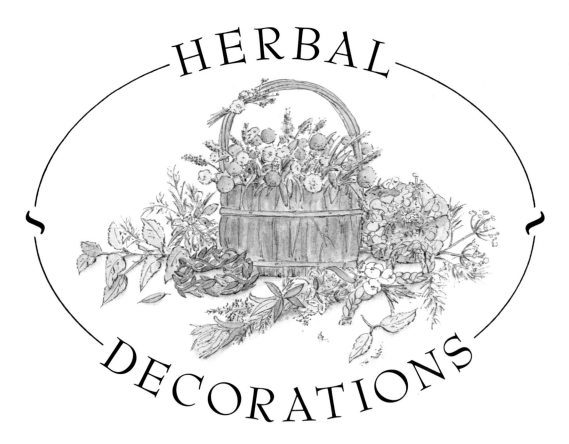

HERBAL DECORATIONS

One of the most delightful aspects of growing herbs is the many attractive ways in which you can display them and appreciate their fragrance indoors. Whether fresh or dried, herbs can be made into striking arrangements, colorful posies, or decorative wreaths and garlands to adorn your home or to present as gifts.

Fresh cut herbs brought straight in from the garden look best in natural, informal arrangements. A mass of summer herbal blooms and leaves in a simple vase can make a truly magnificent display. For added impact, position sweetly scented varieties near a window or in a place where they may be brushed against so their fragrance will waft through rooms.

Simple bunches of herbs hanging to dry look attractive, though they need to be in a warm, dry and dark place if you are drying to preserve them. Once they are dried, hang bunches on walls, from beams or shelves, around a window, or on the back of a door. For extra decorative effect, suspend them from ladders, on rake heads, or from a mesh screen under a high ceiling – anywhere where they will look eyecatching and their scents can be appreciated. Tie small bunches of southernwood, lavender and other moth repellent herbs with ribbon bows and hang them in your closet. Display groups of dried flowers in baskets, earthenware pots, wooden trugs and other suitably natural and complementary containers.

Herbs that you grow indoors can also be used for decorative effect. Evergreen shrubs like rosemary, bay and myrtle may be clipped as miniature topiary pieces, and at Christmas, or on special occasions, you can add color to their branches with ribbon bows and small trinkets.

The following pages show a range of delightful herbal arrangements that should tempt you into trying some floral creativity. Enchant a friend with a herbal posy which is both pretty and aromatic, and composed to bear a message in flower language (see p. 154). Celebrate a festive occasion by making a traditional wreath, or take a practical approach and make a wreath from culinary herbs for the kitchen, sweet-smelling herbs for the bedroom, and pretty, colored herbs that complement your living areas (see p. 156). Use herbs in swags and garlands for their delicate foliage, flowers and fragrance (see p. 158). Arrange dried herbs that will extend the scents and colors of summer into the winter months (see p. 160). Make arrangements of culinary flavoring and garnishing herbs for the dinner table so guests can help themselves to tasty leaves and flowers or simply have their appetites sharpened by their refreshing scents (see p. 162).

A kitchen display
Dried summer herbs in a thyme basket set alongside bottles of herb oils and vinegars make an eyecatching feature in a kitchen corner.

HERBS FOR DECORATIONS

The following plants will add color, interesting shapes and fragrance to arrangements when used fresh.

Those marked with an asterisk (*) also dry well for use in winter displays.

Flowers
*Alliums	*Elecampane	Lily of the valley	Poppies
*Angelica	Flax	Love-in-a-mist	Primrose
*Bergamot	Forget-me-not	Marigold	Pyrethrum
Betony	Foxglove	Marjorams	Rosemary
Borage	Honeysuckle	Meadowsweet	*Teasel
Chamomile	Jasmine	Melilot	Thymes
Columbine	Lady's mantle	Mints	Valerian
Cowslips	*Larkspur	Peony	Violet
Dill	*Lavender	Pinks	*Yarrow

Foliage
*Artemisias (all	Fennel	Myrtle	*Sages
species)	Lungwort	Parsley	Salad burnet
Basils	Marjorams	Pelargoniums	*Santolina
*Bay	Mints	Rosemary	*Thymes
Eucalyptus	Mullein		

Seed heads
*Alexanders	*Fennel	Lovage	*Sorrel
*Alliums	Good King Henry	*Love-in-a-mist	Sunflower
*Angelica	*Hops	*Poppy	*Sweet cicely

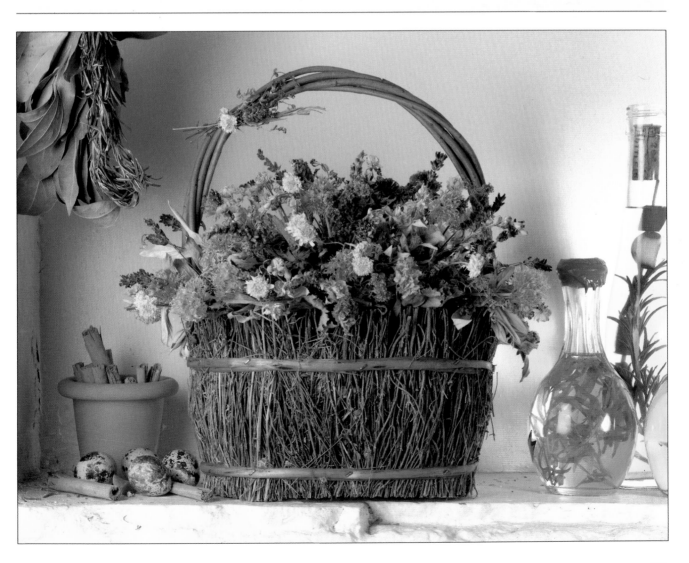

Fresh herbal arrangements

Often thought of as insignificant plants unworthy of inclusion in floral arrangements, herbs offer a wide choice of foliage and flowers as well as their refreshing aromatic qualities.

As the arrangements on these pages show, some herbal flowers have rich, intense colors and intriguing shapes, others are delicate, inviting closer inspection. Use these to add highlights and focal points to arrangements.

Leaves may be feathery, lush, variegated, textured, soft or glossy. They come in all shades of green, and some are evergreen, providing year-round foliage to boost all arrangements. Many, such as the artemisias, have delicate fronds of silvery gray leaves. Fennel provides feathery leaves in green or bronze forms. Varieties of basil and sage offer deep purple-red leaves and there is a range of herbs with yellow variegated leaves,

including some of the highly aromatic mints, marjorams, pelargoniums, lemon balm and golden bay. Include such leaves in arrangements for their shape, form and color as well as their fragrance, which will delight and freshen the senses.

Summer color bowl (opposite)

A fragrant arrangement of summer blooms includes delicate pink honeysuckle, spiky red bergamot, starry blue borage, white double-headed feverfew and sprays of lady's mantle amid sprigs of foliage including rosemary and mints. The simple vase and setting focus attention on the mixed rich colors and delicate shapes of the herbs.

A loose and light display (below)

Frothy sprays of lady's mantle and meadowsweet blossoms, white deutzia flowers, spikes of sorrel buds and feathery fennel leaves give this arrangement a light, airy feel. The gray leaves of artemisia 'Silver King' provide extra highlights and a trailing stem of ivy extends the line of the display.

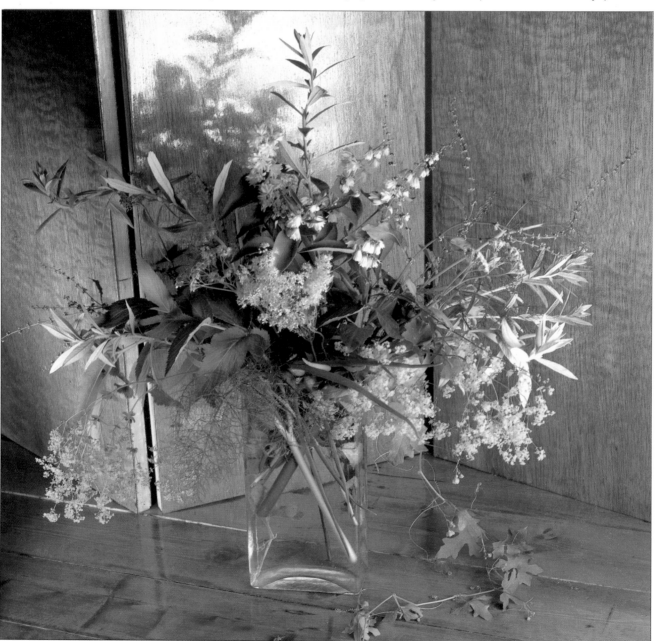

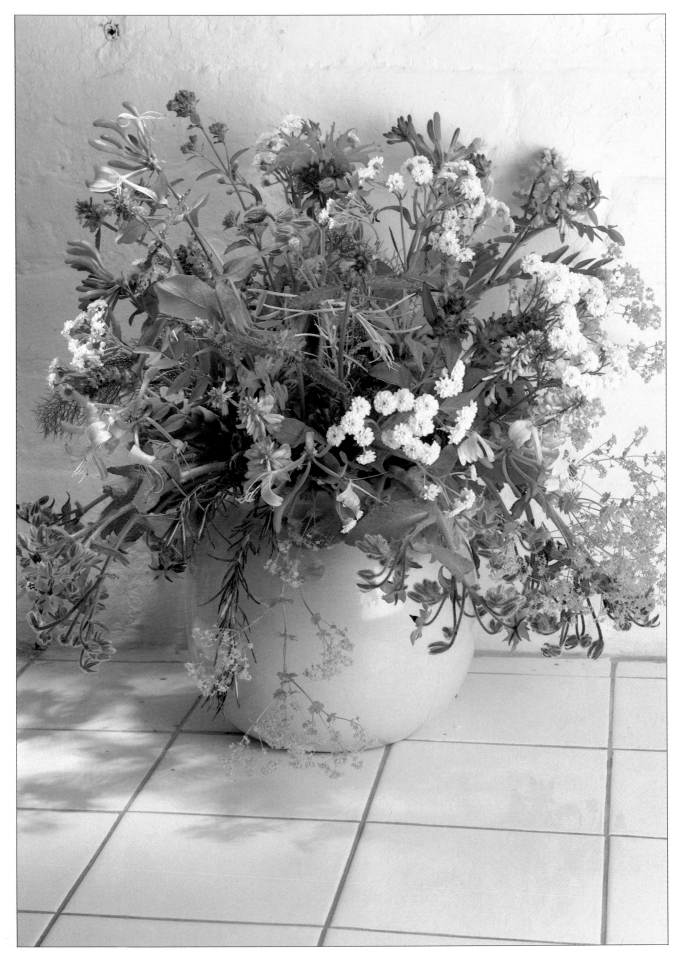

Nosegays

Fragrant posies filled with aromatic herbs and flowers were popular accessories in the sixteenth century, carried through the streets to disguise unpleasant smells and protect the owner from the many virulent diseases that plagued those times. Consequently, they were named nosegays, or more curiously, tussie-mussies.

Apart from their aromatic and disinfectant attributes, nosegays became increasingly popular because they held hidden messages based on the symbolic meanings bestowed on individual plants. This tradition can turn a pretty bouquet into a charming and unique personal gift.

Before making a nosegay, consider its theme and select ingredients for their appearance and symbolism. Start with a central bloom and encircle it with contrasting flowers and leaves. Bind the stems with florist's tape as you go to keep the posy tight. Build up the layers and emphasize the outer rim with a large-leafed herb. Nosegays should stay fresh in water for about a week and can be dried by hanging in a warm, dark place.

The language of plants
A selection of meanings bestowed on some garden plants: agrimony (gratitude); bay (glory); broom (humility); lavender (distrust); lily of the valley (return to happiness); pansy (thoughts); parsley (festivity); poppy (consolation); rue (disdain); sweet basil (good wishes); vervain (enchantment); wormwood (absence).

Birthday nosegay (below)
A pretty arrangement with a garden daisy (innocence) centerpiece surrounded by feathery mugwort (happiness); thyme (courage); angelica (inspiration); southernwood (jesting); marjoram (blushes); pink sweet peas (delicate pleasures). Rounded leaves and flowering sprigs of lady's mantle (protection) form the edging.

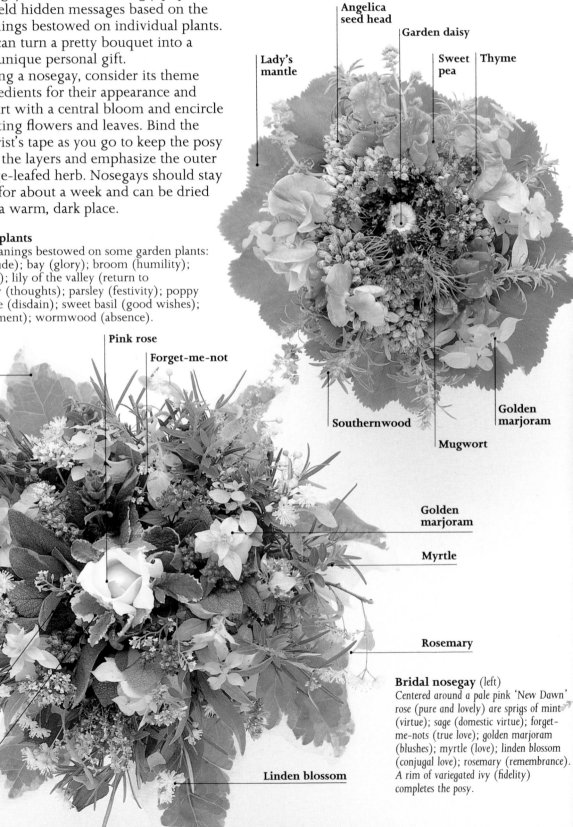

Angelica seed head

Garden daisy

Lady's mantle

Sweet pea

Thyme

Ivy

Pink rose

Forget-me-not

Golden marjoram

Southernwood

Mugwort

Golden marjoram

Myrtle

Rosemary

Sage

Variegated mint

Linden blossom

Bridal nosegay (left)
Centered around a pale pink 'New Dawn' rose (pure and lovely) are sprigs of mint (virtue); sage (domestic virtue); forget-me-nots (true love); golden marjoram (blushes); myrtle (love); linden blossom (conjugal love); rosemary (remembrance). A rim of variegated ivy (fidelity) completes the posy.

154

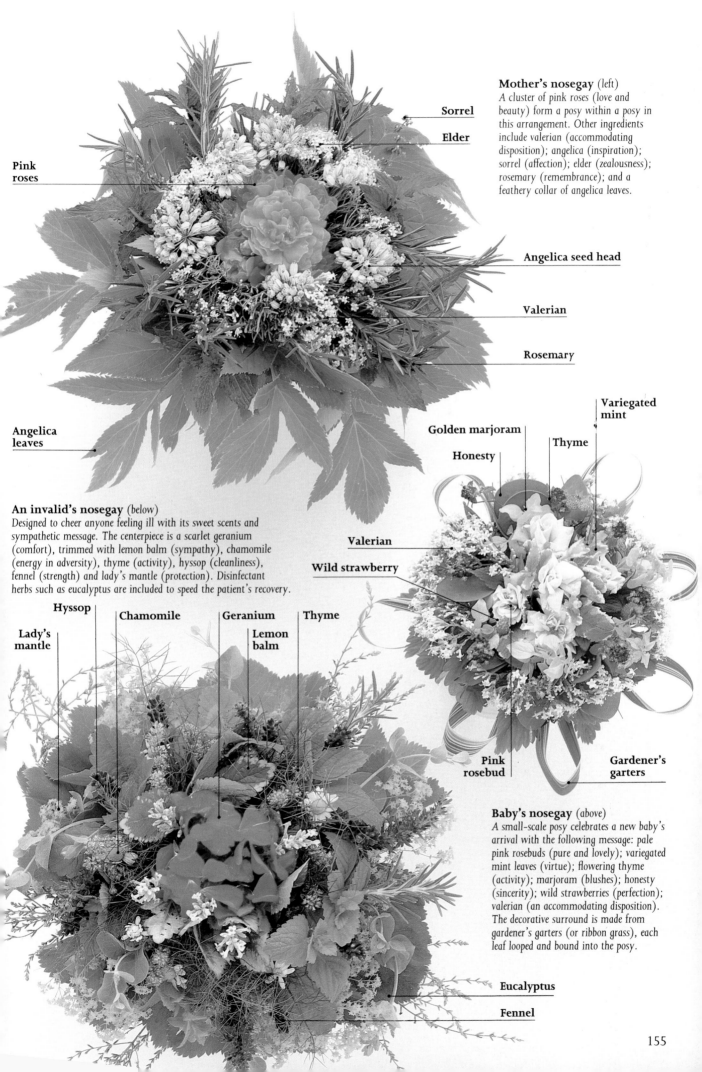

Mother's nosegay (left)
A cluster of pink roses (love and beauty) form a posy within a posy in this arrangement. Other ingredients include valerian (accommodating disposition); angelica (inspiration); sorrel (affection); elder (zealousness); rosemary (remembrance); and a feathery collar of angelica leaves.

Sorrel

Elder

Pink roses

Angelica seed head

Valerian

Rosemary

Angelica leaves

An invalid's nosegay (below)
Designed to cheer anyone feeling ill with its sweet scents and sympathetic message. The centerpiece is a scarlet geranium (comfort), trimmed with lemon balm (sympathy), chamomile (energy in adversity), thyme (activity), hyssop (cleanliness), fennel (strength) and lady's mantle (protection). Disinfectant herbs such as eucalyptus are included to speed the patient's recovery.

Variegated mint

Golden marjoram

Honesty

Thyme

Valerian

Wild strawberry

Hyssop

Chamomile

Geranium

Thyme

Lady's mantle

Lemon balm

Pink rosebud

Gardener's garters

Baby's nosegay (above)
A small-scale posy celebrates a new baby's arrival with the following message: pale pink rosebuds (pure and lovely); variegated mint leaves (virtue); flowering thyme (activity); marjoram (blushes); honesty (sincerity); wild strawberries (perfection); valerian (an accommodating disposition). The decorative surround is made from gardener's garters (or ribbon grass), each leaf looped and bound into the posy.

Eucalyptus

Fennel

155

Wreaths and hangings

One of the most traditional and attractive ways of displaying herbs is in a wreath. Hanging from a wall or door, a wreath adds color and fragrance to any interior. It is also potentially long-lasting and lends itself to an infinite variety of styles.

For the base, which you can make yourself or buy from a florist, use plain or moss-covered wire, plaited raffia or twisted vines. On top of this, wire on bunches of selected herbs. Pick from bay, thyme, sage, lavender, rosemary, savory and artemisias for scent and shape. Fresh material is easier to handle than dry, and you can always make up a wreath and then leave it to dry in a dark, well-ventilated place for later use. For interest, add colorful drying flowers such as yarrow, santolina, roses, bergamot or larkspur; or make a theme wreath like the hanging shown below, using kitchen herbs such as sage, marjoram, parsley, mint and rosemary, adding bunches of spices for extra effect. Expand your repertoire by making seasonal wreaths for spring, summer, autumn or winter, and festive wreaths for weddings, anniversaries and Christmas. The possibilities are endless and always rewarding.

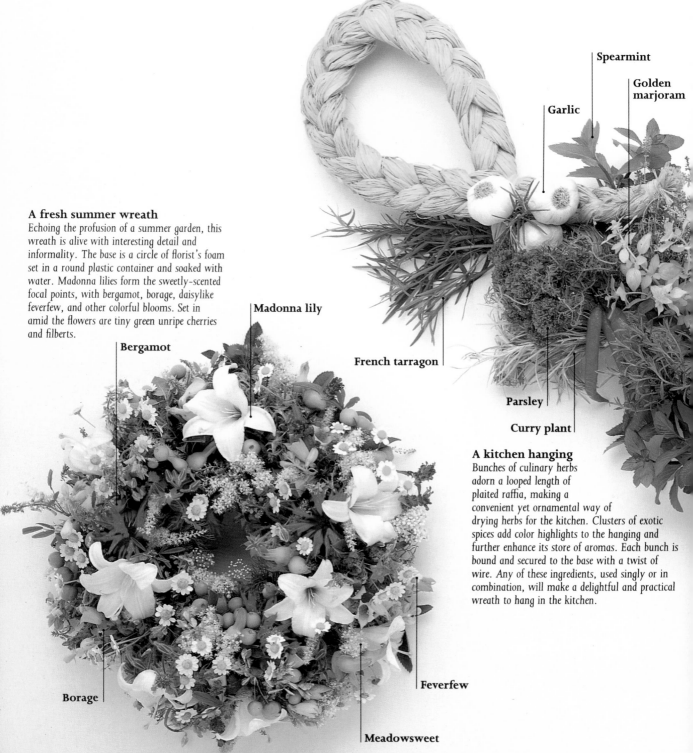

Spearmint

Golden marjoram

Garlic

A fresh summer wreath
Echoing the profusion of a summer garden, this wreath is alive with interesting detail and informality. The base is a circle of florist's foam set in a round plastic container and soaked with water. Madonna lilies form the sweetly-scented focal points, with bergamot, borage, daisylike feverfew, and other colorful blooms. Set in amid the flowers are tiny green unripe cherries and filberts.

Madonna lily

Bergamot

French tarragon

Parsley

Curry plant

A kitchen hanging
Bunches of culinary herbs adorn a looped length of plaited raffia, making a convenient yet ornamental way of drying herbs for the kitchen. Clusters of exotic spices add color highlights to the hanging and further enhance its store of aromas. Each bunch is bound and secured to the base with a twist of wire. Any of these ingredients, used singly or in combination, will make a delightful and practical wreath to hang in the kitchen.

Feverfew

Borage

Meadowsweet

MAKING A FESTIVE WREATH

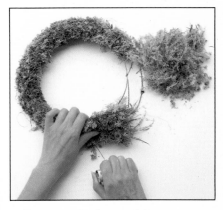

1 Cover a wire base with sphagnum moss, pressing a handful at a time into the frame. Bind on with reel wire, wrapping it over and pulling from underneath. When the base is covered, cut the wire and secure the end by bending it back into the moss.

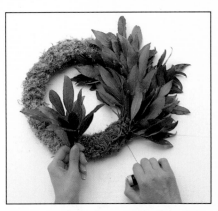

2 Cut small branches of bay to the same length. Place them in overlapping groups all facing the same way and bind in place with wire until the base is covered.

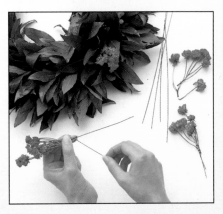

3 Wire together small bunches of rosebuds (or berries): place a medium stub wire against the stems and bend it around about halfway up. Twist over the stems, leaving a length to pin the bunch in place.

Vanilla pods

Rosebuds

Bay

A festive wreath
Simple to make, as the steps at right show, this stunning wreath has a lush covering of traditional bay, with tiny red rosebuds giving rich points of contrasting color, accentuated by the decorative red satin ribbon.

Variegated mint

Hyssop flowers

Bay leaves

Rosemary

age

Chili pepper

Cinnamon

Thyme

Juniper

Garlands

Hanging bunches of dried herbs look attractive in their own right: combined into small posies and wired together to form a thick "rope" of foliage, seed heads and flowers, they can look truly spectacular. A garland of herbs such as the one below will transform any room into a setting suitable for a special event. Using dried herbs gives such a garland long-lasting appeal. Drape it over a fireplace or a mirror, around a picture or window frame, over a door, along shelves or beams.

Choose your ingredients to reflect the occasion, whether it be a wedding, a christening, a seasonal festival or some other celebration. Select items that add color, delicacy, texture and fragrance. Ensure that you have enough materials and assemble them all with the required tools (fine reel wire, scissors, length of string) before you start. Once you are underway, it is very hard to move or put aside the extending length of overlapping posies until the decoration is completed. Experiment with your assembled ingredients, trying out different combinations of color, texture and shapes and seeing how a change in order or composition can alter the overall effect. Once you have settled on your scheme, lay out the herbs in groups within arm's reach so they are easy to combine and wire in position. Add ribbons, baubles and other ornaments as finishing touches.

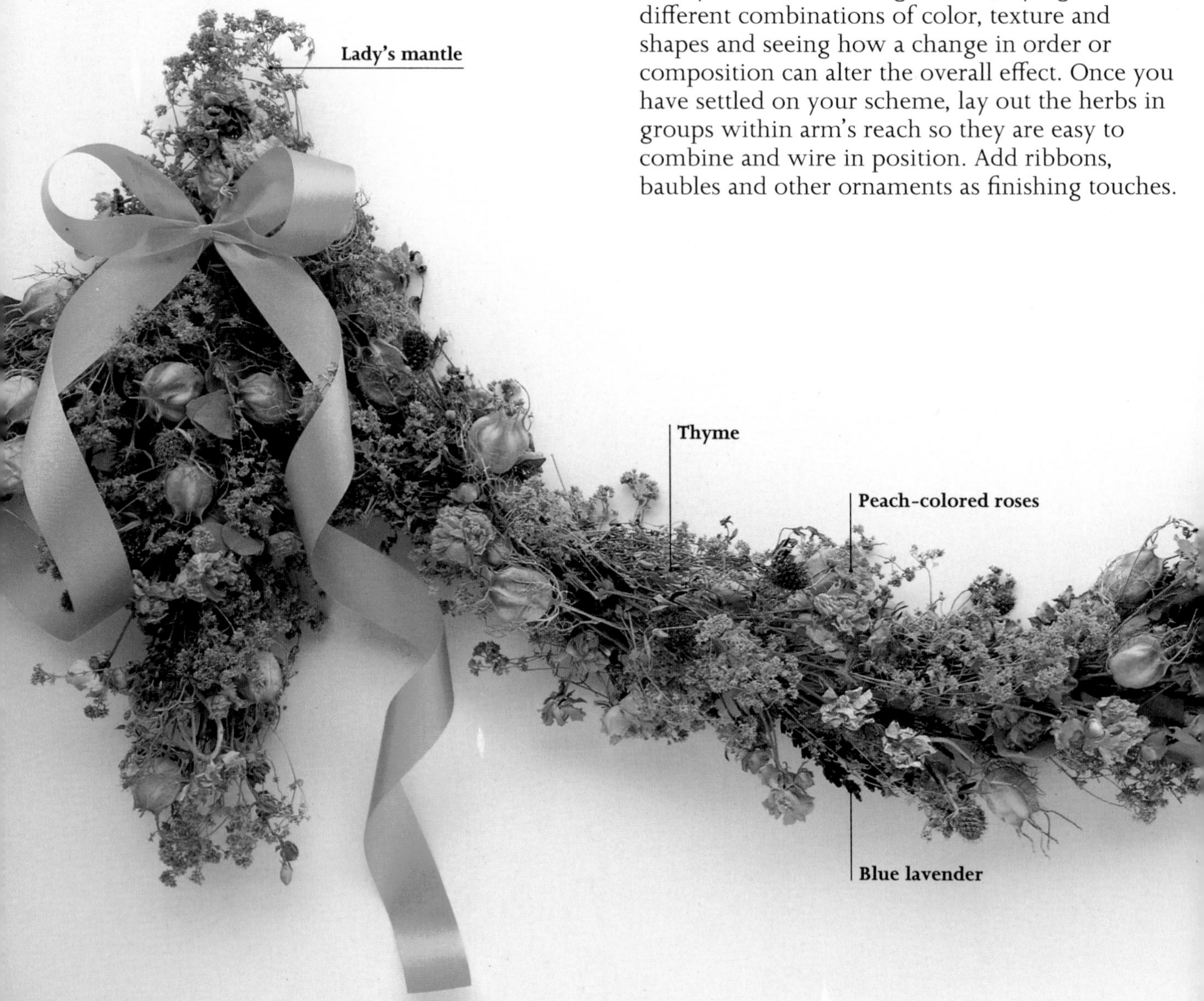

Lady's mantle

Thyme

Peach-colored roses

Blue lavender

Sweet summer garland
Delicately colored and highly fragrant, this striking garland of dried summer herbs makes a spectacular decoration. It is scented with thyme, lavender and eucalyptus. The curled satin ribbons have a softening effect and unite the whole arrangement with their color.

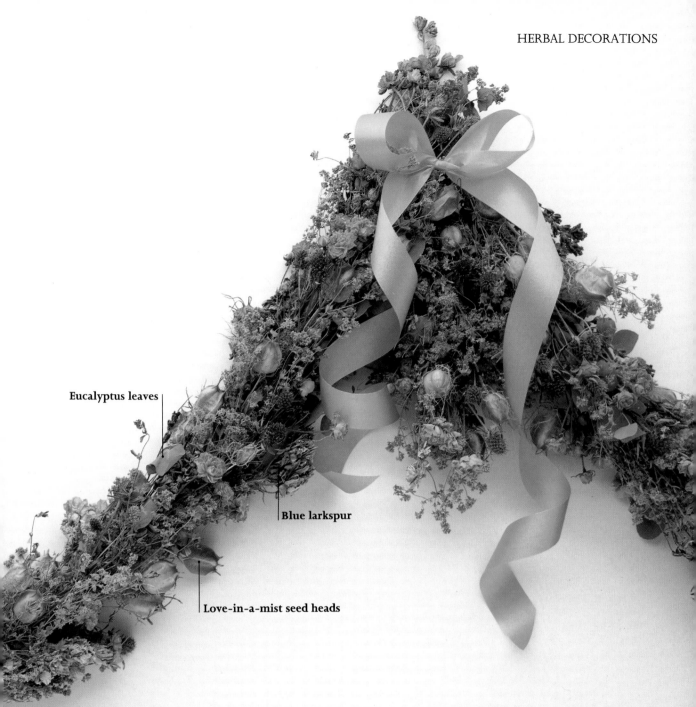

Eucalyptus leaves

Blue larkspur

Love-in-a-mist seed heads

MAKING A GARLAND

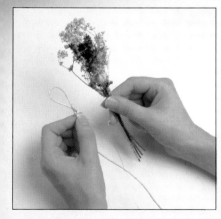
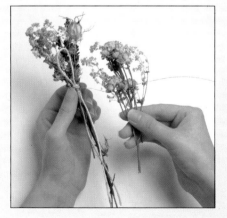
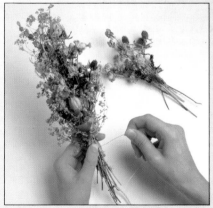

1 Cut string to the required length and knot a loop at one end. Take a length of fine wire and attach one end to the string by wrapping it around a few times. Make up a small bunch from your ingredients and lay it on the string to hide the loop. Bind in place with wire.

2 Turn your hand so the first bunch lies under the string and position a second bunch on top, so it overlaps the stems of the first bunch and covers the string loop. Bind in place by wrapping over the wire, always pulling it tight from underneath after each turn.

3 Keep turning your hand and securing bunches one overlapping the other, always covering the string and the stems of the bunch above. Follow this procedure until you reach the end of the string. Make a hanging loop with the end piece of wire. Finish with ribbons.

Herbal baskets

Baskets make naturally complementary and highly attractive containers for dried herbal displays, particularly as they are constructed from plant materials. The texture of woven stems or branches echoes that of many dried herbs, while the natural colors of baskets show off the range of hues found in dried herbs. Baskets made from the aromatic stems of lavender and thyme are also available, as shown below. Alternatively, attach aromatic stems to a basket's rim or handle to give an arrangement extra appeal.

To arrange dried herbs in a basket, you need to prepare a base which will sit in the container area and hold stems in place, as shown opposite. Select herbs for their colors, shapes and textures so they make striking contrasts or subtle blends. Try to incorporate any handles in your design to add height or extra shape to the arrangement.

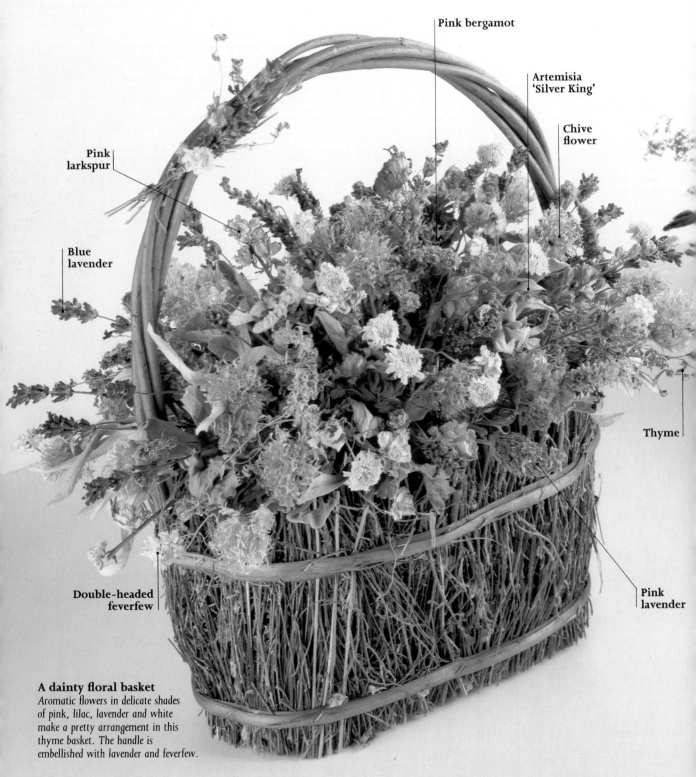

Pink bergamot

Artemisia 'Silver King'

Chive flower

Pink larkspur

Blue lavender

Thyme

Double-headed feverfew

Pink lavender

A dainty floral basket
Aromatic flowers in delicate shades of pink, lilac, lavender and white make a pretty arrangement in this thyme basket. The handle is embellished with lavender and feverfew.

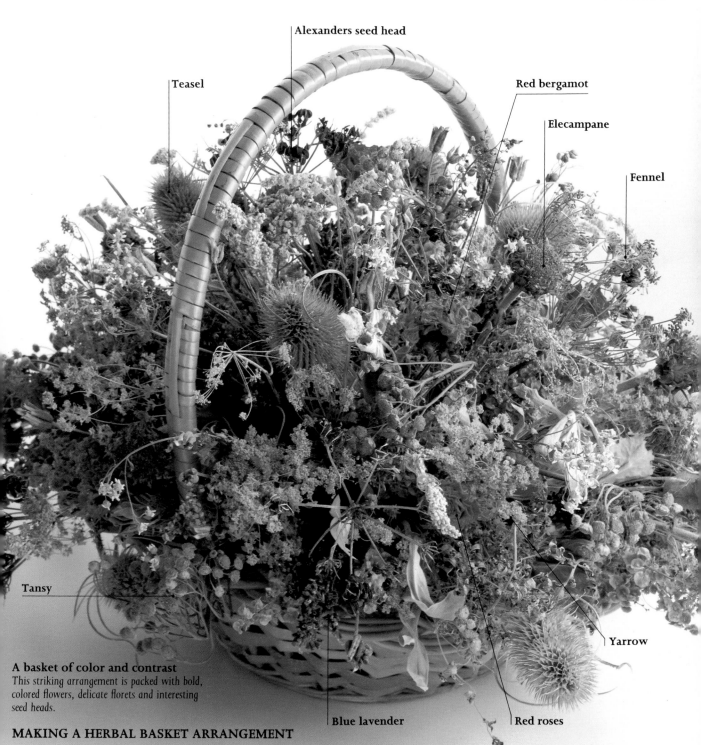

Alexanders seed head

Teasel

Red bergamot

Elecampane

Fennel

Tansy

Yarrow

A basket of color and contrast
*This striking arrangement is packed with bold,
colored flowers, delicate florets and interesting
seed heads.*

Blue lavender

Red roses

MAKING A HERBAL BASKET ARRANGEMENT

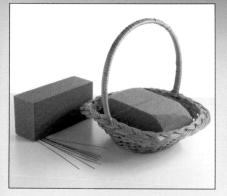

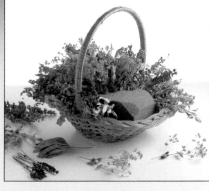

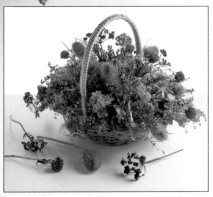

1 Press a block of florist's foam into
the basket. Secure in place with
wire and cut to shape with a sharp
knife so that its surface is slightly
higher than the basket's rim.

2 Form a base of color by lightly
covering the foam with small
flowers and leaves such as artemisia,
thyme, lavender and melilot. Leave
space for the feature plants.

3 Add height, texture and solidity
to the arrangement with larger seed
heads and flowers such as teasel,
alexanders, elecampane, fennel
and bergamot.

Table decorations

Fresh herbal arrangements are the perfect way to decorate a dinner table. Their fragrance awakens the senses, while their flowers and leaves provide color and interest as well as instant garnishing material. For a simple supper party, a spray of parsley, mint, marjoram or thyme by each place setting looks attractive and can be nibbled to freshen the palate betwen courses, to sharpen the appetite or to aid digestion.

The table below is lavishly decorated for a special dinner party. Fresh garnishing herbs are set in pre-soaked, cone-shaped florist's foam. Selected for their colors and flavors, they include mints, parsley, basils, fennel, purple sage, curry plant, rosemary and lemon verbena, which also makes an effective finger freshener after a seafood or fish dish. A fragrant garland made from wired posies of lavender and thymes links the herbal cones and encloses the sumptuous candelabra centerpiece. The effect is stunning, both visually and aromatically.

A herbal dinner table
An arrangement of fresh flavoring herbs sits within reach of each place setting. These are interlinked by a delicate garland of lavender and scented thymes that release their fragrance when touched or brushed against. The central candelabra is covered in dried golden yarrow and contains a colorful central spray of sweetly scented garden flowers.

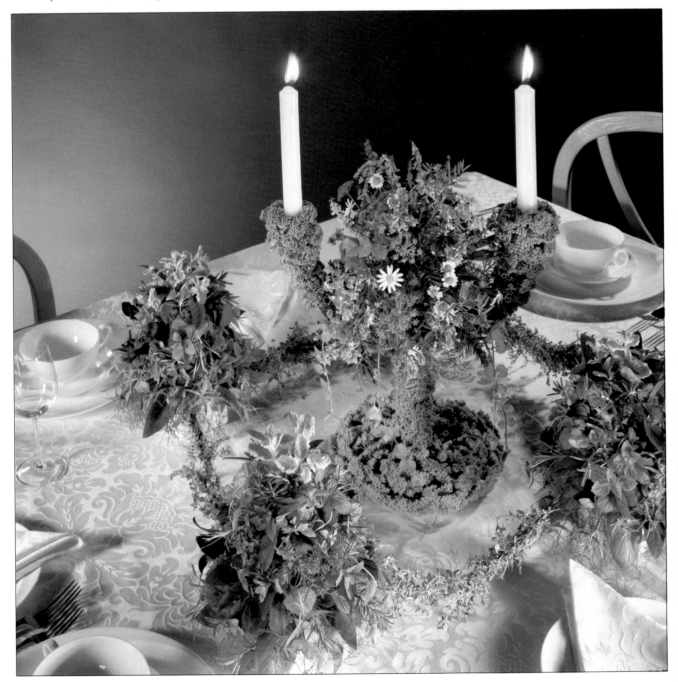

HERBS IN THE KITCHEN

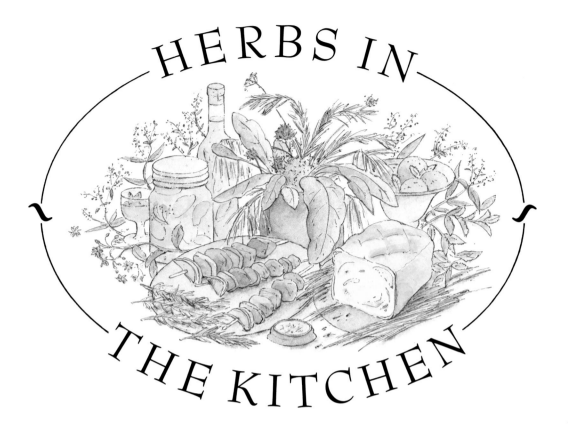

Herbs have been described as the soul of cookery and the praise of cooks. Used judiciously, they can transform a routine meal into a sensuous experience of tangy, spicy, refreshing flavors and crunchy textures. The aromatic leaves of rosemary and thyme delicately permeate cooked dishes; the seeds of dill, fennel and anise add piquancy to fish, salads and vegetables, while the earthy-flavored leaves of lovage and smallage lend body to soups and casseroles.

Many herbs make foods more palatable by easing digestion. Angelica, anise, balm, basil, caraway, coriander, dill, fennel, mint, rosemary and sage have long been eaten for their carminative qualities. The Romans traditionally finished their banquets with small aniseed cakes. Indians frequently serve a plate of roasted seeds at the end of a rich meal. The famous Greek mathematician Pythagoras used to nibble a nutritious mixture of herbs and seeds consisting of poppy and sesame seeds, mallow leaves, sea-onion skin, barley and peas, all mixed to a paste in honey.

Herbs were used to preserve foods: in medieval times meat was wrapped in tansy both to deter flies and to give the flesh a spicy flavor; minty pennyroyal was added to kegs of fresh water on long sea voyages to help keep it sweet. However, the range of edible herbs and the number of ways of using them was much greater in the past than today. A salad for King Henry VIII included over 50 leaves, buds, flowers and roots. Thomas Tusser's sixteenth-century garden plan for farmers' wives recommended the planting of no less than 70 salad and pot herbs. After the Industrial Revolution and the move from the countryside into the towns, herbs became less important in the kitchen. Now, with a fresh interest in the culinary arts, herbs are enjoying a revival.

Most fruit and vegetable growers today tailor their crops to meet the demands of packaging and supermarket shelf life rather than taste, so flavoring herbs and spices must come to the rescue. They enliven any dish, snack or drink. They can also supply extra nutrition to everyday meals, as many herbs, such as parsley, watercress and comfrey, contain a small but rich balance of vitamins, minerals and trace elements.

Using and storing herbs

The emphasis in the following recipes is on fresh herbs. As a guide, 1 teaspoon of a dried herb is equivalent to 1 tablespoon fresh. Always store fresh-cut herbs in a plastic bag in the bottom of the refrigerator. Don't set them in a jar of water in the sun or they will wilt before your eyes. Store dried herbs in dark airtight jars. Try preserving the flavor of herbs in oils and vinegars for use in dressings (see p. 188). Add them to butters, and use them to flavor savory jellies.

The following pages list a selection of useful culinary herbs with guidelines on their attributes and complementary foods.

Popular culinary herbs

ANGELICA
A strong, clean flavor that pierces through heavy syrup makes angelica an excellent candidate for crystallization. Dilute angelica syrup for summer drinks and use to give character to fruit salads and ice cream. Cook leaves with acidic fruits to reduce tartness and sugar consumption.
Angelica and mint sandwich p. 182
Crystallized angelica p. 190
Angelica, mint and sweet cicely yogurt drink p. 191

BASIL
Indispensable for many Mediterranean dishes, the fresh leaf has a sweet, clovelike spiciness and is superb on fresh tomatoes with a little salad oil, and in hot tomato dishes. Basil adds interest to rice salads and combines well with zucchini, beans and mushrooms. It has a powerful enough flavor to stand up to garlic, and together they make the classic pesto sauce. Basil's pungency increases with cooking. The fresh leaves keep their flavor if preserved in oil or vinegar (see p. 188).
Split pea and basil soup p. 166
Crêpes with basil stuffing p. 176

BAY
Bay is one herb that is better dried than fresh. Use it with parsley and thyme to make a bouquet garni. Add a leaf or two to marinades, stock, pâtés, stuffings and curries. When poaching fish, add a bay leaf to the water. A leaf in a storage jar of rice will impart its flavor to the rice. Add at the start of cooking and remove before serving.
Game soup with bay p. 166
Escalope of veal with bay p. 170
Marinated venison fillet p. 170

CHERVIL
Chervil is one of the classic fines herbes much used in French cuisine. It has a delicate flavor and is suitable wherever parsley is used. Chop the fresh leaf into omelettes, salads, dressings and add to chicken before roasting. Add at the end of cooking so its flavor is not lost. Preserve in vinegar and oil (see p. 188).
Carrot and chervil soup p. 166
Chervil-stuffed trout p. 168
Artichokes with ravigote sauce p. 178
Violet herb salad p. 180

CHIVES
Freshly chopped chives lift many foods above the mundane. Sprinkle them on soups, salads, chicken, potatoes, cooked vegetables and egg dishes. Blend chopped chives with butter to garnish broiled meats and fish. Use them in place of raw onion in hamburgers for a milder flavor. Blend with butter (see p. 190), mix in cream cheese, yogurt sauces and baked potatoes. Add at the end of cooking. Chives freeze well but are poor dried.
Sea bass with ginger and chives p. 167
Potato salad with dill and chives p. 182
Cheese balls p. 182
Cheese bread with chives p. 186

CORIANDER
The leaves and ripe seeds have two distinct flavors. The seeds are warmly aromatic and indispensable in tomato chutney and curries. They provide an excellent flavoring for vegetables, especially stir-fried, and in soups, sauces and cookies. The leaves have an earthy pungency, delicious in salads, vegetables and poultry dishes.
Lentil and coriander soup p. 166
Persian chicken with herbs p. 170
Mediterranean vegetables p. 177
Hot salad p. 180

DILL
Frequently described as similar in flavor to caraway, aniseed and fennel, dill is like none of these. It has a totally unique, spicy green taste. Add whole seeds to potato salad, pickles, bean soups, salmon dishes, and apple pies. Ground, they can flavor herb butter, mayonnaise and mustard. The leaves go well with fish, cream cheese and cucumber.
Gravlax p. 168
Potato salad with dill and chives p. 182
Pickled cucumbers p. 188

FENNEL
With its pronounced aniseed flavor, fennel is an excellent digestive and reputed to be a dieting aid. Chop the stems when tender into salads. Stuff the leaves into oily fish such as mackerel, and sprinkle finely chopped on salads and cooked vegetables. Add the seeds to sauces, breads, savory crackers and the water for poaching fish. The swollen bulb of Florence fennel can be eaten raw in salads or cooked.
Fennel soup p. 166
Fennel flan p. 176
Fennel with Roquefort sauce p. 178
Fennel salad with orange p. 180

GARLIC
A strong flavoring for all savory dishes, hot and cold. Rub a clove around a salad bowl to subtly flavor salads; add one or two cloves to dressings and marinades, or make garlic vinegar and oil (see p. 188). Mash with butter and bake in a French loaf or on grilled meat or fish. Insert sliced cloves into cuts of meat before roasting. It can even be baked as a vegetable. The leaves have a lighter flavor.
Pork chops marinated with juniper and garlic p. 173
Mediterranean vegetables p. 177
Spicy eggplant p. 178
Aioli (garlic mayonnaise) p. 182

JUNIPER
The crushed berries of the juniper tree have an aromatic resinous flavor often featured in pâtés, marinades and stuffings for pork, venison and other game. They are a popular flavoring for sauerkraut, sauces, ham and cabbage.
Lamb's kidneys sautéed with juniper p. 173
Pork chops marinated with juniper and garlic p. 173
Cabbage and juniper p. 177
Mulled pears with juniper p. 183

LEMON BALM
Use the refreshing, lemon-flavored leaves fresh in salads; to make a pleasant herbal tea or to give a lemon flavor to Indian tea. Add generously to a white sauce for fish and spread over chicken before roasting. Finely chopped leaves add a lemony sweetness to sauerkraut, mayonnaise, sauces, and stuffings as well as fruit salads and custards. Freeze in ice cubes to add to drinks (see p. 192).
Spicy lemon balm kebabs p. 172
Lemon balm cheesecake p. 185
Sweet herb sorbet p. 185

LOVAGE
The leaves and stems have a meaty flavor, but use sparingly until familiar with their potency. Fresh leaves make an interesting base on which to serve strong-flavoured pâté. Young leaves and blanched stems are good steamed as a vegetable and served with a white sauce. A brew of the leaves is like a yeast-extract broth.
Lovage soup p. 166
Stuffed lovage and grape leaves p. 172
Lovage and lentil roulade p. 174
Lovage seed bread p. 185

MINTS

With their clean, sharp flavors, the mints are an aid to the digestion and can be used individually or blended. Excellent in mint sauce, syrups, vinegar and in teas. Add to new potatoes, to a garlic and cream cheese dip and to a yogurt dressing or drink. Also mix with chocolate cakes, rich desserts and bake with raisins or currants in pastry. Crystallize the leaf for a sweet decoration.

Persian chicken with herbs p. 170
Melon, tomato and mint salad p. 180
Angelica and mint sandwich p. 182
Mint and chocolate ice cream p. 183
Sweet herb sorbet p. 185
Raspberry and mint yogurt drink p. 191
Mint julep p. 192

OREGANO and MARJORAM

Marjoram has a distinctive savory flavor, while oregano is slightly stronger. Both dry well. Marjoram is suitable for thick vegetable soups, pasta, fish, game, beef, chicken, sausages and meat loaf. Tomatoes, zucchini, potatoes and peppers are enhanced by its flavor. It is also used in omelettes and cheese dishes. Oregano is good with pizzas; it can be used like marjoram, but more sparingly.

Oregano cheese pie p. 174
Oregano tomatoes p. 178

PARSLEY

The mild flavor and bright green leaves of parsley make it the most useful and popular kitchen herb. Add it to a bouquet garni with bay and thyme. When cooked, it serves to enhance the flavor of other foods and herbs. To increase its potency, use generous amounts and include the stems, which are more strongly flavored. Feature it in bland dishes and add toward the end of cooking. Use in salads, sandwiches, soups, sauces, mayonnaise and egg dishes. Fry whole sprigs briefly to serve with fish.

Sardines in wine with parsley p. 167
Herby hamburgers p. 173
Green herb omelette p. 174
Mediterranean vegetables p. 177
Green mayonnaise p. 182
Parsley and chive butter p. 190

ROSEMARY

This aromatic resinous leaf aids the digestion of fats, and traditionally is sprinkled on roast lamb and pork or added to chops, pigeon, sausage meats, pâtés and stuffings. Crumble dried leaves and chop fresh, or remove them before serving as they can be tough. Put a whole sprig in the oven to flavor baking bread. Put a sprig in oil or vinegar. Add leaves, presoaked in hot water, to oranges soaked in wine.

Rosemary kebabs p. 172
Sweet herb sorbet p. 185
Rosemary cheese fingers p. 185
Sweet rosemary slices p. 186

SAFFRON

Saffron is our most expensive seasoning, due to the labor required for harvesting the individual stamens. Fortunately, only a pinch is needed to color and flavor a large dish. Good saffron should be less than a year old and a brilliant orange color. It has a strong aroma and a pungent, warmly bitter flavor. When using threads, crush the required number and infuse in hot milk or liquid from the recipe. If using powder (which is easily adulterated), infuse in liquid or add it with the flour for cakes.

Paella p. 167
Mussels in saffron p. 168
Saffron fruit bread p. 186

SAGE

Sage is a strongly flavored, pungent herb which complements strongly flavored foods and aids the digestion of fats. It makes a good flavoring for cheese and cream cheese dips. Use leaves in onion soup, with stewed tomatoes, omelettes, herb scones and bread. Try them in a sage jelly, butter or vinegar (see pp. 188, 190). If dried, sage must be of top quality; otherwise it acquires an unpleasant musty flavor.

Hazelnut and sage pâté p. 174
Leek and sage croustade p. 176
Herb leaf fritters p. 177
Sage oat cakes p. 185

SUMMER and WINTER SAVORY

The two savories have a similar flavor to thyme, with winter savory being marginally milder. Cook with fresh or dried beans and lentils or in a white sauce for bean dishes. Mix with parsley and chives for roasting duck. Sprinkle finely chopped fresh leaves on soups and sauces. Use to flavor vinegar (see p. 188).

Barbecued anglerfish with savory p. 167

SCENTED GERANIUMS (PELARGONIUMS)

The many scented geranium leaves can flavor teas and drinks (see p. 191), cakes, custards, fruit and sorbets. Experiment with them in savory dishes too.

Sweet rice with rose geranium p. 183
Sweet herb sorbet p. 185
Scented geranium leaf sponge p. 186

SORREL

A sharp-flavored leaf with the tangy zest of lemon, sorrel adds piquancy to bland dishes and sauces. Sorrel soup is a classic, and sorrel is often cooked and served like spinach.

Pork and sorrel terrine p. 172
Sorrel and parsnip mousses p. 178

SWEET CICELY

This is a mild-flavored leaf with a hint of aniseed. Add to tart fruit when stewing or making jam to reduce acidity and cut sugar requirements. Use fresh chopped leaves in salads, avocado dressing and cabbage water, and to garnish puddings, cakes, cold drinks and punches. Add green, unripe seeds to fruit salads. Boil the root, slice and serve cold with salad oil or add chopped root to stir-fried dishes.

Sweet cicely baked mackerel p. 167

TARRAGON

An aristocratic herb with a savory flavor and hidden tang; one of the *fines herbes* with chervil and parsley. It is indispensable for Béarnaise and hollandaise sauces, soups, fish dishes and any delicate vegetables. It is particularly good stuffed in a roasting chicken and added to egg dishes.

Tarragon baked chicken p. 172
Tarragon stuffed mushrooms p. 177
Tarragon vinegar p. 188

THYME

Common thyme is used in a bouquet garni with parsley and bay and has a long history of culinary use. It stimulates the appetite and aids digestion of fatty food; useful with meat, shellfish, poultry and game. It is very pungent when fresh, so use with discretion. Try the lemon thymes in fish and poultry dishes.

Sole en croûte with thyme p. 168
Pheasant pot roast with thyme p. 170
Rabbit with mustard and thyme p. 170

Soups

Game soup with bay

4 cups beef stock	1 medium onion,
1 pheasant, partridge,	quartered
pigeon or other game	4 bay leaves
bird carcass	juice of 1 lemon
1 rabbit or hare	salt and black pepper
forequarters	2 fl oz port
1 medium carrot, quartered	

Serves 4–6

1 Place the stock, carcass, forequarters, carrot, onion and bay leaves in a saucepan. Bring to the boil, cover and simmer for about 1 hour until the meat is tender.

2 Strain through a sieve, reserving the carrot, onion and any pieces of meat.

3 Purée the meat, carrot, onion and stock in a blender. Return to a clean pan with the lemon juice, seasoning and port. Reheat and serve with croûtons of bread.

Carrot and chervil soup

2 oz butter	4 cups chicken stock
2½ cups carrots, chopped	salt and black pepper
⅓ cup all-purpose flour	½ cup chopped chervil

GARNISH
cream or plain yogurt   sprigs of chervil

Serves 4–6

1 Melt the butter in a saucepan and gently sauté the carrots for 5 minutes. Stir in the flour, then the stock and seasoning. Bring the soup to the boil, cover and simmer gently for 30 minutes.

2 Allow to cool slightly, then purée the soup in a blender. Return to the pan with the chopped chervil and slowly bring back to the boil. Serve hot or chilled with a swirl of cream or yogurt and sprigs of chervil.

Fennel soup

1 oz butter	2 cups milk
4 bulbs of Florence fennel,	1 bay leaf
sliced	salt and black pepper
1 large onion, chopped	2 egg yolks
4 cups vegetable stock	½ cup light cream

GARNISH
fennel leaves

Serves 8

1 Melt the butter in a large saucepan. Sauté the fennel and the onion to soften; do not brown.

2 Add the stock, milk, bay leaf and seasoning. Bring to the boil, cover and simmer for 30 minutes.

3 Remove the bay leaf, then strain the soup by passing it through a metal sieve.

4 Mix the egg yolks and cream together in a bowl. Whisk in about half a cup of the strained soup. Then add this mixture to the rest of the soup and reheat, taking care not to let it boil, or it will curdle. Garnish with chopped fennel leaves.

Split pea and basil soup

1 tbsp vegetable oil	1 tbsp or cube vegetable stock
1 large onion, chopped	concentrate
1 clove garlic, crushed	1 large potato, diced
8 oz split peas,	4 quarts water
soaked overnight	3 tbsp basil leaves
1 tsp tomato paste	salt and black pepper

GARNISH
½ cup light cream   8 basil leaves

Serves 8

1 Heat the oil in a large saucepan and sauté the onion and garlic for 5 minutes. Add the drained split peas, tomato paste, stock concentrate, potato and water.

2 Bring to the boil, add the basil leaves and seasoning, cover and simmer for 40 minutes, until the peas soften.

3 Allow to cool slightly, then purée the soup in a blender. Return to the pan to reheat for serving. Garnish with a swirl of cream and a basil leaf.

Lentil and coriander soup

1 tbsp vegetable oil	salt and black pepper
1 large onion, chopped	1 tbsp ground
4 oz split red lentils	coriander seeds
2 cups tomato juice	1 tbsp chopped fresh
1 cup water	coriander

Serves 4

1 Heat the oil in a saucepan and sauté the onion for 5 minutes. Add the lentils and sauté for a few minutes.

2 Stir in the tomato juice, water, seasoning and ground coriander. Bring to the boil, cover and simmer for 20 minutes. Serve very hot, sprinkled with fresh coriander.

Lovage soup

For a sharp, lemony soup, try using sorrel instead.

1 oz butter	1 oz all-purpose flour
2 medium onions, finely	2 cups chicken or
chopped	vegetable stock
4 tbsp finely chopped	1 cup milk
lovage leaves	salt and black pepper

Serves 4

1 Melt the butter in a saucepan and gently sauté the onions for 5 minutes until soft. Add the lovage, stir in the flour and cook for 1 minute, stirring constantly.

2 Gradually stir in the stock, cover and simmer gently for 15 minutes. Add the milk and seasoning. Reheat slowly; do not boil the soup or it will curdle.

HERBS FOR SOUPS

General: chervil, garlic, juniper berries, lemon balm, lovage leaf and seed, marjorams, mint, onion (green and bulb), parsley leaf, stem and root, rosemary, savories, smallage, sorrel, tarragon, thyme
Minestrone: basil, rosemary, thyme
Pea: basil, borage, dill, marjoram, mint, parsley, rosemary, savory, thyme
Potato: bay, caraway, parsley
Tomato: basil, dill, marjoram, oregano, tarragon, thyme

Fish

Barbecued anglerfish with savory

1½ lb anglerfish
grated rind and juice of 1 lemon
1 cup olive oil
salt and black pepper
a good handful of winter savory (or rosemary)

Serves 4

1 Remove any bones from the anglerfish and cut the flesh into ½ inch cubes. Lay the cubes in a deep dish.

2 Mix the lemon rind and juice, olive oil and seasoning together in a bowl. Break the winter savory into small sprigs and add to the mixture.

3 Pour this marinade over the fish and leave for 6 hours or overnight in the refrigerator.

4 Thread the anglerfish on to 4 skewers. Cook over a barbecue (or in the broiler) for 5–10 minutes, turning often and using the marinade for basting. Serve on a bed of boiled rice and accompany with a green salad.

Sardines in wine with parsley

3 tbsp olive oil
16 sardines, cleaned
2 cloves garlic, crushed
4 tbsp chopped parsley
1 tbsp lemon juice
½ cup white wine

Serves 4

1 Heat the oil in a deep frying pan and add the sardines, garlic, parsley, lemon juice and wine.

2 Simmer for 5–6 minutes or until cooked. Serve hot with French bread or cold as an appetizer.

Sweet cicely baked mackerel

Fennel leaves also work well in this recipe.

2 oz butter
8 oz onion, thinly sliced
1 clove garlic, crushed
2 oz fresh ginger, grated
1 cup finely chopped sweet cicely
4 mackerel, about 8 oz each, or 2 larger fish, cleaned

Serves 4

1 Preheat the oven to 350°F.

2 Melt the butter in a pan and gently sauté the onion for about 5 minutes. Add the garlic, ginger and sweet cicely and sauté until soft but still moist.

3 Cut deep slits diagonally from head to tail on both sides of the mackerel.

4 Divide the onion and sweet cicely mixture between the fish and spoon it into the cavities.

5 Lay the fish in a baking dish. Bake for 15 minutes, or 25 minutes if the fish are larger.

6 If you like, you can crisp the fish by browning for about 2 minutes on each side either in the broiler or over a barbecue.

Sea bass with ginger and chives

2 lb sea bass
salt
1 tbsp soy sauce
1 tsp sesame oil
1 tbsp grated fresh ginger
4 tbsp chopped chives

Serves 6

1 Put the fish into a pan of boiling salted water to cover. Simmer for 5 minutes. Drain and arrange on a serving dish.

2 Mix the soy sauce, oil and ginger together and pour over the fish. Sprinkle with the chopped chives and serve with plain boiled rice or new potatoes.

Paella

Any kind of shellfish can be used in this dish, although squid and mussels are traditional.

4 tbsp olive oil
4 chicken drumsticks or other small portions, about 3 oz each
½ cup red pepper, cut into strips
2 large tomatoes, skinned and chopped
1½ cups Valencia or short grain rice
4 baby squid, ink sacs and eyes removed
8 oz unshelled shrimp or 8 jumbo shrimp or langoustines
1 lb mussels, scrubbed and cleaned
¼ tsp saffron, infused in 2 tbsp hot water
4 cups water

Serves 4

1 Heat the oil in a large paella dish or heavy frying pan and gently fry the chicken until golden brown. Remove the chicken from the pan.

2 Add the pepper and tomatoes to the pan and fry for a few minutes. In stages, add the rice, squid, shrimp, mussels, saffron and finally the water, mixing well all the time. Return the chicken pieces to the pan and bring to the boil.

3 Cover and simmer for 30 minutes or until the water has been absorbed and the rice is fluffy. If the water evaporates before the rice has cooked, add more water. However, if the rice has cooked and there is still water, boil rapidly until the rice is dry. Each grain of rice should be separate, so stir with a fork only when absolutely necessary. Serve from the pan and accompany with a crisp green salad.

HERBS FOR FISH

General: alexanders, basil, bay, caraway, chervil, chives, dill, fennel, lemon balm, lemon thyme, lovage, marjoram, mint, parsley
Baked or grilled: all the above, savory, tarragon, thyme
Oily fish: fennel, dill
Salmon: dill seed, rosemary
Seafood: basil, bay, chervil, chives, dill, fennel seed, marjoram, rosemary, tarragon, thyme
Soups: bay, lovage, sage (though this should be used sparingly), savory, tarragon, thyme

Mussels in saffron

4–5 lb mussels	1 oz butter
1 tbsp olive oil	$\frac{1}{4}$ cup all-purpose flour
1 tbsp rolled oats	$\frac{2}{3}$ cup milk
2 small onions, sliced	$\frac{1}{4}$ tsp saffron, infused
2 tbsp finely	in 1 tbsp hot water
chopped parsley	$\frac{3}{4}$ cup dry breadcrumbs
$\frac{1}{3}$ cup dry white wine	

Serves 4–6

1 Soak the mussels for about 2 hours in a bowl of fresh water with the rolled oats added to plump them up. Carefully scrub all the mussels under running water and remove their beards.

2 Heat the oil in a large saucepan and sauté the onion until soft. Add the parsley, mussels and wine. Cover the saucepan and leave the mussels to steam open (about 5 minutes), stirring occasionally. As the mussels open, remove them from the pan.

3 Preheat the oven to 400 °F.

4 Melt the butter in a saucepan and stir in the flour to make a roux. Add the milk and liquid from the cooked mussels and the saffron infusion. Stir well to make a smooth sauce and remove from the heat.

5 Stir the cooked mussels into the sauce, then pour into a deep, square, ovenproof dish. Sprinkle with breadcrumbs and bake for about 10 minutes. Serve with garlic bread.

Sole en croûte with thyme

4 fillets of sole	$\frac{2}{3}$ cup dry white wine
1 oz butter	8 oz puff pastry
salt and black pepper	1 egg, beaten

STUFFING

1 oz butter	2 cups fresh breadcrumbs
1 medium onion, finely	$\frac{1}{2}$ cup raisins
chopped	1 tbsp chopped thyme
$\frac{2}{3}$ cup mushrooms,	1 egg, beaten
finely chopped	salt and black pepper

Serves 4

1 Preheat the oven to 325 °F.

2 Put the sole fillets in a baking dish, dot with butter, season and pour over the wine. Bake gently for about 15 minutes. Drain, retaining the fish juices.

3 Melt the butter and sauté the onion. Add the finely chopped mushrooms and fry for a few minutes until just soft.

4 Mix the onion and mushrooms with the rest of the stuffing ingredients and set aside.

5 Raise the oven temperature to 375 °F.

6 Divide the puff pastry into four portions. Roll out each one to the size of a small plate. Place one sole fillet with a quarter of the stuffing on each round of pastry. Roll over, moisten the pastry edges with beaten egg and seal.

7 Brush with beaten egg and bake for about 20 minutes, or until golden brown. Delicious served with a thyme-flavored cream sauce.

Gravlax

2 lb fresh salmon	black pepper
$\frac{1}{3}$ cup sugar	$\frac{1}{3}$ cup dill leaves
$\frac{1}{3}$ cup coarse or kosher salt	

SAUCE

2 tbsp French mustard	salt and black pepper
1 tsp clear honey	$\frac{1}{2}$ cup olive oil
1 egg yolk	2 tbsp chopped
2 tbsp white wine	dill leaves
vinegar	

Serves 6

1 Cut the salmon in half lengthways and remove all the bones.

2 Mix together the sugar, salt and black pepper. Rub the mixture over the fish.

3 Place a layer of dill in the bottom of a dish and lay half the salmon, skin side down, on the dill. Cover with more dill and lay the other half of salmon on it skin side up. Coat with the rest of the dill and any of the remaining sugar mixture.

4 Cover the dish with Saran Wrap and a weighted plate. Leave in a cool place for 24 hours.

5 Make the sauce by putting all the ingredients except the oil and dill in a bowl and beating with a whisk. Slowly beat in the oil and then add the chopped dill.

6 Scrape the marinade off the salmon. Slice the flesh away from the skin, across the grain, and serve with the sauce and a garnish of lemon and dill leaves.

Chervil stuffed trout

2 oz butter	juice and rind of 1 lemon
$\frac{1}{2}$ cup onion, finely	1 cup of chopped chervil
chopped	salt and black pepper
2 cups fresh	4 trout, about 8 oz
breadcrumbs	each, or 1 large fish,
1 cup mushrooms,	2–4 lb, gutted
finely chopped	and cleaned

Serves 4

1 Preheat the oven to 350 °F.

2 Melt the butter and gently sauté the onion until golden but not brown.

3 Combine the breadcrumbs, mushrooms, lemon rind and juice, chervil and seasoning in a large bowl. Add the cooked onion and mix together.

4 Divide the stuffing mixture between the trout, spooning it into each stomach cavity. Put a knob of butter on top of each fish and then wrap in a square of lightly greased kitchen foil. Bake for 15 minutes.

5 Remove the fish from the oven, open the foil and broil or barbecue for 5 minutes on each side.

Clockwise from the top: Chervil stuffed trout; Sole en croûte with thyme; Mussels in saffron; Gravlax.

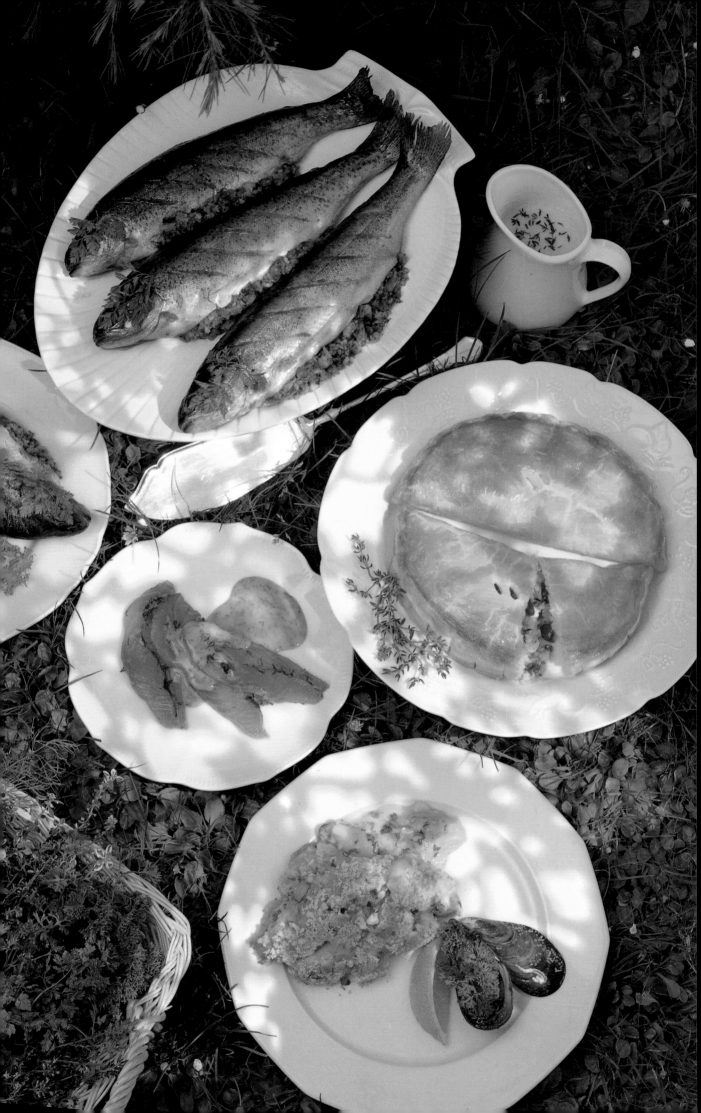

Meat

Pheasant pot roast with thyme

This is a succulent way of cooking any type of game; just adjust the cooking time accordingly.

2 tbsp vegetable oil	4 oz small whole
1 pheasant	mushrooms
2 oz bacon, cut	1 medium onion,
into 2 in pieces	thickly sliced
8 oz carrots, cut	6 large sprigs of thyme
into 2 in chunks	$\frac{1}{4}$ cup all-purpose flour
4 oz celery, cut into	1 cup red wine
2 in lengths	1 cup water
	salt and black pepper

Serves 4

1 Preheat the oven to 350 °F.

2 Heat the oil in a heavy casserole and quickly brown the pheasant on all sides. Remove from the casserole and set aside.

3 Add the bacon to the casserole and fry until lightly browned. Add the carrots, celery, mushrooms, onion and 3 sprigs of thyme and gently sauté until browned.

4 Stir in the flour, then add the red wine and water. Stir well and gently bring to the boil. Add the pheasant and remaining thyme. Season to taste.

5 Cover and pot roast for $1\frac{1}{2}$ hours. When cooked, remove the pheasant from the casserole and place it on a serving dish. Strain the sauce into a sauce boat.

Rabbit with mustard and thyme

The mustard and thyme coating forms a delicious crust. For chicken try savory or chives instead of thyme.

2 tbsp dry mustard	salt and black pepper (optional)
$\frac{1}{4}$ cup all-purpose flour	about 3 fluid oz water
1 tbsp chopped thyme	1 rabbit, cut up

Serves 4

1 Preheat the oven to 350 °F.

2 Mix the dry mustard, flour and thyme together in a bowl. Season if liked. Gradually add the water, mixing the mustard and flour to a smooth paste. Using a pastry brush or the back of a spoon, spread the paste all over the surfaces of the rabbit pieces.

3 Arrange the pieces on a greased baking dish. Bake for $1-1\frac{1}{2}$ hours or until tender. Serve hot or cold.

HERBS FOR GAME AND POULTRY

Venison: bay, juniper, lovage seed, rosemary, sage, savory, sweet marjoram
Rabbit/Hare: basil, bay, lovage seed, marjoram, rosemary, sage
Pigeon: juniper berries, rosemary, thyme
Chicken: chervil, chives, fennel, lemon balm, marjoram, mint, parsley, savory, tarragon, thyme
Duck: bay, rosemary, sage, sweet marjoram, tarragon
Goose: fennel, sage, sweet marjoram,
Turkey: parsley, sage, sweet marjoram, tarragon, thyme

Marinated venison steaks

MARINADE

1 cup wine vinegar	1 branch parsley
1 cup red wine	6 tarragon leaves
3 tbsp olive oil	1 tsp juniper berries
3 bay leaves	1 small onion, chopped
1 branch thyme	
4 venison steaks	1 tbsp flour
1 oz butter	1 fluid oz brandy

Serves 4

1 Boil all the marinade ingredients together for 5 minutes. Allow to cool.

2 Place the steaks in a deep ovenproof dish. Pour the marinade over and leave to steep for 24 hours, turning from time to time.

3 Remove from the marinade and fry in butter for about 10 minutes. Keep warm while you make a sauce.

4 Stir the flour into the butter, then gradually stir in about half of the marinade mixture and the brandy. Pour over the steaks and serve.

Escalope of veal with bay

1 oz butter	4 dried bay leaves
1 small onion, finely chopped	1 cup dry white wine
4 veal escalopes, about	$\frac{1}{2}$ cup light cream
4 oz each	salt and black pepper

Serves 4

1 Melt the butter in a large frying pan and sauté the onion for about 5 minutes until soft.

2 Add the veal escalopes and crush the bay leaves over them. Turn the escalopes over and add the wine to the pan. Cook, uncovered, for 5 minutes. Pour in the cream and stir well. Season to taste. Serve on a bed of rice.

Persian chicken with herbs

4 oz butter	$\frac{1}{4}$ cup chopped mint
2 medium onions, sliced	$\frac{1}{4}$ cup chopped
1 boiling chicken	coriander leaves
2 cups chicken stock	$\frac{1}{3}$ cup walnuts, chopped
salt and black pepper	$\frac{2}{3}$ cup orange juice
1 cup chopped parsley	grated rind of 2 oranges
1 cup chopped chives	2 eggs, beaten (optional)

Serves 4–6

1 Melt 1 oz of the butter in a large pan and sauté the onions until golden.

2 Add the chicken to the pan with the stock and seasoning. Cover and simmer for 1 hour until tender.

3 Melt the remaining butter in a pan and lightly cook the parsley, chives, mint and coriander to flavor the butter. Add to the chicken, then stir in the chopped walnuts, orange juice and rind. Simmer for 30 minutes.

4 If liked, stir in the beaten eggs just before serving. Accompany with noodles or rice.

Clockwise from the top: Spicy lemon balm kebabs (p. 172);
Rosemary kebabs (p. 172); Stuffed lovage and grape leaves (p. 172); Pork
and sorrel terrine (p. 172); Persian chicken with herbs.

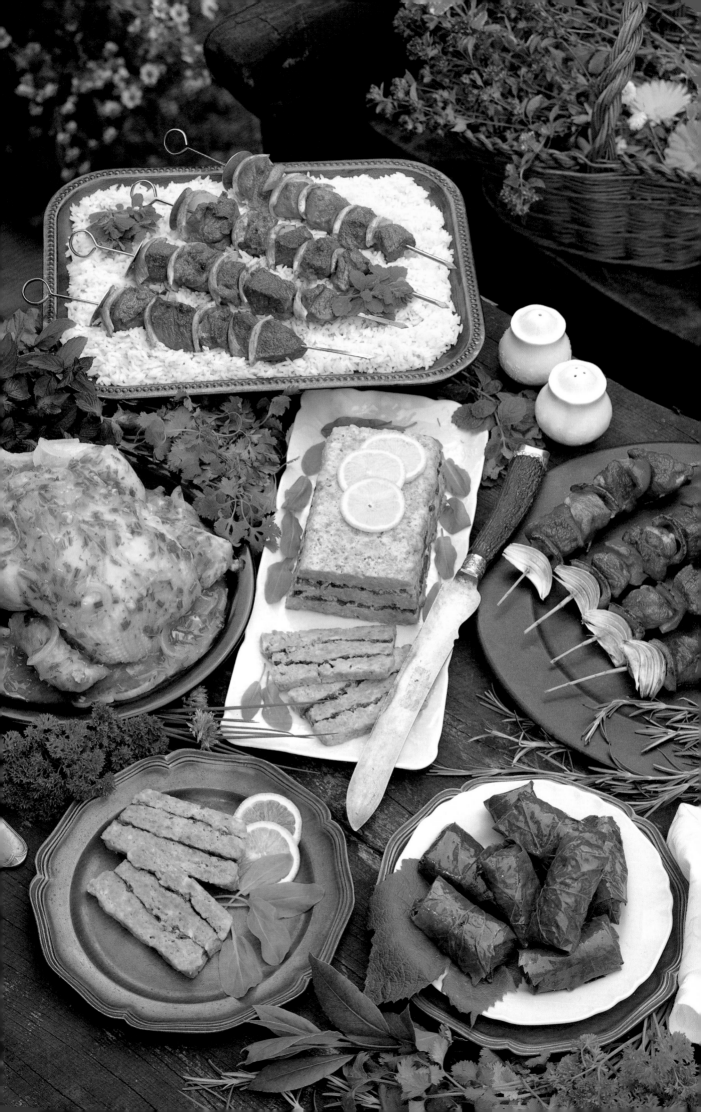

Tarragon baked chicken

Parsley, chives, thyme or chervil can be substituted for the tarragon.

8 chicken thighs or drumsticks, 3 oz each	2 tbsp chopped tarragon
2 oz butter	salt and black pepper

Serves 4

1 Preheat the oven to 375 °F.

2 To remove the bones from the chicken pieces, use a sharp knife and run it downward between the bone and the flesh until the bone comes loose. Gently twist the bone with your hands and it will come out easily.

3 Soften the butter a little and work to a paste with a wooden spoon. Mix in the tarragon and seasoning.

4 Divide the flavored butter between the chicken pieces, filling each cavity with a generous amount. Seal the open ends of each chicken piece using a wooden cocktail stick or small skewer.

5 Lay the pieces in a 9 inch square ovenproof dish and cover with foil. Bake for 40 minutes, removing the foil for the last 10 minutes. The chicken can also be finished off over a barbecue.

Spicy lemon balm kebabs

1 clove garlic	1 large onion, sliced into chunks
1 leg of lamb, about 3 lb, boned and cut into 1 in cubes	2 good handfuls of lemon balm leaves

MARINADE

2 fl oz wine vinegar	1 tbsp brown sugar
1 tsp ground coriander	1 tbsp mango chutney
1 tsp ground cumin	2 bay leaves
$\frac{1}{2}$ tsp chili powder	2 chilis (optional)
1 tsp ground turmeric	salt and black pepper

Serves 6

1 Rub the surface of a deep dish with the peeled and cut clove of garlic. Arrange the lamb cubes in the dish. Cover with a layer of onion and top with the lemon balm leaves.

2 For the marinade, boil the vinegar, coriander, cumin, chili, turmeric, brown sugar, chutney and bay leaves together for 5 minutes. Leave to cool. Pour the cooled marinade over the meat. Add the chilis and seasoning. Cover and leave overnight in the refrigerator.

3 Drain the lamb and onion pieces and thread them on metal skewers. Barbecue or broil for 15–20 minutes until browned, basting with the marinade. Discard the bay leaves before serving. Serve with hot garlic bread or on a bed of rice, accompanied by a crisp green salad.

Rosemary kebabs

To make a marinade for 1 lb cubed lamb or pork, mix 4 tablespoons olive oil, the juice of 2 lemons and the grated peel of 1 lemon, a crushed garlic clove and 4 sprigs of rosemary, or 2 teaspoons dried leaves. Marinade the meat for at least 4 hours, then thread it on skewers, or woody rosemary stalks, alternating it with chunks of red and green pepper and onion. Use the marinade to baste the meat as it grills.

Pork and sorrel terrine

1$\frac{1}{2}$ lb lean pork	2 cloves garlic
2 cups fresh breadcrumbs	salt and black pepper
	about 60 sorrel leaves,
1 medium onion	washed and drained

Serves 8

1 Grind the pork with the breadcrumbs, onion and garlic. Mix very well and season to taste.

2 Preheat the oven to 375 °F.

3 Grease a 2 lb loaf pan and press a third of the pork mixture into the base. Next make a layer of half the sorrel leaves. Add another third of the pork mixture, then the rest of the sorrel leaves, pressing each layer down well. Finish with the remaining pork mixture.

4 Cover with foil and stand the tin in a roasting pan half filled with water. Bake for 1$\frac{1}{2}$ hours.

5 Let it cool in the pan; slice and serve with hot toast.

Stuffed lovage and grape leaves

about 8 large stalks of lovage	1 tsp chopped rosemary
1 tbsp olive oil	salt and black pepper
1 small onion, finely chopped	8 oz lean ground lamb
2 oz pine nuts	8 grape leaves
1 oz raisins	

Serves 4

1 Cut the lovage leaves as close to the small groups of leaves as possible and lay them in a large heatproof dish. Cover with boiling water, leave for 10 minutes, drain and rinse under cold water. Set aside to cool.

2 Preheat the oven to 400 °F.

3 Heat the oil in a large saucepan and gently sauté the onion for about 5 minutes until soft. Add the pine nuts, raisins, rosemary and seasoning. Remove from the heat and leave to cool.

4 Mix the lamb into the cooled onion mixture.

5 Lay out the grape leaves and put 2–3 lovage leaves on each one.

6 Place about 1 tablespoon of the lamb stuffing on the leaves and roll them up. Place the rolls in a greased 8 inch square ovenproof dish. Cover and bake for about 30 minutes.

HERBS FOR MEAT
Beef: basil, bay, caraway seed, chervil, lovage seed, marjoram (pot roasts), mint, oregano, parsley, peppermint, rosemary, sage, savory, tarragon, thyme
Lamb: basil, chervil, cumin, dill, lemon balm, lovage seed, marjoram, mints, parsley, rosemary, savory, thyme
Pork: chervil, coriander, fennel, lovage seed, marjoram, rosemary, sage, savory, thyme
Liver: basil, dill, marjoram, sage, tarragon
Ham: juniper berries, lovage, marjoram, mint, mustard, oregano, parsley, savory

Lamb's kidneys sautéed with juniper

8 lamb's kidneys	1 tsp tomato paste
2 tbsp vegetable oil	2 tbsp dry sherry
4 oz small whole	1 cup meat stock
mushrooms	1 dried bay leaf
6 juniper berries, crushed	salt and black pepper
2 tbsp all-purpose flour	

Serves 4

1 Using a sharp knife, skin the kidneys, cut them in half lengthways and remove the cores.

2 Heat the oil in a large frying pan and gently sauté the kidneys and mushrooms for 2–3 minutes. Add the juniper berries and gently sauté for 2–3 minutes. Remove the mushrooms and kidneys, leaving the juniper berries in the pan.

3 Stir the flour into the remaining juices and add the tomato paste, sherry, meat stock, bay leaf and seasoning. Heat through, stirring.

4 Strain the sauce through a sieve and make up to 1½ pints with water.

5 Return the liquid to the pan with the mushrooms and kidneys. Retrieve the juniper berries from the sieve and add to the pan. Simmer for 20 minutes, uncovered, stirring occasionally.

Baked ham with marigold glaze

Marigold (calendula) petals and violets were commonly used in ham and meat glazes in the seventeenth century.

5 lb ham

GLAZE

¼ cup brown sugar	salt and black pepper
½ tsp dry mustard	⅓ cup dry
4 tbsp milk	breadcrumbs
1 cup marigold	
(calendula) petals	

Serves 12

1 First, soak the ham for 24 hours in cold water. Change the water at least two or three times, keeping the ham covered.

2 Preheat the oven to 350 °F. Wrap the ham in kitchen foil, enclosing it completely. Stand it in a roasting pan containing about 1 cup water. Bake, allowing 45 minutes per pound, turning halfway through the cooking time.

3 When cooked, leave the ham to stand for 30 minutes. Remove the foil and cut off the rind while it is still warm.

4 Score the fat into diamond shapes and replace the ham in the roasting pan, this time without water.

5 Mix all the glaze ingredients together and spread across the ham. Increase the oven temperature to 400 °F and bake for a further 10 minutes.

Pork chops marinated with juniper and garlic

2 tbsp olive oil	4 pork chops, ¾ in
6 juniper berries, crushed	thick, about 8 oz each
2 cloves garlic, crushed	¼ cup all-purpose flour
salt and black pepper	1 cup dry cider

Serves 4

1 Mix the oil, juniper berries, garlic and seasoning together in a bowl.

2 Lay the pork chops in the base of a shallow dish and cover them with the marinade, making sure all the surfaces are coated. Cover and leave for at least 3 hours, preferably overnight.

3 Drain the chops and reserve the marinade.

4 Heat a large frying pan and add the reserved marinade. When hot, add the pork chops and cook over a moderate heat for about 10 minutes on each side. To test if the chops are cooked, insert a sharp knife between the thickest part of the meat and the bone; all traces of pink should have gone. Remove the chops from the pan.

5 Leave the frying pan over the heat and stir the flour into the remaining juices. Add the cider and bring to the boil. Return the chops to the sauce in the pan. Heat through and serve.

Herby hamburgers

1 lb lean ground beef	black pepper
1 egg, lightly beaten	1 tsp soy sauce
2 tsp equal parts basil, sweet	1 large onion, minced
marjoram, thyme and	2 tbsp butter
lovage or smallage leaves	approx ¼ cup
1 tbsp chopped parsley	breadcrumbs
½ tsp salt	

Serves 4

1 Mix the meat, egg, herbs, salt and pepper and soy sauce together in a large bowl.

2 Sauté the onion in the butter until golden. Stir into the stuffing mixture. Add enough breadcrumbs to hold the mix together.

3 Shape into flattened patties and broil or barbecue until cooked through (about 5 minutes each side). Serve on a seeded bun with crisp lettuce, fresh tomato, and mayonnaise.

HERBS FOR CASSEROLES
Borage, bay, chicory, chives, coriander seed, dill seed, fennel, garlic, good King Henry, lemon balm, lovage, marjorams, mint, oregano, parsley, sage, savory, smallage, thyme

HERBS FOR MARINADES
Basil, bay, coriander seed and leaves, cumin, dill, fennel, garlic, juniper berries, lemon balm, lovage, mint, onion greens and bulbs, parsley stems, rosemary, tarragon

Savory main dishes

Green herb omelette

6–8 eggs	3 tbsp chopped herbs,
2 leeks, washed and chopped	such as tarragon,
4 spring onions, chopped	coriander, chives,
4 oz spinach, washed	chervil, dill
and chopped	1 tbsp chopped walnuts
3 tbsp chopped parsley	salt and black pepper

Serves 4

1 Heat the oven to 350 °F.

2 Beat the eggs in a large bowl. Add the chopped vegetables, herbs and walnuts. Season to taste and mix the ingredients together thoroughly.

3 Butter a large ovenproof dish and pour in the mixture. Cover and bake for 30 minutes. Remove the cover and bake for a further 15 minutes, or until the top is golden. Serve hot or cold.

Lovage and lentil roulade

The lovage can be replaced by spinach, sorrel or any other leafy herb.

2 oz bacon, chopped	2 oz margarine
6 oz split red lentils	$\frac{1}{3}$ cup all-purpose flour
1 small onion, finely	1 cup milk
chopped	2 eggs, separated
1 cup water	salt and black pepper
1 tbsp tomato paste	$\frac{1}{3}$ cup dry breadcrumbs
4 oz lovage leaves	

Serves 6

1 Place the bacon, lentils and onion in a saucepan and cover with the water. Simmer, uncovered, for 15 minutes. Add the tomato paste and simmer for a further 15 minutes until the mixture has thickened and absorbed the liquid.

2 Place the lovage leaves in a pan with just a sprinkling of salt, no water. Cover and cook for 5 minutes.

3 Preheat the oven to 400 °F.

4 Melt the margarine in a pan, add the flour and cook for 2–3 minutes, stirring until smooth. Gradually add the milk and simmer for 2 minutes, stirring to make a smooth sauce. Remove from the heat and add the egg yolks to the sauce.

5 Purée the cooked lovage and add to the sauce. Season to taste.

6 Whisk the egg whites until stiff and fold into the lovage mixture.

7 Grease and line an 11 inch jelly roll tin and spread the lovage mixture into the tin. Bake for 25 minutes until golden and well risen.

8 Scatter the breadcrumbs onto a sheet of greaseproof paper and turn out the cooked lovage mixture on to it.

9 Spread over the lentil filling, then roll up like a jelly roll. Return to the oven and bake for a further 10 minutes. Serve hot or cold.

Hazelnut and sage pâté

1 cup hazelnuts	$\frac{1}{3}$ tsp black pepper
$\frac{1}{4}$ cup sesame seeds	1 tbsp chopped sage
8 oz cream cheese	2 tbsp olive oil
2 cloves garlic, crushed	about 4 tbsp milk
$\frac{1}{3}$ tsp salt	

Serves 4–6

1 Preheat the oven to 350 °F.

2 Place the hazelnuts and sesame seeds on separate baking trays. Lightly roast in the oven for 5–10 minutes. When the nuts are cool, rub off the skins.

3 Grind the nuts and seeds together until they resemble fine crumbs. Or, if you prefer a coarse pâté, grind half the nuts and seeds finely and half coarsely.

4 Beat the cream cheese, garlic, salt, pepper, sage and oil together in a bowl.

5 Add the nut and seed mixture, combining well. Add the milk to give a moist consistency. The mixture needs to be fairly wet as the nuts will absorb some liquid.

6 Serve chilled in ramekins or on small individual salads with toast.

Oregano cheese pie

PASTRY

2 cups all-purpose flour	4 oz butter, cut
pinch of salt	into pieces

FILLING

8 oz ricotta cheese	2 tbsp chopped oregano
1 tbsp chopped onion	7 oz tomato paste
2 oz Parmesan	2 oz black olives,
cheese, grated	pitted and sliced
2 eggs	4 oz Mozzarella
black pepper	cheese, thinly sliced
2 tbsp chopped parsley	1 large green pepper,
1 tbsp olive oil	deseeded and sliced
1 clove garlic, crushed	a little beaten egg

Serves 6

1 For the pastry, sift the flour and salt into a bowl. Rub in the butter until the mixture resembles fine breadcrumbs. Add enough water to bind to a dough.

2 Roll out half the dough and use to line an 8 inch greased deep pie dish.

3 Preheat the oven to 400 °F.

4 For the filling, mix together the ricotta, onion, Parmesan, eggs, plenty of black pepper and parsley.

5 Heat the oil in a small pan and sauté the garlic with the oregano. Stir in the tomato purée and olives.

6 Spread half the ricotta mixture on the pastry base, cover with half the Mozzarella slices, then half the tomato mixture and half the pepper slices. Repeat.

7 Roll out the remaining dough to make a lid. Seal the edges. Brush the top of the pie with beaten egg and slash 4 times with a knife because the pie rises during cooking. Bake for 30–40 minutes.

Clockwise from top right: Tagliatelle with marigold sauce aurore (p. 176); Oregano cheese pie; Green herb omelette; Herb leaf fritters (p. 177).

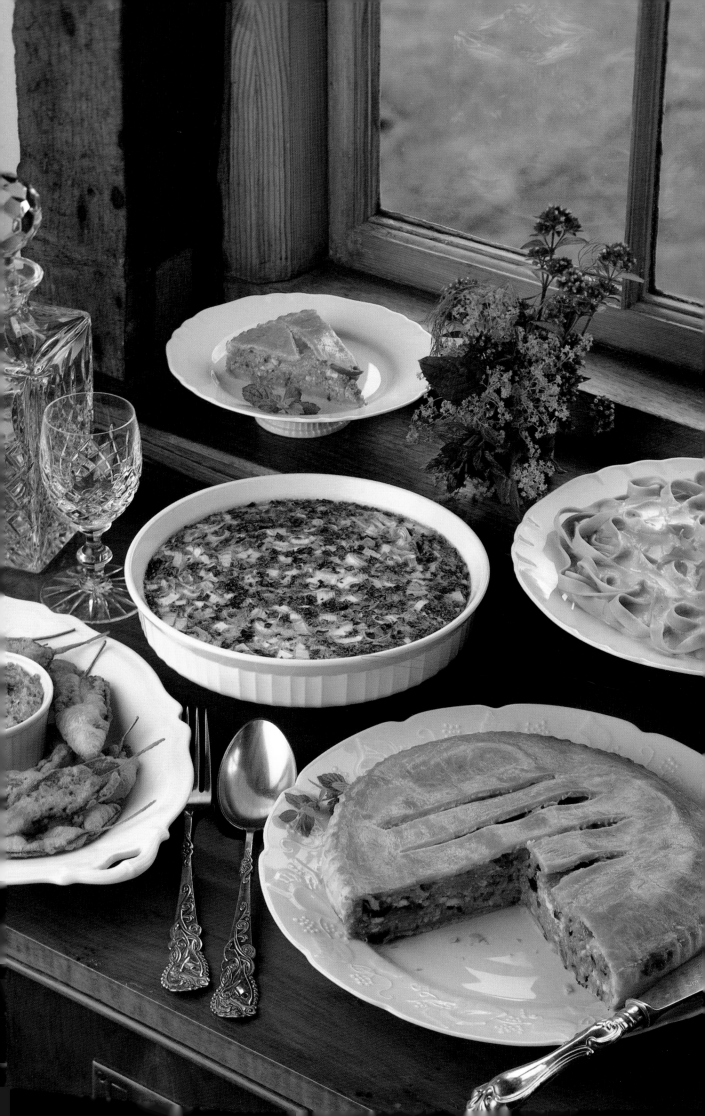

Tagliatelle with marigold
sauce aurore

1½ cups milk	1 bay leaf
1 large onion, quartered	4 oz butter
4 tbsp marigold	¾ cup all-purpose flour
(calendula) petals,	1½ cups cheese, grated
fresh or dried	salt and black pepper
2 large carrots, sliced	8 oz tagliatelle verde
lengthwise	

Serves 4

1 Place the milk, onion, marigold petals, carrots and bay leaf in a saucepan. Cover and simmer gently for about 10 minutes, until the carrots are soft.

2 Pour through a sieve into a jug and reserve the carrot and onion pieces.

3 Melt the butter in a pan, add the flour and cook for 2–3 minutes, stirring until smooth. Gradually add the flavored milk and simmer for 2 minutes, stirring to make a smooth sauce.

4 Press the cooked carrot and onion through a sieve and add to the sauce. Fold in the cheese and seasoning.

5 Cook the tagliatelle in a pan of boiling salted water until al dente. Serve topped with the marigold sauce.

Leek and sage croustade

2 cups fresh breadcrumbs	1 tsp rosemary,
¾ cup mixed	chopped
chopped nuts	1 tsp oregano
1 clove garlic, crushed	2 oz butter
1 tsp basil	1 cup cheese, grated

SAUCE

2 oz butter	2 tomatoes, skinned and
4 leeks, washed and finely	chopped
chopped	2 tbsp chopped sage
¼ cup all-purpose flour	salt and pepper
1 cup milk	

Serves 6

1 Preheat the oven to 350 °F.

2 Mix the breadcrumbs, nuts, garlic and herbs together in a bowl. Mix in the butter with your fingertips, then stir in the cheese. Press this mixture into an 8 inch quiche dish. Bake for 20 minutes until golden.

3 For the sauce, melt the butter in a saucepan and fry the leeks for about 10 minutes until soft. Stir in the flour, then add the milk and cook for 5 minutes, stirring. Add the tomatoes, sage and seasoning.

4 Spread the leek sauce over the cooked croustade. Bake for a further 20 minutes.

HERBS FOR EGGS AND CHEESE

Eggs, general: basil, chervil, chives, dill, parsley, tarragon
Deviled eggs: the above, marjoram, rosemary
Scrambled eggs and omelettes: the above, sweet marjoram, oregano
Cheeses, hard: caraway, dill seed, rosemary, sage
Cheeses, soft: caraway, chervil, chives, dill seed, fennel, marjoram, mints, rosemary, sage, savory, thyme
Fondues: basil, garlic, mint
Welsh rarebit: basil, parsley, sweet marjoram, tarragon

Fennel flan

PASTRY

1 cup all-purpose flour	3 oz butter, cut
pinch of salt	into pieces

FILLING

2 tbsp vegetable oil	2 tbsp chopped
1 large onion, chopped	fennel leaves
1 clove garlic, crushed	4 eggs
1 bulb Florence fennel, sliced	1 cup light cream
1 tbsp fennel seeds	salt and black pepper

Serves 6

1 For the pastry, sift the flour and salt into a bowl. Mix in the butter with your fingertips until the mixture resembles fine crumbs. Add enough water to bind to a dough. Roll out to line an 8 inch quiche dish.

2 Preheat the oven to 350 °F.

3 For the filling, heat the oil in a pan and sauté the onion and garlic for about 5 minutes until soft. Remove and drain on kitchen paper.

4 Repeat with the fennel.

5 Spread the onion and fennel over the pastry base. Scatter the fennel seeds and leaves on top.

6 Beat the eggs with the cream, season well and pour over the filling.

7 Bake for 30 minutes. Serve hot or cold.

Crêpes with basil stuffing

BATTER

¾ cup all-purpose flour	2 eggs
⅓ cup beer	2 oz butter, melted
⅓ cup milk	salt

FILLING

1 oz butter	8 oz cream cheese
1 small onion, finely chopped	2 eggs, beaten
1 clove garlic, crushed	1 tbsp shredded basil
8 oz mushrooms, chopped	salt and black pepper

TOPPING

3 tbsp grated	½ cup light cream
Parmesan cheese	

Serves 4

1 Put all batter ingredients in a blender and blend for about 1 minute. Leave to stand for at least 1 hour.

2 For the stuffing, melt the butter in a pan and sauté the onion and garlic for about 5 minutes. Add the mushrooms and sauté for 1 minute. Leave to cool. Mix with the remaining filling ingredients. Chill.

3 Preheat the oven to 350 °F.

4 For the crêpes, melt a little butter in a small frying pan. Add about 2 tbsp of batter and swirl round the pan. Cook for about 2 minutes until the underside is golden, then turn the crêpe and cook the other side for about 1 minute. Put the crêpe on a paper towel. Use the remaining batter to make 7 more crêpes.

5 Fill the 8 crêpes with the cream cheese and mushroom mixture. Roll up and place in an ovenproof dish. Sprinkle with Parmesan cheese and pour over the cream. Bake for 20 minutes.

Vegetable side dishes

Herb leaf fritters

Any of the stronger-tasting herb leaves can be used. Salad burnet leaves have a delicate shape and good flavor, or try sage, basil or sorrel.

20–30 herb leaves, depending on size   oil for deep frying

BATTER
¾ cup all-purpose flour   4 tbsp warm water
pinch of salt   1 large egg white
2 tbsp olive oil

Serves 4

1 Carefully rinse and dry the herb leaves.

2 For the batter, mix the flour and salt together in a bowl. Blend in the oil and water until smooth and creamy. Leave to stand for 1–2 hours in a cool place.

3 Whisk the egg white until stiff, then fold it carefully into the batter.

4 Heat the oil until a drop of batter crisps and browns quickly but does not burn. Dip the leaves, one at a time, into the batter. Fry, several at a time, for 2–3 minutes until golden brown.

5 Carefully remove the fritters and drain on kitchen paper. Keep warm in the oven until all the fritters are cooked. Serve immediately.

Cabbage and juniper

1½ lb cabbage   1 clove garlic, crushed
1 tbsp olive oil   8 juniper berries, crushed
1 onion, finely chopped   salt and black pepper

Serves 4–6

1 Preheat the oven to 400 °F.

2 Remove and discard the outer leaves from the cabbage and cut out the center stalk. Finely shred the cabbage, then rinse in a colander. Drain well.

3 Heat the oil in a flameproof casserole and gently fry the onion and garlic for about 10 minutes until soft. Stir in the juniper berries, then add the cabbage and mix well. Season to taste.

4 Cover with a tight-fitting lid. Bake for about 35 minutes. Check that the cabbage is cooked but still crisp before serving.

Tarragon stuffed mushrooms

1 lb large mushrooms   2 tbsp finely
3 cups fresh   chopped tarragon
breadcrumbs   2 eggs
2 cloves garlic, crushed   salt and black pepper
1 small onion, very finely   1½ cups dry breadcrumbs
chopped   oil for deep frying

Serves 4–6

1 Wipe the mushrooms clean. Carefully remove the stalks without damaging the caps. Finely chop the stalks and set aside.

2 Place the fresh breadcrumbs in a bowl and add the garlic. Stir in the onion, tarragon, 1 egg, seasoning and chopped mushroom stalks. Mix very well to form a soft stuffing.

3 Divide the mixture between the hollows of the mushroom caps, pressing it in well.

4 Beat the remaining egg in a dish and dip each stuffed mushroom into it.

5 Place the dry breadcrumbs in a dish and dip the egg-coated mushrooms into them, ensuring that they are evenly coated.

6 Heat about 4 cups oil in a heavy pan. Deep-fry the mushrooms for 4 minutes in about 4 batches. Drain on kitchen paper. Serve immediately with an herb mayonnaise (p. 182).

Mediterranean vegetables

⅓ cup olive oil   8 oz okra, trimmed
2 cloves garlic, chopped   4 oz onion, sliced
8 oz potato, cubed   1 tbsp coriander, chopped
8 oz green beans   juice of 1 lime
8 oz zucchini, sliced   juice of 1 lemon

GARNISH
2 tbsp chopped parsley

Serves 4

1 Heat the oil in a large saucepan and sauté all the vegetables and the coriander for about 5 minutes.

2 Add the lime and lemon juices, then cover and cook gently for 30 minutes, stirring occasionally to prevent the mixture from sticking to the bottom of the pan. Garnish with parsley.

HERBS FOR VEGETABLES	
Artichokes: bay, savory, tarragon **Asparagus:** chervil, chives, dill, lemon balm, salad burnet, tarragon **Avocado:** dill, marjoram, tarragon **Brussels sprouts:** dill, sage, savory **Cabbage:** borage, caraway, dill seed, marjoram, mint, oregano, parsley, sage, savory, sweet cicely, thyme **Carrots:** chervil, parsley **Cauliflower:** chives, dill leaf and seed, fennel, rosemary **Celeriac:** chervil, parsley, tarragon **Green beans:** dill, marjoram, mint, oregano, rosemary, sage, savory, tarragon, thyme **Lentils:** garlic, mint, parsley, savory, sorrel **Mushrooms:** basil, dill, lemon balm, marjoram, parsley, rosemary, salad burnet, savory, tarragon, thyme	**Onions:** basil, marjoram in soup, oregano, sage, tarragon, thyme **Peas:** basil, chervil, marjoram, mint, parsley, rosemary, sage, savory **Potatoes:** basil, bay, chives, dill, lovage, marjoram, mint, oregano, parsley, rosemary, savory, thyme **Sauerkraut:** dill, fennel seed, lovage, savory, tarragon, thyme **Spinach:** borage, chervil, marjoram, mint, rosemary for soup, sage, sorrel, tarragon **Tomatoes:** basil, bay, chervil, Chinese chives, chives, dill seed, garlic, marjoram, mint, oregano, parsley, sage, savory, tarragon **Turnips:** dill seed, marjoram, savory **Zucchini:** basil, dill, marjoram, rosemary, tarragon

Spicy eggplant

2 large eggplants
1 tbsp olive oil
1 tsp cumin seeds
1 tsp fennel seeds
1 lb tomatoes, skinned and chopped

1 inch fresh ginger, grated
4 cloves garlic, crushed
1 tsp ground coriander
1 tsp ground cardamom
1 cup water
salt and black pepper

GARNISH
fresh coriander leaves

Serves 4

1 Wipe the eggplants, remove the stalks and cut into finger-sized pieces. Fry them in the oil for about 5 minutes until brown. Drain on paper towels.

2 Fry the cumin and fennel seeds for about 2 minutes, stirring all the time, until they turn a shade darker. Stir in the chopped tomatoes, grated ginger, crushed garlic, coriander, cardamom and the water. Simmer for about 20 minutes until the mixture is a thick sauce.

3 Return the eggplant pieces to the pan and heat through. Garnish with coriander leaves.

Artichokes with ravigote sauce

4 artichokes

SAUCE
mixed bunch of parsley, tarragon, watercress
a bunch of chervil
a few chives
1 tbsp capers

2 cornichons finely chopped
4 tbsp olive oil
1 tbsp tarragon vinegar
a little lemon juice

Serves 4

1 Wash the artichokes and soak in salted water to clean. Trim the stalks close to the base.

2 Place the artichokes in a large pan of boiling salted water and simmer for about 30 minutes until cooked. Remove the artichokes and drain upside down.

3 For the sauce, finely chop all the herbs. Add the capers and cornichons, then the oil, vinegar and lemon.

4 Transfer the sauce to individual pots. To serve, dip the artichoke leaves into the sauce.

Oregano tomatoes

4 large tomatoes
2 oz butter
1 tbsp chopped fresh oregano or 1½ tsp dried oregano

1 clove garlic, crushed
black pepper
pinch of salt
2 tbsp grated Parmesan cheese

Serves 4

1 Cut the tomatoes in half horizontally and place in a shallow flameproof dish.

2 Beat the butter with the oregano, garlic, pepper, salt, and Parmesan in a bowl. Spread the mixture over the cut side of each tomato.

3 Broil the tomatoes under medium heat for about 5 minutes until the topping is just turning golden.

Sorrel and parsnip mousses

1 lb parsnips, peeled and cut into large pieces
about 36 sorrel leaves
2 oz butter
⅓ cup all-purpose flour

1 cup milk
1 egg, separated
1 tbsp chopped chives
salt and black pepper

Serves 6

1 Place the parsnips in a saucepan, cover and simmer for 20 minutes until tender.

2 Preheat the oven to 375 °F.

3 Very quickly dip each sorrel leaf into a bowl of boiling water to blanch. Use these leaves to line the bases and sides of 6 ramekin dishes. (You will need about 6 leaves for each dish.)

4 When the parsnips are cooked, drain and mash them into a smooth purée.

5 Melt the butter in a pan, add the flour and cook for 2 minutes, stirring until smooth. Gradually add the milk and simmer for 2 minutes, stirring to make a smooth, thick sauce.

6 Beat the egg yolk into the sauce. Whisk the egg white in a bowl until soft peaks form.

7 Mix the sauce and parsnip together. Add the chives and seasoning. Fold in the egg white.

8 Divide the mixture between the lined ramekin dishes. Place the dishes in a deep roasting pan half filled with hot water.

9 Bake for 50 minutes, or until golden and puffy. Turn out and serve hot.

Fennel with Roquefort sauce

4 bulbs of Florence fennel

SAUCE
1 oz butter
¼ cup all-purpose flour
1 cup mixed milk and fennel stock

¾ cup Roquefort cheese, grated
black pepper
1 tbsp plain yogurt

GARNISH
1 tbsp chopped parsley
1 tbsp chopped fennel leaves

Serves 4

1 Halve the fennel bulbs vertically, put in a saucepan and cover with water. Bring to the boil and simmer for about 15–20 minutes or until tender. Drain, reserving ¾ cup of the cooking liquid.

2 For the sauce, melt the butter, add the flour and cook for 2 minutes, stirring until smooth. Gradually add the milk and stock and simmer for 2 minutes, stirring to make a smooth sauce.

3 Add the grated cheese and black pepper to taste. Do not allow the sauce to boil. Stir in the yogurt and cook gently for a few minutes, stirring.

4 Place the fennel in a serving dish and pour over the Roquefort sauce. Garnish with the parsley and fennel.

Clockwise from the top: Artichokes with ravigote sauce; Oregano tomatoes; Fennel with Roquefort sauce; Sorrel and parsnip mousses.

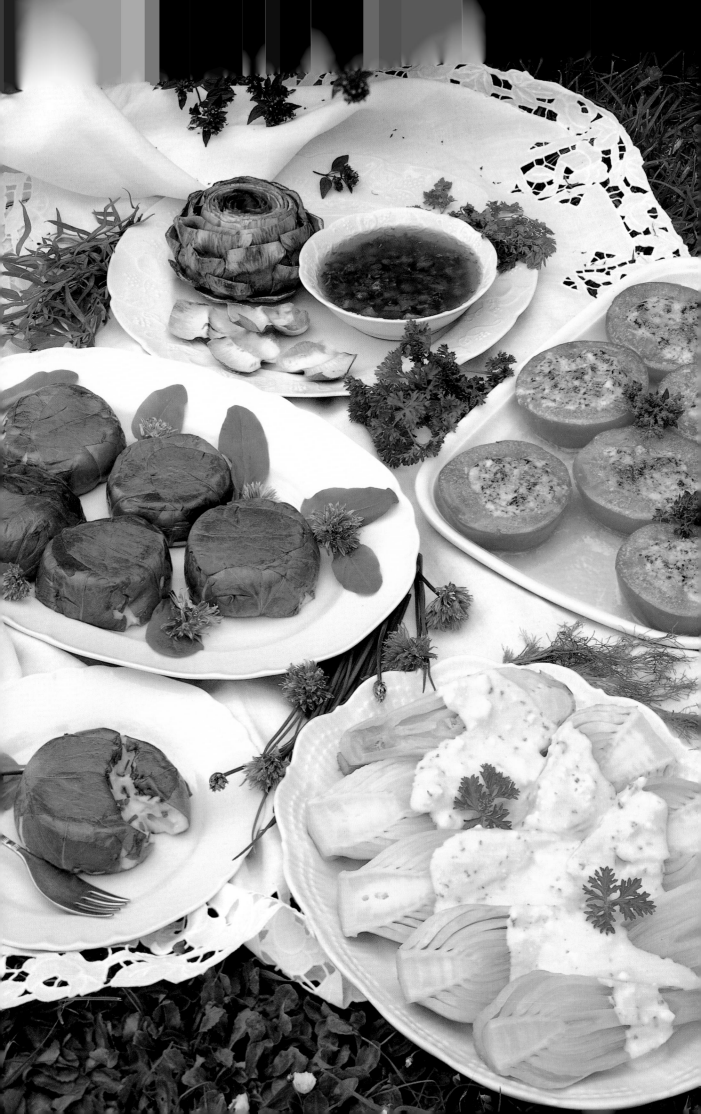

Salads and snacks

Salad herbs can be divided into three groups. First are those selected for their crunchy texture and mild flavor, so any amount can be used. These include the ornamental lettuces, forced endive, and blanched leaves such as dandelion and summer purslane. Second are the flavoring herbs. This includes most of the savory leaves and seeds listed in the box below, as well as pickled herbs and buds. Use these in small quantities, as they can taste sharp. The third group consists of herb flowers, which have subtle flavors and are employed more for their beauty than taste. Be selective: a hodgepodge of every flower will diminish the impact of one or two. Try to keep within one range of colors – say blue borage and sage flowers, or golden calendula and gold variegated lemon balm.

Melon, tomato and mint salad

Try replacing the mint with lemon balm or fresh basil leaves for a different combination.

8 oz canteloupe or ogen melon	$\frac{1}{2}$ cup finely chopped mint
8 oz firm tomatoes, cut into thin wedges	1 cup plain yogurt
6 oz cucumber, peeled and grated	salt and black pepper

GARNISH
mint leaves

Serves 4

1 Cut the melon flesh into balls with a ball cutter. Alternatively, cut the melon into cubes.

2 Combine the melon, tomato and cucumber in a large salad bowl.

3 Stir the mint into the yogurt to make a dressing, then pour over the salad. Season to taste, and garnish the dressed salad with mint leaves.

Fennel salad with orange

1 bulb of Florence fennel, thinly sliced	1 bunch of watercress
1 lettuce	fennel leaves, chopped

DRESSING

$\frac{1}{2}$ cup olive oil	1 tsp fennel seeds
juice of 1 large orange	salt and black pepper
1 tsp French mustard	

Serves 6

1 First make the dressing. Put all the ingredients in a jar with a lid and shake well. Leave to stand for at least 30 minutes.

2 Arrange the fennel, lettuce and watercress in a salad bowl. Scatter with the fennel leaves.

3 Shake the dressing, then pour over the salad just before serving.

Hot salad

2 onions	grated rind and juice of 1 large lemon
2 radishes	
2 large carrots	1–2 chilis, chopped (seeded if preferred)
1 large tomato, chopped	
1 small lettuce, shredded	salt and black pepper
bunch of fresh coriander, chopped	

Serves 4–6

1 Grate the onions, radishes and carrots and place in a salad bowl.

2 Add the remaining ingredients and toss together well. Add extra lemon juice to taste.

Violet herb salad

1 head of endive	1 tbsp chopped parsley
1 tbsp finely chopped celery	1 tbsp chopped chervil
	2 olives, finely chopped
1 tbsp finely chopped, tender fennel stalks (peeled if necessary)	salad dressing to taste
	petals of 30 sweet violets

Serves 4

1 Separate the endive leaves and place in a salad bowl. Add the remaining salad ingredients, including the herbs, and gently mix well.

2 Add the dressing and toss the salad. Sprinkle on the sweet violet petals.

Sweet anise salad

3 red apples	2 bananas, sliced
3 tbsp lemon or orange juice	$\frac{3}{4}$ cup walnuts, coarsely chopped
1 tsp sugar	$\frac{1}{2}$ cup mayonnaise
6 oz anise stalks, sliced	lettuce leaves

GARNISH
parsley

Serves 4

1 Core the apples and dice, leaving the peel on. Reserve some apple to use as a garnish.

2 Mix the lemon juice and sugar together in a bowl, then toss the apple in the mixture.

3 Add the anise stalks, banana and walnuts to the apple. Mix in the mayonnaise and chill.

4 Serve the salad in a lettuce-lined salad bowl and garnish with the reserved apple and parsley.

SALAD HERBS

General: alexanders, angelica, arugula, basil, borage leaves, caraway, chervil, chicory, Chinese chives, chives, coriander leaves, corn salad, dill, fennel, lemon balm, lovage, marjoram, mint, mustard seedlings, nasturtium leaves, orach, parsley, purslane (summer and winter), salad burnet, savory, smallage, sorrel, sweet cicely, tarragon, thyme, watercress.
Floral additions: bergamot, borage, calendula, chives, nasturtium, primrose, rose petals, sweet rocket, violet.

Clockwise from the top: Mixed flower and leaf salads; Hot salad; Melon, tomato and mint salad; Herb spread sandwiches (p. 182); Fennel salad with orange.

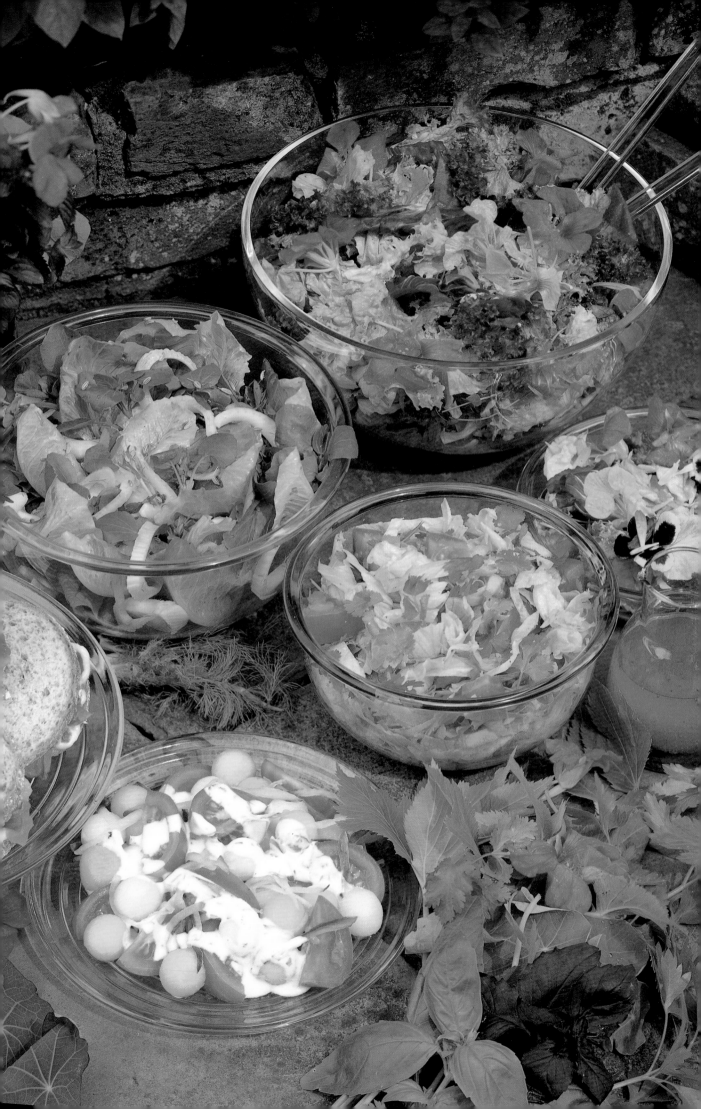

Potato salad with dill and chives

4 medium potatoes	finely chopped or
1 tbsp chopped onion	1 tsp dill seed
1 tbsp chopped parsley	3 tbsp mayonnaise
1 tbsp chopped chives	1 tbsp cream or yogurt
1 flowering head of dill	salt and black pepper

Serves 4

1 Boil the potatoes in their skins until just tender. Cool, peel and slice them.

2 Sprinkle on the onion, parsley, chives and dill.

3 Blend the mayonnaise and cream, season with salt and pepper. Add to the potato mixture and stir gently. Leave to stand a few hours so the flavors mingle.

Cheese balls

8 oz cream cheese	herbs: chives, parsley,
1 cup finely chopped	rosemary, sage, thyme

Shape the cheese into plum-sized balls and then roll them in the chopped herbs. Serve with salads, on hot vegetables or as a spread.

Herbal vinaigrette

One of the simplest dressings to make and one that is infinitely variable. Select herbs from those listed to vary the emphasis. Substitute a herbal oil or vinegar for extra pungency.

3 tbsp olive oil	3 tbsp fresh chopped
1 tbsp wine vinegar	herbs (basil, chervil, chives,
$\frac{1}{4}$ tsp mustard	dill seed, lemon balm,
salt and black pepper	marjoram, rosemary, salad
1 clove garlic, crushed	burnet, tarragon, thyme)

Makes about $\frac{1}{2}$ cup

Mix all the ingredients together in a jar or bottle and shake well.

Green mayonnaise

Use the following herbs, either singly or in combination: garlic, lemon balm, lovage, salad burnet, tarragon, thyme.

1 egg yolk	2 tbsp chopped parsley
1 cup olive oil	1 tbsp selected herbs
1 tbsp wine vinegar	

Makes 1 cup

1 Beat the egg yolk for a minute or so, then start adding the oil, drop by drop, beating continuously.

2 When over half the oil has been added and the mixture has started to thicken, beat in the vinegar.

3 Add more oil drop by drop until it thickens again, then slowly pour in the rest. (If the mixture refuses to thicken, or curdles, break a fresh egg yolk into a clean basin and slowly beat in the first mixture.)

4 Stir in the chopped herbs.

Aioli (garlic mayonnaise)

1 egg yolk	salt and black pepper
1 cup olive oil	4 cloves garlic
1 tbsp wine vinegar	

Makes 1 cup

1 Make up the mayonnaise as described before.

2 Crush or pound the garlic in a pestle and mortar. Mix into the mayonnaise.

Tartare sauce

1 cup mayonnaise	3 shallots finely
(see above)	chopped
2 tbsp chopped green	$\frac{1}{2}$ tsp mustard
herbs (chervil, chives,	1 tbsp capers, chopped
parsley, tarragon)	

Makes 1 cup

Mix all the ingredients together.

Horseradish sauce

2 tbsp wine vinegar	$\frac{1}{2}$ tsp black pepper
1 tsp sugar	4 tbsp finely grated
$\frac{1}{2}$ tsp salt	horseradish
1 tsp mustard	3 tbsp cream

Makes about $\frac{2}{3}$ cup

1 Heat the vinegar in an enamel pan. Add the sugar, salt, mustard and pepper and stir over low heat for 2 minutes.

2 Add the horseradish and heat for 2 minutes more. Leave to cool, then blend in the cream. Chill to serve.

HERB SPREADS

These make a delicious snack served with crackers, bread or vegetable crudités.

Mix equal quantities of mayonnaise with chopped chervil, chives, coriander, dill, fennel, nasturtium petals, parsley, tarragon. The following mixture is a favorite.

Angelica and mint sandwich

Choose a variety of mint with a clean spearmint flavor such as Moroccan mint or red raripila spearmint.

a good handful of fresh	1–2 tbsp mayonnaise
young angelica leaves	2–4 slices of wholewheat
a good handful of fresh	or rye bread
mint leaves	

Serves 2

1 Pass the leaves through a food mill or chop very finely by hand. Mix the two herbs together.

2 Toast the bread, then spread 2 slices with mayonnaise.

3 Sprinkle a thick layer of the herb mixture on top. Cover with a slice of toast or leave open. Cut into quarters and serve.

Desserts

Gooseberry and elderflower cream

1 lb fresh washed gooseberries	1 cup sugar (or to taste)
$\frac{1}{2}$ cup water	2 oz butter
5 elderflower heads or	3 eggs, beaten
1 tbsp orange-flower water	whipped cream for topping

DECORATION
borage flowers

Serves 4

1 Cook the gooseberries and elderflowers in the water until soft. Remove the flowers and purée the fruit.

2 Return the mixture to the saucepan. Add the sugar and heat to dissolve. (At this stage, the mixture can be strained, bottled and kept in the freezer as a delicious syrup for serving on fruit dishes or diluted with club soda as a summer drink.)

3 To make the cream dessert, stir in the butter until melted. Cool a little and slowly add the beaten eggs, stirring constantly until thick. Do not boil.

4 Spoon into serving glasses, top with cream and garnish with borage flowers.

Rose layered dessert

1 cup loosely packed scented rose petals, white heels removed	2 tbsp mincemeat
	4 tbsp rose petal jam (see p. 190)
4 bananas, mashed	juice of 2 oranges
approx. 4 oz chopped dates (equal volume to banana)	small carton whipped cream

DECORATION
crystallized rose petals   sweet cicely seeds (optional)

Serves 4

1 Cover a dish with pink and red rose petals.

2 Mix the banana, dates and mincemeat and make a layer over the petals, leaving the petals protruding around the edge. Cover with a layer of rose petal jam.

3 When ready to serve, pour over the orange juice. Add a layer of whipped cream and garnish with crystallized rose petals and sweet cicely seeds.

Mulled pears with juniper

4 firm pears	$\frac{1}{4}$ cup dark brown sugar
$\frac{2}{3}$ cup red wine	
$\frac{2}{3}$ cup fresh orange juice	4 juniper berries, crushed

Serves 4

1 Either peel the pears whole, leaving the stalks intact, or peel, core and quarter them.

2 Mix the red wine, orange juice, brown sugar and juniper berries together in a saucepan. Bring to simmering point.

3 Add the pears and simmer, uncovered, for 15 minutes, or 25 minutes if the pears are whole. Turn and baste from time to time.

Sweet rice with rose geranium

$\frac{1}{2}$ cup round-grain rice	1 oz dry coconut
2 cups milk	2 oz flaked almonds
8 scented rose geranium leaves	2 oz raisins
	$\frac{1}{4}$ cup soft brown sugar

Serves 6

1 Mix the rice and milk together in a saucepan. Add 4 geranium leaves to the pan. Cover and simmer very gently for 30 minutes.

2 Remove from the heat and take out the leaves. Preheat the oven to 375 °F.

3 Add the coconut, almonds, raisins and sugar to the milk mixture, stirring well.

4 Transfer the mixture to a large 8 inch ovenproof dish. Arrange the remaining geranium leaves across the top. Bake for 45 minutes.

Mint and chocolate ice cream

1 cup mint leaves, preferably spearmint	3 oz semisweet chocolate
	2 eggs, separated
$\frac{1}{3}$ cup superfine sugar	1$\frac{1}{3}$ cups heavy cream

DECORATION
mint leaves   1 oz semisweet chocolate

Serves 6

1 Mix the mint leaves with half of the sugar and chop as finely as possible.

2 Set a bowl over a pan of simmering water and melt 2 oz of the chocolate. Remove from the heat. Add the egg yolks and whisk until creamy. Leave to cool.

3 Whip the cream until soft peaks form, then fold in the chopped mint. Fold the whipped mint cream into the cooled chocolate mixture. Freeze the mixture in a 2 quart ice-cube tray.

4 When the ice cream becomes crisp at the edges, whisk for 2 minutes. Return to the freezer, then whisk the ice cream every 45 minutes until it is just set.

5 Whisk the egg whites until soft peaks form. Fold in the remaining sugar, then fold carefully into the frozen ice cream. Finally grate the remaining 1 oz chocolate and stir into the ice cream. Return the ice cream to the freezer until completely set.

6 Serve decorated with mint leaves dipped in melted chocolate (leave to set on wax paper).

HERBS FOR DESSERTS
General: angelica, aniseed, bergamot, elderflower, lemon balm, lemon verbena, pineapple sage, rosemary, saffron, sweet cicely leaves and green seeds
Custards: bay, lemon thyme, mint, rose petals, scented geraniums (pelargoniums)
Fruit salads: aniseed, lemon balm, mints, rosemary, sweet cicely leaves and green seeds
Fruit compotes: dill, mint with pears; aniseed, caraway, coriander, dill with apples; savory with quinces; angelica, sweet cicely with acidic fruits

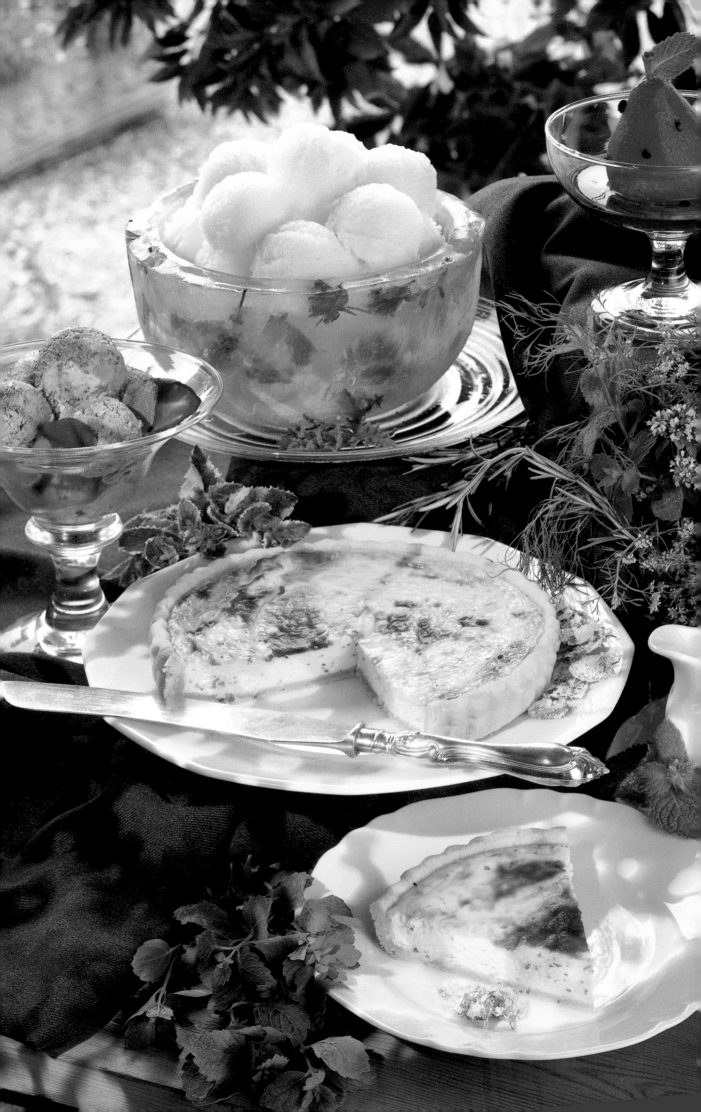

Lemon balm cheesecake

PASTRY

1 cup all-purpose flour   3 oz margarine, cut
pinch of salt   into pieces

FILLING

2 oz margarine   2 eggs, beaten
2 tbsp honey   6 tbsp very finely
12 oz cream cheese   chopped lemon balm

Serves 6

1 Preheat the oven to 400 °F.

2 For the pastry, sift the flour and salt into a bowl. Rub in the margarine with your fingertips until the mixture resembles fine breadcrumbs. Add enough water to make a soft dough. Roll out to line a 7 inch quiche dish. Bake blind for 15 minutes.

3 For the filling, beat the margarine, honey and cream cheese together in a bowl until soft and creamy. Beat in the eggs and fold in the lemon balm. Reduce the oven temperature to 350 °F.

4 Pour the filling into the pastry case. Bake for 45 minutes until the filling is golden and set. Serve with whipped cream or yogurt.

Sweet herb sorbet

$\frac{1}{2}$ cup superfine sugar   lemon balm, scented
1 cup water   geranium or rosemary)
$\frac{1}{4}$ cup spearmint   juice of 1 lemon
leaves (or apple mint,   1 egg white

DECORATION

spearmint leaves

Serves 4

1 Place the sugar in a saucepan and add the water. Bring to the boil, stirring, until the sugar is dissolved.

2 Chop the herb leaves and add to the pan. Cover, then remove from the heat. Leave to infuse for 20–30 minutes. Test for flavor; if it is too light, bring to the boil again then leave to infuse for 15 minutes.

3 Strain the liquid and add the lemon juice. Transfer the mixture to an ice-cube tray and freeze for 2–3 hours.

4 When the sorbet is semifrozen, whisk the egg white until stiff and fold it into the mixture. Return to the freezer for a further 3–4 hours or until frozen.

5 Serve the sorbet in individual dishes, and decorate each serving with extra herb leaves.

Breads, cakes and biscuits

Lovage seed bread

Try with poppy seeds or sweet cicely seeds instead.

$\frac{1}{2}$ oz fresh yeast $2\frac{1}{2}$ cups strong white flour
$\frac{1}{2}$ tsp sugar   1 tbsp vegetable oil
$1\frac{3}{4}$ cups warm water   1 medium onion, grated
2 tsp salt   1 tbsp lovage seeds
$2\frac{1}{2}$ cups wholewheat flour

Makes about 14 rolls or two 1 lb loaves

1 Mix the yeast, sugar and warm water together in a bowl. Leave in a warm place until frothy.

2 Mix the flours, salt and oil together in a bowl. Add the yeast and onion, kneading to make a soft dough.

3 Knead lightly on a floured surface for 10 minutes until the dough is smooth and elastic. Place the dough in a bowl, cover with a damp cloth and leave to rise in a warm place for about $1\frac{1}{2}$ hours until doubled in size.

4 Turn out the dough onto a floured surface and knead for about 5 minutes. Shape into rolls or loaves and place on a baking tray or greased loaf pans.

5 Brush the dough with a little water and sprinkle with the lovage seeds. Leave to prove for 20 minutes.

6 Preheat the oven to 450 °F.

7 Bake for 10 minutes, then reduce the oven temperature to 400 °F for a further 5–20 minutes. Turn out on to wire racks to cool.

Rosemary cheese fingers

2 oz butter   1 egg, beaten
2 cups oat flakes   1 tbsp chopped rosemary
$1\frac{1}{2}$ cups cheddar   pinch of cayenne
cheese, grated   salt

Makes 12 slices

1 Preheat the oven to 350 °F.

2 Melt the butter in a saucepan. Place the remaining ingredients in a bowl and mix in the butter.

3 Press the mixture into a greased 8 inch square pan. Bake for 30–40 minutes. Cut into fingers.

Sage oat cakes

1 oz lard $\frac{1}{2}$ tsp dried sage
$\frac{1}{3}$ cup boiling water $\frac{1}{2}$ tsp bicarbonate of soda
3 cups medium oatmeal   pinch of salt

Makes 8 slices

1 Preheat the oven to 350 °F.

2 Place the lard and water in a small pan and heat until the lard has melted. Cool.

3 Mix the oatmeal, sage, bicarbonate of soda and salt together in a bowl. Stir in the cooled liquid and mix to a soft dough, adding a little more water if necessary.

4 Pat the dough into a round bottomless pan about 8 inches in diameter. Place on an ungreased baking tray.

5 Bake for about 40 minutes. Cut into 8 wedges, then leave to cool slightly before turning on to a wire rack.

Clockwise from top center: Sweet herb sorbet; Mulled pears with juniper (p. 183); Lemon balm cheesecake; Mint and chocolate ice cream (p. 183).

Cheese bread with chives

½ oz fresh yeast or
1 oz dried yeast and
1 tsp sugar
¼ cup water
3½ cups all-purpose flour
¾ cup wholewheat flour
pinch of salt

1 cup water, heated
to blood temperature
2 oz butter
2½ cups cheese, grated
3 tbsp chopped chives
1 egg, beaten

Makes one 2 lb loaf

1 Put the yeast into a cup and stir in the ¼ cup water. If using dried yeast, add the sugar. Leave in a warm place until frothy.

2 Put the flours and salt into a large bowl. Pour the yeast mixture into the center of the flour and mix together well with a knife, adding some of the warm water. Add the rest of the water, then knead the dough for 2 minutes.

3 Form the dough into a ball and sprinkle with flour. Cover the dough with a damp cloth and leave to rise in a warm place for 1½–2 hours until doubled in size.

4 Knead the dough lightly. Roll into a rectangle and dot with butter. Fold into 3, then roll out to the same size again. Sprinkle with the cheese and chives to within 1 in (2.5 cm) of the edge. Roll up from the short end, like a jelly roll.

5 Place in a greased bread pan and score the top with a sharp knife. Leave to prove in a warm place for about 30 minutes.

6 Preheat the oven to 425 °F.

7 Brush the loaf with beaten egg. Bake for 35–40 minutes. Best eaten when warm.

Sweet rosemary slices

2 eggs
⅔ cup soft brown sugar
few drops vanilla essence
1 cup all-purpose flour
1 tsp baking powder
pinch of salt
1 tbsp rosemary leaves
or 2 tsp dried

8 oz raisins and
candied fruit, such as
angelica, glacé cherries
or candied pineapple
1 cup pecan
nuts, chopped, or
¾ cup sunflower seeds

Makes 24 slices

1 Preheat the oven to 375 °F.

2 Beat the eggs in a bowl, then gradually add the sugar and vanilla essence. Mix well.

3 Sift in the flour, baking powder and salt. Add the rosemary leaves, then fold in the fruit and nuts.

4 Spoon the mixture on to a greased and floured 8 inch baking pan and spread evenly.

5 Bake for 30 minutes. Remove from the pan while still warm. Allow to cool, then cut into squares.

HERBS FOR BREADS
Aniseed, basil, caraway, chives, dill, fennel, lovage seed, poppy seed, rosemary, sunflower seed, thyme

Saffron fruit bread

1 cup milk, warmed
1 oz fresh yeast
1 tsp sugar
¼ tsp saffron
powder or strands
½ cup boiling water
3½ cups all-purpose flour

4 oz butter
⅓ cup superfine sugar
6 oz currants or raisins
4 oz chopped
candied peel
1 tsp dried thyme

Serves 10

1 Place the milk in a bowl and dissolve the yeast and the 1 teaspoon of sugar in it. Leave in warm place for about 10 minutes until frothy.

2 Steep the saffron in the boiling water, then leave the mixture to cool.

3 Sift the flour into a large bowl. Mix in the butter with your fingertips. Add the rest of the sugar, the currants or raisins, peel and thyme, mixing well.

4 Add the yeast liquid and saffron liquid to the flour mixture. (Strain the saffron mixture if using strands.) Mix until smooth with a wooden spoon; it should look like a very thick batter.

5 Pour the batter into a greased and lined 10 inch round cake pan. Cover with a damp cloth and leave in a warm place for about 1 hour until the mixture rises to the top of the tin.

6 Preheat the oven to 375 °F.

7 Bake the bread for 1 hour. Leave to cool in the pan. Slice and serve with butter.

Scented geranium leaf sponge

20 scented geranium leaves
8 oz butter
1¼ cups superfine sugar

4 eggs, beaten
1½ cups self-rising
flour, sifted

DECORATION
scented geranium leaves   icing sugar

Serves 6

1 Grease and line two 8 inch cake pans. Arrange the geranium leaves on the lining paper.

2 Preheat the oven to 375 °F.

3 Cream the butter and sugar together in a bowl until light and fluffy. Add the beaten eggs, a little at a time, to the creamed mixture, beating well. Fold in the flour.

4 Divide the mixture between the prepared pans. Bake for 20–25 minutes until golden.

5 Turn out of the pans and cool on wire racks. Remove the leaves and lining paper.

6 Sandwich the sponges with a filling: sweet geranium jelly and whipped cream are excellent. Arrange some geranium leaves on top of the sponge, then sift over some icing sugar. Carefully remove the leaves before eating.

Clockwise from top center: Saffron fruit bread; Cheese bread with chives; Sage oat cakes (p. 185); Herb butter (p. 190); Sweet rosemary slices; Cheese balls (p. 182); Scented geranium leaf sponge.

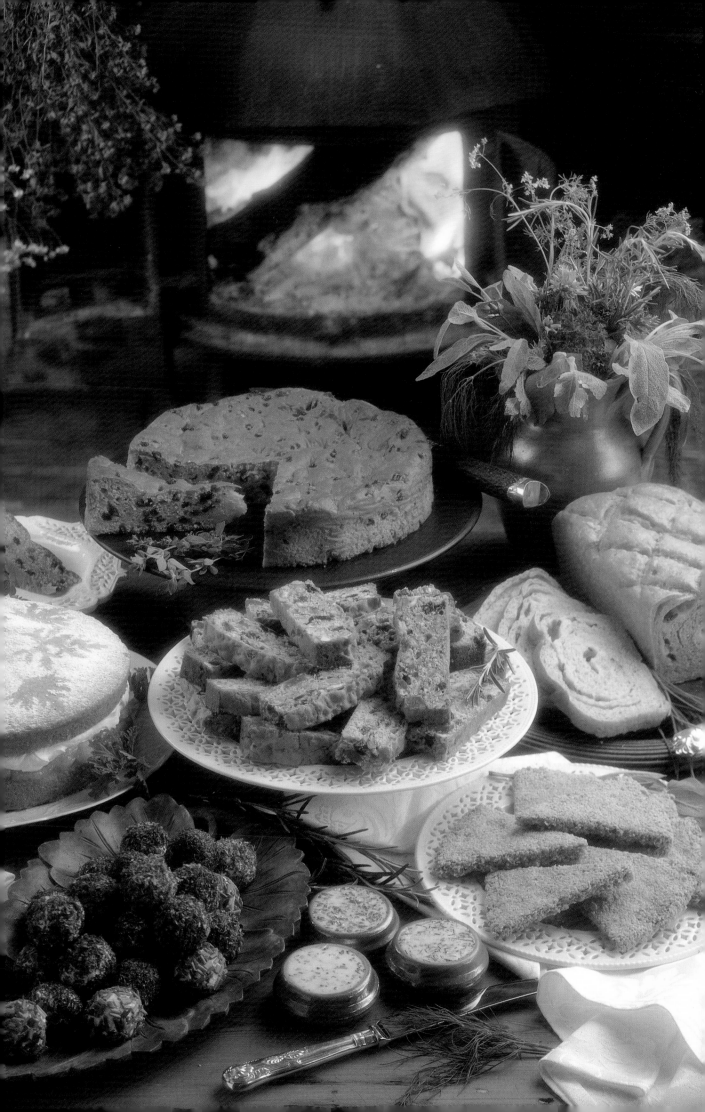

Preserves

HERBAL OILS

To make an herb oil, loosely fill a clear jar with freshly picked herbs and cover with unheated safflower or sunflower oil. (Any oil can be used but avoid strongly flavored ones.) Cover with cheesecloth and place on a sunny window sill. Allow to steep for 2 weeks, stirring daily. Strain through the cloth, and check the flavor. If it is as strong as you wish, bottle and label. If you want a stronger flavor, repeat the process with fresh herbs. Use herb oils in salad dressings, marinades, for browning meats and softening vegetables.

For sweet oils, use almond oil with scented flowers.

HERBS FOR OILS
Savory: basil, garlic, fennel, marjoram, mint, rosemary, tarragon, thyme, savory **Sweet:** clove pinks, lavender, lemon verbena, rose petals

HERBAL VINEGARS

Use cider or wine vinegar as a base. Bruise the freshly picked herbs and loosely fill a clean jar. Pour on warmed but not hot vinegar to fill the jar and cap with an acid-proof lid. Set in a sunny window and shake daily for 2 weeks. Test for flavor; if a stronger taste is required, strain the vinegar and repeat with fresh herbs. Store as it is or strain through cheesecloth and rebottle. Add a fresh sprig to the bottle for identification and visual appeal. Use in salad dressings, marinades, gravies and sauces.

Tarragon vinegar

Follow the above instructions and add a sliced clove of garlic to the steeping tarragon and vinegar. Remove the garlic after one day and replace with 2 cloves for the remaining 2 weeks. Strain and bottle.

Floral vinegars

Floral vinegars are made in the same way and are used with fruit salads and in some cosmetic recipes. Select from the list below, removing stems and any green or white heels from the petals.

HERBS FOR VINEGARS
Basil, bay, chervil, dill leaves, fennel, garlic, lemon balm, marjoram, mint, rosemary, savory, tarragon, thyme

FLOWERS FOR VINEGARS
Carnations, clover, elderflowers, lavender, nasturtiums, primroses, rose petals, rosemary flowers, thyme flowers, sweet violets

Blended vinegars

With imagination and skill many other interesting flavors can be created using the method described above.
Try the following savory combinations:
1 part tarragon to 2 parts lemon balm
1 part basil to 2 parts salad burnet
1 part each of tarragon, basil, chives and 2 parts each of lemon thyme and salad burnet and 1 clove garlic.
1 part each crushed seed of anise, caraway, celery, coriander, cumin, dill, salad burnet and 1 clove garlic.

Floral bouquet vinegars: Follow the method described for savory blends using these combinations:
1 part lavender flowers to 1 part lemon verbena
1 part lavender flowers to 3 parts rose petals
1 part each clove pinks and rosemary, 2 parts each rose petals and elderflowers.

Pickled horseradish

Pick good-sized roots, wash and scrape off the skin. Mince in a food processor or grate and pack loosely into small jars. Cover with salted vinegar made from 1 teaspoon salt to 1 cup vinegar. Seal and leave for about a month before using.

Pickled alexanders buds

Pick young, dry buds and pack loosely in a small earthenware jar. Cover with boiling white wine vinegar and seal. Leave at least 2 weeks before using. Try this with green seeds of sweet cicely or dry elderflowers, picked as the flowers open.

You can adapt this recipe to make a sweet pickle using flowers such as rosebuds, violets, rosemary blooms or cowslips. Follow the same procedure but sprinkle sugar over each layer.

Pickled nasturtium seeds

These can be used as a substitute for capers. Pick nasturtium seeds on a dry day while they are still green. Steep in brine made from $\frac{1}{2}$ cup of salt to 1 quart of water for 24 hours. Remove and dry the seeds, then pack into small jars. Make a strong spiced vinegar to fill the jars, using white wine vinegar and salt and a selection from tarragon leaves, mace, nutmeg, shallots, garlic, peppercorns and horseradish slices. Pour the hot vinegar into the jars, then seal and leave for about a month. After opening the jar, use up the contents quickly.

Pickled cucumbers

about $2\frac{1}{2}$ lb small cucumbers, 3–5 inches long	$\frac{1}{3}$ cup coarse salt
	6 peppercorns
2 cloves garlic	1 cup white wine vinegar
2 dill flower heads with leaves	3 cups water

Makes approx. 2 quart jars

1 Scrub the cucumbers and soak overnight in salted cold water. Drain.

2 Place 1 clove garlic and a dill flower head in each sterilized jar.

3 Either leave the cucumbers whole or cut in quarters lengthways. Pack them into the jars.

4 Place the salt, pepper, vinegar and water in a saucepan and bring to the boil. Pour over the cucumbers. Seal, label and date. Store in a cool place for 6 weeks before using. Keep in the refrigerator once the jars have been opened.

From left to right: Savory herb jelly (p. 190); Rose petal jam (p. 190); Tarragon vinegar; Thyme oil; Basil oil; Lemon verbena vinegar; Lavender vinegar; Pickled cucumbers.

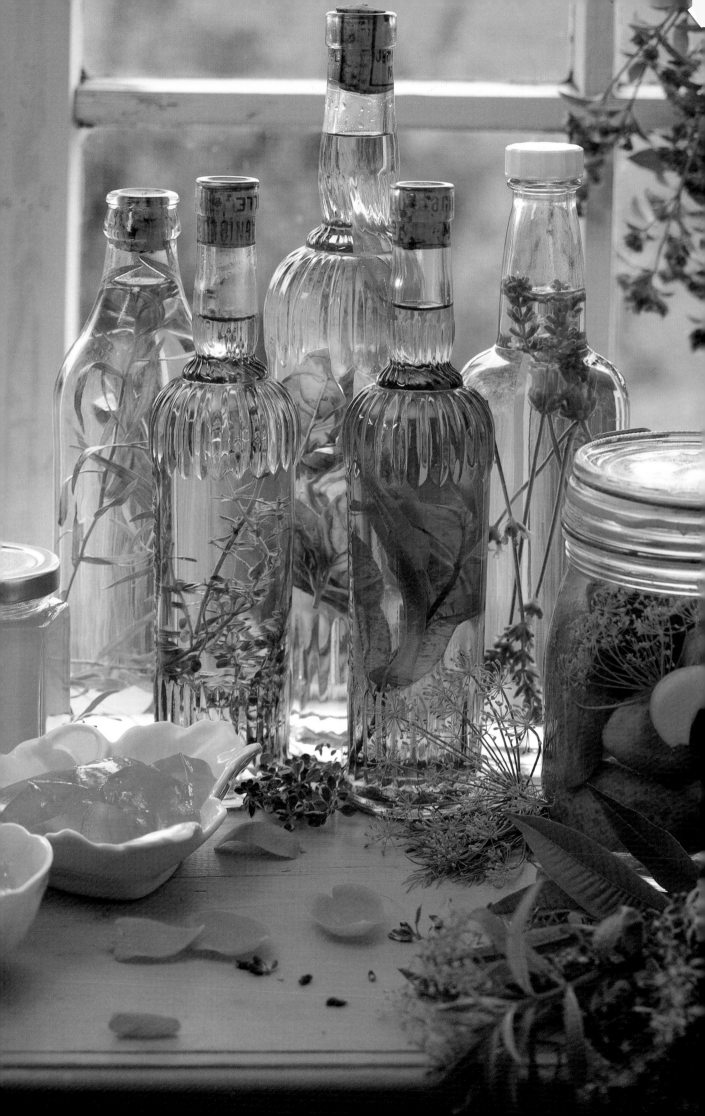

HERB BUTTERS

Herb butters are a delicious way of adding the full flavors of fresh herbs to savory snacks and dishes. Spread on sandwiches, toast and crackers; use to add piquancy to grilled meats and fish, and vegetables.

Try the blend below or make up your own. Choose from well-flavored herbs such as chervil, chives, garlic, parsley, rosemary, sage, salad burnet, tarragon and thyme.

Follow the same method, substituting soft cheeese for the butter to make a flavorsome spread.

Parsley and chive butter

2 tbsp chopped parsley juice of 1 lemon
1 tbsp chopped chives salt and black pepper
8 oz butter,
slightly softened

1 Beat the herbs into the butter and then add the lemon juice and seasoning. Mix until smooth.

2 Chill before serving. Shape in a mold if desired. Store in a cool place, or freeze in an ice-cube tray for handy portions.

JELLIES

The flavor of most aromatic herbs can be captured in a jelly to serve with cold meats, pâté, game, roasts, salads and sandwiches, and even to garnish soups and vegetables. An apple or crab-apple jelly makes a suitable base.

Savory herb jelly

4 lb tart cooking 1 cup wine vinegar
apples or crab apples, a good handful of fresh herbs
roughly chopped 1 cup sugar per cup
4 cups water of juice

Makes about 4 lb

1 Boil the cooking apples with the water and vinegar in a large preserving pan. Add the fresh herbs and simmer. Cook until the apples are soft. Strain through a jelly bag overnight.

2 Measure the juice, return to the saucepan and add the sugar. Stir to dissolve the sugar, then boil until setting point is reached, taking care not to let it boil over. Allow to cool a little for 10 minutes.

3 Pour into clean, sterilized jars and add a few leaves as decoration, if desired. Seal, label and date. Store in a cool, dark cupboard.

Sweet jelly

Follow the same procedure for sweet jellies but omit the vinegar and use 5 cups water.

HERBS FOR JELLY
Savory: basil, mint, rosemary, sage, savory, thyme
Sweet: bergamot, marigold (calendula), lavender flower petals, lemon balm, lemon verbena, scented geranium leaves (rose, apple, peppermint, lemon), sweet violet

Rose petal jam

1 lb heavily scented 2½ cups superfine sugar
red or pink rose petals juice of 2 lemons
2 cups water 1 tbsp rosewater

Makes approx. 2 × 1 pint jars

1 Remove the bitter white base from each petal. Rinse and drain the petals.

2 Bring the water to the boil in a large, heavy saucepan. Reduce to simmering point, then add the rose petals. (The mixture will froth up considerably so do not have the pan more than half full.) Simmer gently for 5 minutes, until the petals are soft.

3 Add the sugar and lemon juice. Bring back to the boil and simmer for about 30 minutes, stirring until the sugar has dissolved and the mixture begins to thicken. Add the rosewater.

4 Allow the mixture to bubble up well. When the bubbles have turned more to foam, test for setting point. To do this, first remove the pan from the heat. Put a spoonful of the jam on a cold saucer, allow to cool and push the surface; if it wrinkles it is ready.

5 Allow the jam to cool slightly, then pour into sterilized jars, label and seal.

CRYSTALLIZED FLOWERS AND LEAVES

Crystallized flowers and leaves can make wonderful decorations for cakes, desserts and summer drinks. The method is time-consuming but relaxing. Pick leaves or flowers on a sunny, dry day. Remove stalks and the white bases from petals, then commence.

Lightly beat an egg white until it starts to foam. Dip each flower or leaf into the egg white to coat, then dip it into a dish of caster sugar. Once coated, place on a sheet of wax paper on a wire cooling rack. Cover with another sheet of paper and place in a very low oven with the door left ajar. Store in an airtight tin when dry.

Flowers to crystallize

Borage, cowslips, lavender, lilac, pinks, primroses, rose petals, rosemary, sage

Leaves to crystallize

Bergamot, lemon balm, lemon verbena, mint

Crystallized angelica

1 lb angelica stalks 1 cup water
2½ cups sugar

1 Wash the stalks and cut them in 3 inch lengths. Boil in a little water until tender.

2 Drain, remove the outer skin and place in a shallow dish. Sprinkle the sugar, cover and leave on for 2 days.

3 Transfer into a pan with the water. Bring to the boil, stirring all the time. Simmer until all the syrup is absorbed and the stalks are clear. Drain and cool.

4 Sprinkle the stems with sugar to coat. Spread them out on a cake rack and allow to dry thoroughly. Store in airtight containers.

Herbal drinks

HERBAL TEAS

Teas made of aromatic leaves, flowers or roots steeped in boiling water are the most ancient and the most commonly consumed liquid after pure water. Most herb teas are infused: the leaves or flowers are put into a warm teapot, boiling water is poured over and the tea is brewed for 3–5 minutes. Alternatively, add 1 teaspoon of dried or 3 teaspoons of fresh herb to a cup of boiling water. Grind or pulverize seeds and root just before use and then make into a decoction; simmer 1 tablespoon of crushed root or seeds in 2 cups of boiling water until the water is reduced to 1 cup. This takes from 5–20 minutes, depending on the herb and herb part used.

Many people find herb teas bland by comparison with coffee and black tea but there are some intermediate steps you can take. Mix China tea with herbs or, to supply some of the "bite" we get from from regular tea and coffee, add dried leaves of raspberry, strawberry, or lady's mantle, which have a high tannin content.

Start with herbs which have strong, familiar flavors: anise, chamomile, lemon verbena, linden blossom, mint, rose hip and sage are all refreshing.

China tea blends

Infuse the herbs for 5 minutes in 2 cups boiling water, and strain before drinking.

Herbal "Earl Grey"

1 tsp China tea	3 tsp fresh young bergamot leaves

Spicy geranium

1 tsp China tea	(Also try 3 cloves with
1 stick cinnamon	rose geranium leaves)
3 apple geranium leaves	

Hibiscus

A pleasant lemony flavor with a beautiful amber-ruby color. Also refreshing as an iced tea.

1 tsp China tea	1 tsp hibiscus flowers

YOGURT DRINKS

These are nutritious, easy to digest and refreshing to drink. They can be savory or sweet.

Raspberry and mint yogurt drink

1 cup plain yogurt	1 tbsp raspberry syrup
$\frac{1}{2}$ cup mineral water	1 tsp mint syrup
3 oz raspberries or	

DECORATION
2 sprigs of mint

Serves 2

1 Purée all the ingredients in a blender.

2 Pour the drink into 2 glasses and decorate each with a sprig of mint. Serve chilled.

Angelica, mint and sweet cicely yogurt drink

2 cups plain yogurt	4 medium sweet
1 cup mineral water	cicely leaves
1 medium angelica leaf	1 tsp mint syrup

DECORATION
4 sprigs of mint

Serves 4

1 Purée all the ingredients in a blender.

2 Pour the drink into 4 glasses and decorate each with a sprig of mint. Serve chilled.

SYRUPS

Herb and fruit syrups are a convenient way of capturing a seasonal crop for year-round use. They can be diluted for drinks, poured over ice creams and desserts, and used as a base for jellies and sorbets.

Spearmint, lemon verbena, rose petals, apple, lemon or rose geranium, elderflowers, rose hips and all soft fruit and berries are suitable. For hips and fruit, leave in the jelly bag overnight to collect the juices.

Peppermint syrup

4 cups loosely packed	green food color
peppermint leaves	(optional)
white sugar	

1 Place the leaves in a saucepan with just enough water to cover. Simmer for 30 minutes.

2 Strain through a jelly bag for 1 hour.

3 For each cup of liquid, add 1 cup of sugar. Place the mixture in a pan and simmer for 15 minutes. Add food color, if using.

4 Bottle, label and date. Alternatively, freeze in convenient portions.

Lemon verbena and lime cordial

10 lemon verbena leaves	1 oz sugar
juice of 1 lemon	2 cups water
$\frac{1}{4}$ cup lime juice	

DECORATION
lemon verbena leaves	slices of lime
slices of lemon	

Makes about 2 cups

1 Either finely chop the lemon verbena leaves or pound in a pestle and mortar.

2 Place all the ingredients in a saucepan and heat until the sugar is dissolved, stirring. Leave to cool in the refrigerator for 2–3 hours or overnight.

3 Strain the drink and serve with ice cubes in tall glasses or a jug, decorated with lemon verbena leaves and lemon and lime slices.

HERBS AND ALCOHOL

Herbs have long been used to improve the flavor of alcoholic drinks. Some of the most exotic and revered liqueurs derive their character from herbal ingredients. Many of these are produced in monasteries and their recipes are a closely guarded secret. However, we know that benedictine and chartreuse both contain a huge range of herbal flavorings; crème de menthe is flavored with mint, and Kümmel with caraway and cumin. You can make your own by steeping a handful of fresh herb leaves in two cups of brandy or kirsch, following the method on p. 193.

Many aperitifs also contain herbs: anise flavors Pernod; wormwood flavors vermouth; and a range of bitter herbs characterize Campari.

Herbs make attractive garnishes in drinks and cocktails. Try freezing borage flowers or mint leaves in ice cubes to add to summer drinks.

HERBS FOR WINE CUPS
Angelica leaves (bestow a Muscatel flavor), bergamot leaves and flowers, borage leaves and flowers, clary sage leaves, lemon balm leaves, lemon verbena leaves, mint leaves (all varieties), rosemary leaves, salad burnet leaves, sweet woodruff leaves

From left to right: Loving cup; Herbal tea (p. 191); Spicy geranium tea (p. 191); Raspberry and mint yogurt drink (p. 191); Hock cup (p. 193); Lager cup (p. 193); Angelica, mint and sweet cicely yogurt drink (p. 191).

Mint julep

½ cup water	juice of 1 lemon
4 tbsp chopped mint leaves	1 cup club soda
	½ cup whisky
2 tbsp sugar	sprigs of mint

1 Bring the water to the boil and pour over the mint. Stir in the sugar until it dissolves. Leave to cool.

2 Add the lemon juice then strain. Just before serving, pour in the club soda and the whisky. Add a sprig of mint to each glass as decoration.

Loving cup

2 lemons	3½ cups water
6 sprigs of lemon balm	½ bottle dessert wine
6 sprigs and flowers of borage or viper's bugloss	½ cup good brandy
	1 bottle champagne or
½ cup sugar	sparkling dry white wine

DECORATION
borage flower ice cubes

1 Remove the thin rind (zest) from one of the lemons with a zester. Peel and thinly slice the lemons.

2 Put the lemon balm, borage, sliced lemon, lemon zest and sugar into a jug. Stir in the water, wine and brandy. Cover and chill for 1 hour.

3 Chill the champagne and mix in just before serving. Decorate with borage flower ice cubes.

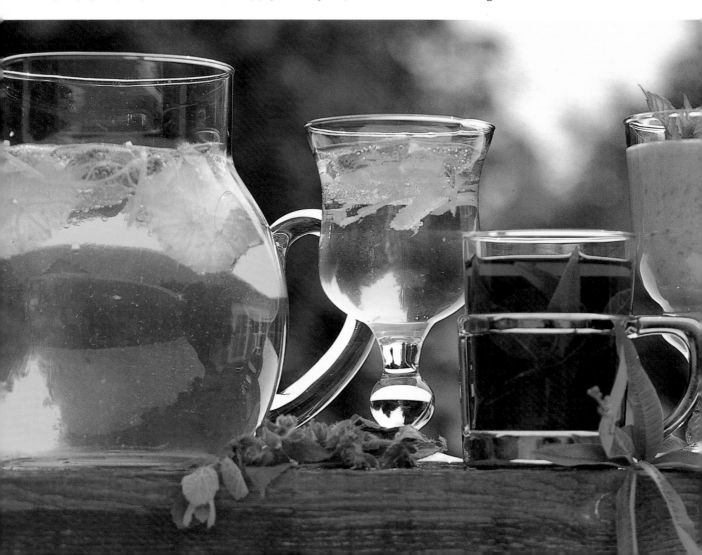

Four flower liqueur

4 cups brandy, vodka, kirsch or white eau de vie	8 oz clove pink petals
	8 oz orange blossoms or 3 oz dried orange blossoms
1 in piece cinnamon stick	
2 cloves	8 oz sweet violet flowers
8 oz scented rose petals, white heels removed	sugar to taste

Makes about 4 cups

1 Put the alcohol, spices and flowers in a large glass jar with a tight-fitting lid or cork. Place in a sunny or warm position to infuse for 1 month.

2 Filter through coffee filters. Add sugar, stirring until dissolved. Bottle in strong glass or pottery.

Hock cup

1 bottle hock (German dry white wine)	benedictine
6 cups club soda	finely grated rind of 1 lemon
1 liqueur glass brandy	finely grated rind of 1 orange
½ liqueur glass curaçao or	12 young salad burnet leaves
	sprinkling of calendula petals

1 Chill the hock and club soda for 1 hour.

2 Place the brandy, liqueur, lemon and orange rind and salad burnet leaves in a jug. Pour in the chilled hock, add the club soda and decorate with calendula petals. Serve immediately.

Lager cup

thinly peeled rind of 1 lemon	juice of 2 lemons
a few mint leaves	1 tbsp superfine sugar
pinch of grated nutmeg	crushed ice
2 tbsp vodka	1 cup club soda
½ cup water	3½ cups lager

Makes about 4 cups

1 Put the lemon rind, mint, nutmeg and vodka in a jug. Cover and steep for 20 minutes.

2 Add the water, lemon juice and sugar. Strain and add some crushed ice, the club soda and lager.

Elderflower fizz

Elderflowers must be picked on a dry, sunny day, as the yeast is mainly in the pollen.

5 quarts water	2 tbsp cider or wine vinegar
3½ cups sugar	
juice and thinly peeled rind of 1 lemon	12 elderflower heads

1 Bring the water to the boil. Pour into a sterilized container; add the sugar, stirring until dissolved.

2 When cool, add the juice and rind of the lemon, vinegar and elderflowers. Cover with several layers of cheesecloth and leave for 24 hours.

3 Filter through cheesecloth into strong bottles. This drink is ready after 2 weeks. Serve chilled.

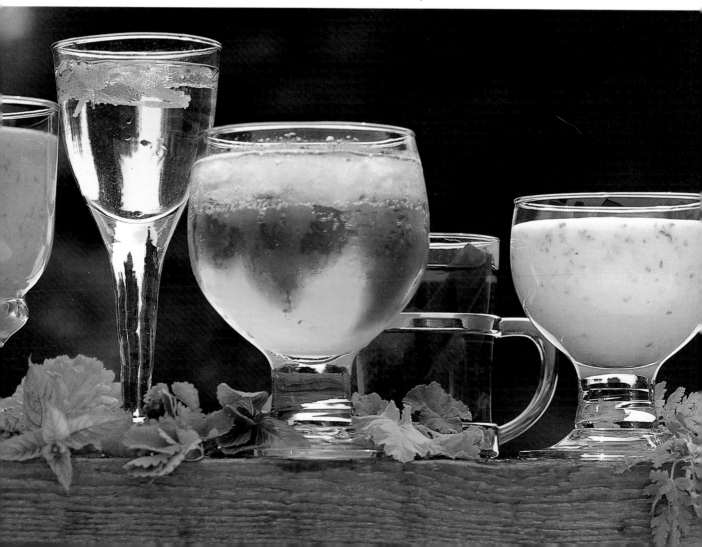

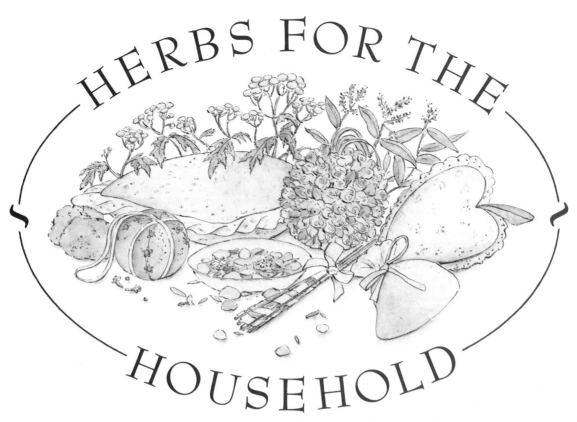

HERBS FOR THE HOUSEHOLD

In days gone by, herbs were central to the household economy. As well as being used to flavor and preserve food, and to make medicines for people and livestock, herbs were incorporated in roof thatch; used to cover floors; to clean, polish and disinfect utensils; and to sweeten and purify musty air.

Each nation used its native plants with creative ingenuity, and many still do. The Chinese use bamboo to make food, medicine, clothing, paper and pens, musical instruments and the intriguing bamboo wife – a basketwork cylinder designed to bring solace on hot summer nights, as the sleeper embraces it and receives the cooling breezes that pass through its frame. To give another example, North American Indians use birch bark to make canoes, baskets, documents, snowshoes, medicine, syrup, tea and – as the bark prevents decay – to wrap meat and embalm the dead.

Tudor stillroom
In Tudor England so many activities centered around processing and preserving herbs that a special room, the stillroom, was set aside for this purpose. Here a small still made spirits for medicinal purposes as well as floral waters, like lavender water, to scent the laundry. Herbs were dried and tucked into clothes chests to protect and perfume linen, or added to wax to make aromatic furniture polish. Roots and seeds of angelica were dried for burning on a chafing pan to disinfect a room. Leaves and berries were collected to dye wool.

Favorite and valued recipes were passed along from mother to daughter taking the form of "A household book of receipts," and new skills were always welcomed. When a certain Mistress Dinghen arrived in England from Holland in the sixteenth century, Elizabethan ruffs were in vogue. She found many customers who were willing to pay her to teach them the art of making and using perfumed starch.

Perhaps the most pleasurable stillroom activity for the lady of the household was the blending of herbs, flowers and spices to make potpourri. She would escape to her warm and private stillroom, rich in sweet and pungent aromas, and gather together the aromatic leaves and flowers dried through the summer, remembering the day and the circumstances when each was picked; then she would measure and blend until she had created a mixture that pleased her.

Modern uses
It is not only historical interest or nostalgia that makes the idea of using herbs attractive to us today. Herbal dyes are still unsurpassed for subtlety of color, and aromatic herbs contain antiseptic oils useful in cleaning.

But beyond this, the fresh fragrance of herbs has a way of pushing our thoughts past the strictly utilitarian. To fold sheets scented with lavender water or to polish furniture with sweet marjoram-scented wax makes a chore into a pleasure. Perhaps it reminds us of the seasons or gives us a sense of continuity with the past. Whatever the reason, herbalists through the ages have told us that fresh sweet scents will lift our spirits, and modern research confirms this assertion.

Herbal household products

HERBS FOR CONTROLLING PESTS

Herbs can be used effectively to keep unwanted insects and mice at bay. They have the advantage over chemical poisons of being completely safe, which is especially important in the kitchen and other places where food is kept.

Ants Place sprigs of pennyroyal, rue or tansy on shelves or in cupboards to deter ants. Disturb the leaves occasionally to release more scent. This doesn't kill ants, but it encourages them to go away.

Flies Many herbs help to deter flies, including elder, lavender, mint, mugwort, peppermint, pennyroyal, rue and southernwood (but see also p. 210). Use them in arrangements, wreaths or potpourri. Hang pieces of sticky elecampane root around windows and doors.

Fleas and lice Burn the leaves of common fleabane (*Pulicaria dysenterica*), ploughman's spikenard (*Inula conyza*), mugwort or wormwood on an open fire over low embers, to destroy fleas and lice. Encourage the fumes to fill the room but try to avoid breathing them.

Mice Mint and tansy in your store cupboard will deter mice.

Preserving wraps Wrap dried nettle leaves around stored apples and pears, root vegetables and moist cheeses to preserve them and keep off pests. The wraps will keep vegetables and fruit skins smooth and moist for 2 or 3 months. Wrap figs in mullein leaves to preserve them.

Strewing In the Middle Ages, herbs were often strewn on the floor to repel fleas, lice, moths and insect pests. They also masked unsavory smells and provided insulation against the cold in winter and the heat in summer. This practice is unsuitable today, but sprigs of herbs can be placed under doormats or carpets, or perhaps on the porch. Choose from the following:

balm, basil, chamomile, costmary, cowslip, daisies, fennel, germander, hop, marjoram, meadowsweet, mint, pennyroyal, pine, rose, rosemary, sage, southernwood, sweet flag, sweet woodruff, tansy, thuja, thyme, sweet violet or winter savory.

Wasps Burn dried leaf of *Eupatorium cannabinum* to drive away wasps.

Weevils Place a few bay leaves in flour and rice bins, and among dried pulses, to prevent weevils.

HOUSE CLEANING

These herbal products make polishing and cleaning an aromatic pleasure. They are also kinder to your skin and to the environment than many chemical household cleansers.

Lemon disinfectant Mix 6 drops of essential oil of lemon with 1 teaspoon of isopropyl alcohol (to aid dispersal), and add to 2 quarts of tepid water (hot water would make the oils evaporate too quickly). You can also use essential oils of tea tree, thyme, orange, bergamot, juniper, clove, lavender, niaouli, peppermint, rosemary, sandalwood or eucalyptus – listed in descending order of their antiseptic powers.

Rosemary disinfectant Simmer some leaves and small stems for 30 minutes in water; the less water, the more concentrated the disinfectant will be. Strain and use to clean sinks and bathrooms or to give a fresh scent to rooms. Add dishwashing detergent to get rid of grease on surfaces. Store any excess in the refrigerator for up to one week. Disinfectants can also be made with the leaves and flowering stems of eucalyptus, juniper, lavender, sage and thyme, and with angelica roots.

Scouring pad The precursors of steel wool, horsetail stems (*Equisetum arvense* or *E. hyemale*) have a fine sandpaper surface of silica crystals which will clean pots and pans. Rub a handful of dried, leafless stems on surfaces, then rinse to remove any residual green stains.

Metal polish Make a strong infusion of fresh horsetail, using 1 ounce to $2\frac{1}{2}$ cups of water. Soak for at least 2 hours, then simmer in the same water for 15 minutes and strain. Pour the infusion over metal articles and soak them for 5 minutes. Remove the articles and allow them to dry slowly; then polish with a soft cloth. If the article is too large to soak, simply wipe it with a cloth dipped in the solution, allow it to dry, then polish with a soft cloth.

Sweet marjoram furniture wax

4 oz beeswax	1 tbsp olive oil-based soap
$2\frac{1}{2}$ cups turpentine	essential oil of sweet
$1\frac{1}{2}$ cups strong infusion of sweet marjoram	marjoram (optional)

1 Grate the beeswax into the turpentine and leave to dissolve, which may take a few days. Alternatively, warm the beeswax and turpentine carefully over a flameless heat until the wax melts. Turpentine can easily burst into flames, so it's safest to warm it over boiling water.

2 In a separate pan, bring the infusion to boiling point and stir in the grated soap until melted.

3 Allow both mixtures to cool, then blend slowly, stirring until it resembles thick cream. Stir in a few drops of essential oil. Pour into a wide-mouth container and label.

Leaves of mock orange, lemon balm, lemon verbena, or rosemary, or lavender flowers, can be used instead of sweet marjoram.

Sweet cicely polish Pound aromatic, fresh, soft sweet cicely seeds in a mortar. Pick up a handful in a cloth and rub on wood as a polish.

Herbal dyes

Plant dyes are unsurpassed for richness and subtlety of color, and often have an individual fragrance too. They are created by boiling fresh or dried pigment plants in water; the material is then put in the dye bath, as described on p. 198. Dyes take best on wool and silk, but can be used on unbleached cotton or linen with a more complex process; they do not color synthetics, except rayon. The white fleece, spun wool, silk cloth and silk thread shown here have been dyed with light-fast and wash-fast herbal colors. Each batch has been dyed in the same dye bath and displays the range of tones obtainable on different materials.

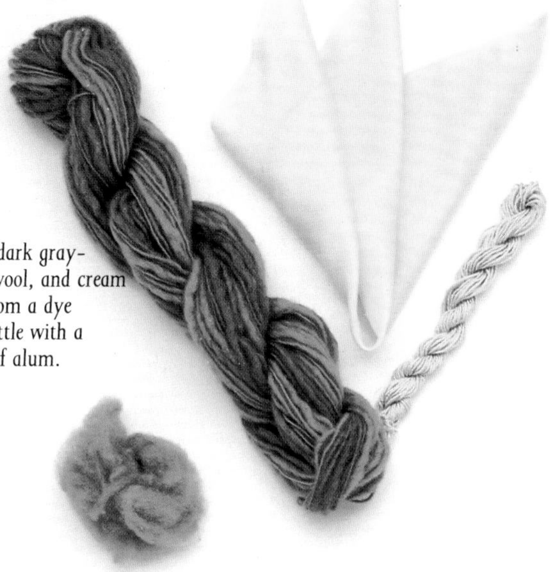

Nettle
Shades of dark gray-green on wool, and cream on silk, from a dye bath of nettle with a mordant of alum.

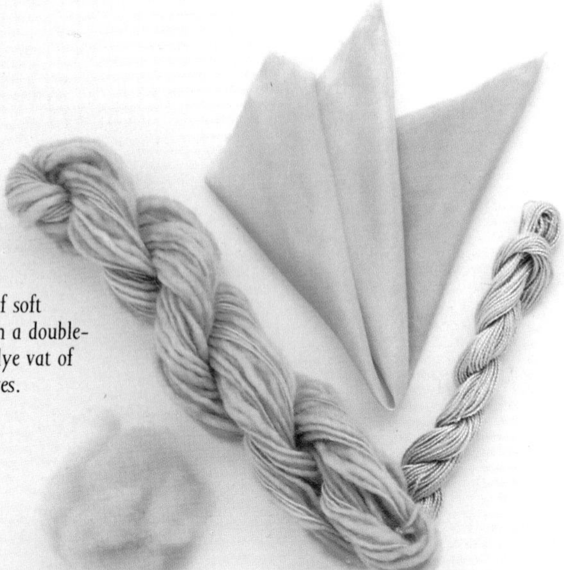

Woad
A range of soft blues from a double-strength dye vat of woad leaves.

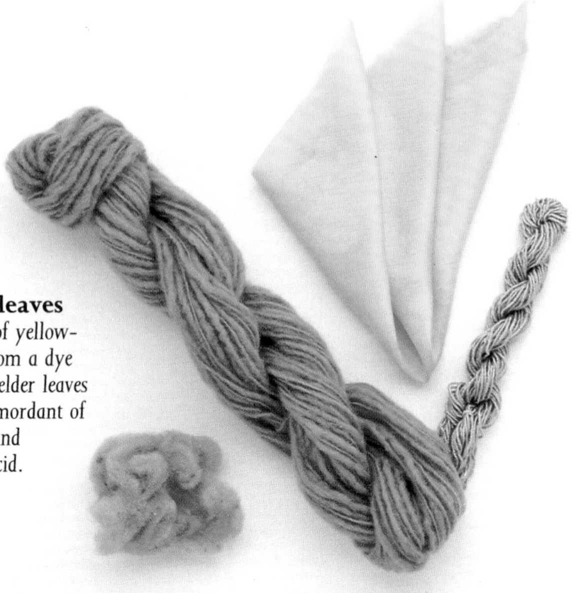

Elder leaves
Shades of yellow-green from a dye bath of elder leaves with a mordant of copper and acetic acid.

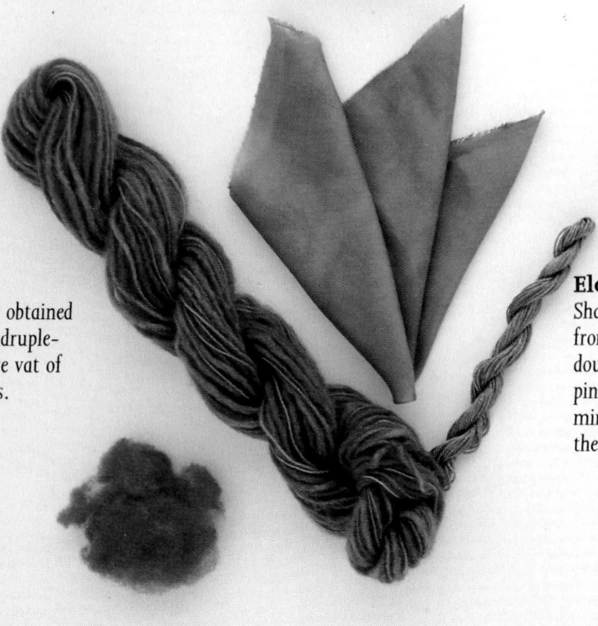

Woad
A rich blue obtained from a quadruple-strength dye vat of woad leaves.

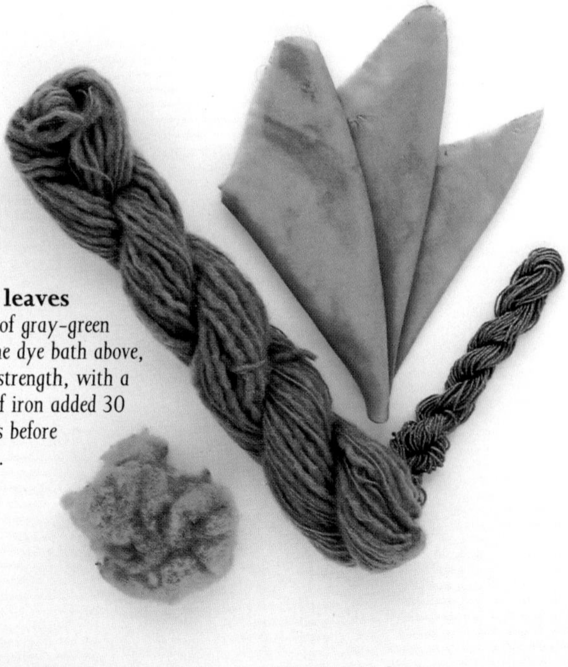

Elder leaves
Shades of gray-green from the dye bath above, double strength, with a pinch of iron added 30 minutes before the end.

Bramble shoots
Shades of oatmeal from a dye bath of bramble shoots with a mordant of alum and cream of tartar.

Alkanet root
Shades of pink-brown from a dye bath of alkanet root with acetic acid.

**Weld
(Dyer's rocket)**
Soft green-yellows from a dye bath of weld plant with a mordant of copper and acetic acid.

Onion skins
Rich browns from a dye bath of red onion skins with a mordant of copper and acetic acid.

Chamomile
Bright yellow-gold from a dye bath of dyer's chamomile flowers with a mordant of alum and cream of tartar.

Madder root
Rich russet-red from a dye bath of madder root with a mordant of alum and cream of tartar.

Making herbal dyes

No two batches of herbal dyes will be identical: the final color depends on the plant variety used, how much sunlight the plant received when growing, the chemicals in the water, the type of pan used (iron, copper and aluminum can alter the color), the mordant, or fixative (see the box at right), and the immersion time. This unpredictability restricts large-scale commercial use of herbal dyes but adds interest to home experiments.

There is an optimum time to pick each herb, usually when it is about to flower, or for roots, in autumn (see p. 269). Use the same weight of herb as the weight of wool to be dyed; for silk, use twice the weight.

EQUIPMENT FOR HOME DYEING

Glass rod or wooden dowels
Pestle and mortar
Pillowcase or muslin bag
Rubber gloves
Sink or buckets for rinsing
Stainless steel or unchipped
enamel bath or large pan to use as a dye bath
Thermometer
Water, soft or filtered, or rainwater
Weighing scale

PROCEDURE FOR DYEING

Dyeing with herbs is a time-consuming but fascinating process. The fabric must be prepared to receive the dyes, which involves scouring and mordanting, and the dyes have to be extracted from the herbs. The process is explained below.

Avoid exposing wool and silk to sudden changes in temperature. For instance, when lifting wool from a hot bath, don't put it on a cold surface. Always handle wool very gently. To dry wool at any stage for storage, tumble dry in a muslin bag on a no-heat program; always dry away from direct heat. If you dry wool after scouring, you must wet it again in 6 quarts of water at 120–125 °F with a drop of dishwashing detergent for an hour before mordanting.

Scouring

Soak wool for several hours or overnight in 5 gallons of water at 120–125 °F with 1 tablespoon of liquid detergent or a proprietary scouring agent to remove oil. Squeeze the wool gently, remove, then repeat. Give a final rinse in warm water with $\frac{1}{4}$ cup of vinegar. Follow the same procedure for silk but have the water at 195 °F.

Mordanting

Dissolve the mordant in a little hot water, then stir into 5 gallons of water at 120–125 °F. Submerge the wet wool. Take an hour to bring to the boil and simmer at 180–200 °F for a further hour. Immerse silk at 140 °F and steep for 24 hours. Then rinse and dye immediately in a prepared dye bath.

MORDANTS

Color is influenced by the choice of mordant. A mordant (from the Latin *mordere*, to bite) is used to help "fix" the dye. Some common mordants are listed below; they are available from pharmacies or dye suppliers. Quantities recommended are for use with 1 pound of dry wool:

● **Alum** (aluminum potassium sulfate); 1 oz. Often combined with cream of tartar (tartaric acid); $\frac{3}{4}$ oz. Alum gives bright, clear colors.
● **Iron** (ferrous sulfate); $\frac{1}{8}$ oz. Dulls and deepens colors and is called a "saddening" agent. Use alum first, add wool to the dye bath, simmer for 45 minutes, remove the wool, add the iron, replace the wool and simmer for a further 30 minutes.
● **Copper** (copper sulfate); $\frac{1}{2}$ oz with 1 cup vinegar gives a blue-green tint to colors. Copper is poisonous, so handle it with care.
● **Chrome and tin**; Chrome gives color depth and greater permanence, and tin brightens tones. Both are poisonous and require careful handling.

Dye bath

Chop or crush the plant material. Place loosely in a muslin bag and soak in 5 gallons of tepid soft water overnight. Then simmer at 180–200 °F for about 1–3 hours, until the desired color is reached. Remove the herbs, cool the liquid to hand heat, and gently add the wool. Take 1 hour to return to a simmer and simmer for a further hour. Leave to cool to hand heat, then remove the wool or silk and rinse in warm, tepid and finally cold water. Leave silk to cool overnight, then rinse. Hang to dry.

Woad (or indigo) dye bath

(for 1 pound wool)
Woad and indigo require a different process to yield their rich blue dyes. Pick 4 pounds of fresh leaves, chop and boil in 20 quarts of water for 7 minutes. Strain, squeeze the leaves and discard. Cool the liquor and add a few drops of liquid ammonia. Aerate by whisking or pouring liquid from one bucket to another for 10–15 minutes until the froth becomes pale blue. Warm the liquor until hand hot. Sprinkle 2 teaspoons of sodium dithionite (obtainable from a pharmacist or craft shop) over its surface to remove oxygen; do not stir. This turns the dye yellow. Leave to stand for 30 minutes to cool to room temperature.

Wet the wool in water with a pinch of sodium dithionite, then slide it very gently into the dye so no air enters. Soak for 20 minutes. Remove gently and catch any drips with a cloth so they will not oxidize the water. Shake out and hang the wool for 10–15 minutes and watch it turn blue. Add more sodium dithionite and repeat 3 to 6 times. Finally, wash in soapy water at the same temperature, rinse and dry.

DYE HERB CHART

The chart below provides a selection of dye-yielding herbs and tells you which part of the plant to use ("whole plant" means all the parts above ground), and which mordant combination to use for specific colors.

COMMON NAME	BOTANIC NAME	PLANT PART USED	MORDANT	COLOR
Agrimony	Agrimonia eupatoria	flowering tops	alum	butter yellow
Alkanet	Anchusa officinalis	root	acetic acid	soft pink-brown
Bearberry	Arctostaphylos uva-ursi	dried leaves	alum	violet gray
Bearberry	Arctostaphylos uva-ursi	dried leaves	iron	charcoal black
Blackberry	Rubus species	young shoots	alum	creamy fawn
Bloodroot	Sanguinaria canadensis	root	alum	reddish orange
Bracken	Pteridium aquilinum	young shoots	alum	yellowish green
Coltsfoot	Tussilago farfara	whole plant	alum	green-yellow
Comfrey	Symphytum officinale	fresh green plant	alum	yellow
Chamomile, dyer's	Anthemis tinctoria	flowers	alum & cream of tartar	bright yellow
Chamomile, dyer's	Anthemis tinctoria	flowers	copper, acetic acid	olive
Dog's mercury	Mercurialis perennis	plant tops	alum	grayish yellow
Dyer's greenweed	Genista tinctoria	flowering tops	alum	yellow
Elder	Sambucus nigra	leaves	alum & cream of tartar	greenish yellow
Elder	Sambucus nigra	leaves	copper, acetic acid	olive (pinch of iron for gray green)
Elder	Sambucus nigra	berries	alum, salt	purple
Heather	Calluna vulgaris	young tips	alum	yellow
Heather	Calluna vulgaris	fresh branches	alum, pinch of iron	green
Horsetail	Equisetum arvense	fresh sterile stems	alum	creamy yellow
Juniper	Juniperus communis	crushed berries, fresh	alum	strong yellow
Juniper	Juniperus communis	crushed berries, dried	alum, cream of tartar, copper	olive-brown
Lady's bedstraw	Galium verum	roots	alum	coral pink
Madder	Rubia tinctorum	roots	alum, cream of tartar	rich tomato red
Marigold	Calendula officinalis	petals	alum, cream of tartar	pale yellow
Meadowsweet	Filipendula ulmaria	roots	alum	black
Nettle	Urtica dioica	whole plant	alum, cream of tartar, pinch of iron	greeny gray
Nettle	Urtica dioica	whole plant	copper	soft gray green
Onion	Allium cepa	skins	alum, cream of tartar	orange
Onion	Allium cepa	skins	copper, acetic acid	deep brassy yellow (tan on silk)
Parsley	Petroselinum crispum	fresh leaves, & stems	alum	cream
Privet	Ligustrum vulgare	leaves, young shoots	alum	strong yellows
Privet	Ligustrum vulgare	ripe berries	alum	grayish green
Safflower	Carthamus tinctorius	flowers	alum	yellows & tan
St John's wort	Hypericum perforatum	flowers	alum	beige
Sorrel	Rumex acetosa	whole plant	alum	grayish yellow
Sorrel	Rumex acetosa	roots	alum	soft pink
Tansy	Tanacetum vulgare	flowering tops	alum	mustard yellow
Turmeric	Curcuma longa	powdered root	alum	gold-orange
Walnut	Juglans regia	leaves	no mordant	creamy fawn
Walnut	Juglans regia	green husks & shells	no mordant	light to dark browns
Weld	Reseda luteola	whole plant	alum	lemon yellow
Weld	Reseda luteola	whole plant	copper, acetic acid	green-yellow
Woad	Isatis tinctoria	leaves	sodium dithionite, ammonia	blue
Yew	Taxus baccata	heartwood chips	alum	orange-brown

Herbal papers

Paper can be scented with herbs, decorated with herbs, have herbs embedded in its fibers and even be made exclusively from herbs.

The cellulose in plants forms the raw material for paper, and herbs such as nettles, chamomile, dandelions and fennel all yield fibrous pulps. However, successful paper-making from herbs requires dedication, time and space. A simpler route is to recycle existing paper, adding herb leaves and petals when mixing the pulp, as described on p. 202. Some results are shown here. Each sheet of recycled herb paper will have its own character; no two are ever alike. Even the two surfaces have distinctive qualities, one being smooth and one having more texture, allowing scope for endless experimentation.

Use these textured herbal papers for mounting drawings or photographs; as a base for pressed herb and flower collages, or for charcoal, crayon or watercolor work.

You can also enhance your personal letters by adding the fragrance of lavender or a herb sachet to a box of writing paper. For a more subtle effect, scent ink as described on p. 203.

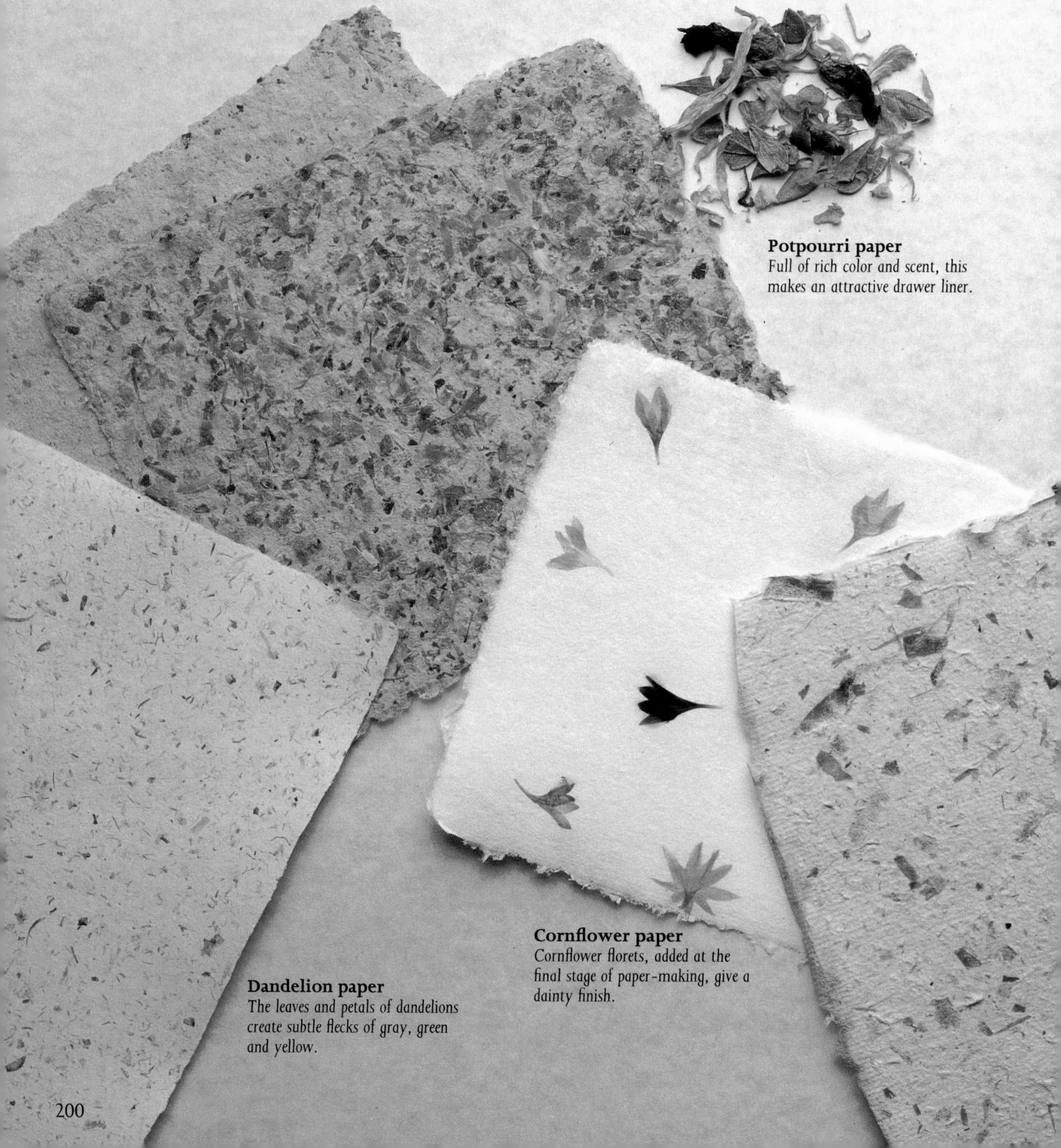

Potpourri paper
Full of rich color and scent, this makes an attractive drawer liner.

Cornflower paper
Cornflower florets, added at the final stage of paper-making, give a dainty finish.

Dandelion paper
The leaves and petals of dandelions create subtle flecks of gray, green and yellow.

Lavender paper
Scent a box of writing paper with grains of lavender or other sweet-smelling herbs.

Scented ink
Add fragrance to ordinary ink with a decoction of lavender, rosemary or lemon verbena.

Sunflower stem paper
The pale gold fibers of dried sunflower stems are embedded in the pulp.

Fern paper
Dried fern leaves add an earthy accent to a delicate paper.

Onion skin paper
Crushed onion skins add subtle tints of mauve and burgundy.

Petal paper
Delicate petals from lavender, rose and other garden flowers make a colorful addition.

Hop vine paper
A fine-textured paper with silver-gray speckles.

Making herbal papers and ink

The Chinese invented paper-making around 105
A.D. using flax with tree bark, and paper is still
made from the cellulose fibers of plants. Excellent
herbs are flax, straw, nettles and rush. Others of
use are bamboo, broom, chamomile, cow parsley,
dandelion, dill, fennel, iris, mullein, pampas grass,
sunflower and most cereal grasses.

EQUIPMENT

For making plant pulp
3 gallon bucket
Pestle and mortar or mallet
12 quart stainless steel or
galvanized pan
Rubber gloves

Wooden spoon
Metal sieve
Strong nylon net bag
Blender

For making paper
Large plastic basin
Wooden frames, $8\frac{1}{2} \times 11$ or
$8\frac{1}{2} \times 14$ inches square, with
waterproof joints and strong
net stapled taut

One extra frame
of the same size, without
netting
Newspapers

Preparing plant pulp

3 gallons fresh herbs   2 tbsp caustic soda
1 quart water

1 Gather a 3 gallon bucketful of herbs and cut or tear
them into 1–2 inch square pieces. Crush thick pieces
with a mallet or a pestle and mortar to speed the
breakdown process.

2 Put 1 quart cold water into a stainless steel pan and
stir in the caustic soda, using a wooden spoon. Avoid
breathing the fumes, wear rubber gloves and rinse off
any splashes with cold water immediately. Add the
herbs, cover with extra warm water if necessary and
mix well. Simmer for $1\frac{1}{2}$–2 hours, or until the plant
fibers feel soft.

3 Rinse the plants thoroughly to remove all traces of
caustic soda. Then strain them through a metal sieve.

4 Gather the pulp (much reduced) into a net bag and
rinse in water, squeezing the fibers repeatedly for
several minutes.

5 Blend $2\frac{1}{2}$ tablespoons of the fibers with 3 cups water
for 20 seconds. The more finely the plant fibers are
blended, the finer the paper will be. This pulp can be
used as it is or added to recycled paper pulp.

6 Writing paper needs to be treated or "sized" to
receive ink. Mix $\frac{1}{5}$ teaspoon cold-water laundry starch
with a little water and stir into the pulp.

Recycled paper pulp

You can use old papers to make fresh paper, which
you can then embellish with herbal additives or
mix with plant pulp. Try absorbent papers such as
newspaper, wallpaper, blotting paper or computer
printout. Soak small pieces of paper overnight in
warm water. Blend $2\frac{1}{2}$ tablespoons paper with
3 cups water for 15 seconds. "Size" as above.

Making paper

pulp (recycled paper, plant or mixed)

optional additions
flowers, petals, stalks, essential oil

1 Fill the plastic basin with pulp to just below the rim.

2 Place the empty wooden frame over a netted frame,
hold together and dip vertically into the basin. Tilt to
horizontal below the water, and raise slowly, keeping
the frame horizontal.

3 Lay on newspaper to drain. Remove the empty top
frame, scatter on petals or leaves for decoration and
leave the pulp to dry.

4 When completely dry, slide a palette knife under the
sheet to loosen it from the frame. Clean the frame and
reuse, following the same process.

Scented paper

Scent paper by storing it with aromatic herbs in an
enclosed space. Lay lavender bundles or envelopes
of your favorite herb blend in a box of writing
paper. Wallpaper absorbs scent well and can be
used to line drawers. Slip thin muslin bags of
potpourri laced with extra essential oils between
layers of drawer-lining paper, roll up and cover
with plastic wrap for 6 weeks to scent.

Paper decorations

Press flowers of borage, daisy, forget-me-not,
primrose or sweet violet; leaves of alpine lady's
mantle, chervil, pelargonium or salad burnet; or
sprigs of lemon thyme, rosemary or myrtle
between sheets of blotting paper or newsprint in a
heavy book. When they are dried, use a small
amount of latex-based glue to fix the herbs to
writing paper, greeting cards and gifts.

MAKING INK

Black ink is made from pigments that are dark and
contain tannin which prevents fading. These can
be found in oak galls (formed by some oak trees)
and in the bark of blackthorn, alder and dogwood.
A red ink can be made from field poppy petals, as
described opposite. Alternatively, you can scent
inks with fragrant herbal infusions.

Scented oak gall ink

This recipe is adapted from an eleventh-century recipe.

8 oz bruised oak galls
$2\frac{1}{2}$ quarts boiling
water or herbal decoction
a few drops of essential oil

a few drops of tincture of myrrh
$1\frac{1}{2}$ oz gum arabic
3 oz sulfate of iron
(ferrous sulfate)

1 Steep the galls in water for 24 hours. Strain.

2 Add essential oil to the tincture of myrrh, then add
the gum arabic.

3 Stir this with the sulfate of iron into the gall
infusion. Bottle and label.

Scented ink

Give ink a sweeter fragrance with an infusion of strongly scented herbs.

1 oz dried aromatic flowers or leaves (lavender flowers; lemon verbena, rose geranium, rosemary, or sweet myrtle leaves)
½ cup water
1 small bottle of ink

1 Immerse the herbs in the water, bring to the boil and simmer for 30–45 minutes, covered. Take care that the mixture does not boil dry, but reduce the decoction to make about 4 teaspoons of strong-smelling dark liquid.

2 Strain, allow to cool and mix with the ink.

Red ink

Take 1 cup field poppy petals and pour on a small amount of boiling water, just enough to cover the petals. Steep overnight. Add 15 percent isopropyl alcohol to preserve. Strain and bottle.

Herbal toys and trinkets

Children and adults alike will love these scented beads and quaint, fragrant toys. They are fun to make, whatever your age, and are excellent gifts.

Aromatic beads

(makes 75 pea-sized beads)
Paint the finished beads or tint them with food coloring to make them more decorative.

1½ tbsp each of powdered orris root, sweet flag and basil
1 tbsp each of powdered gum benzoin, cinnamon and mace
½ tsp ground cloves
½ nutmeg, freshly grated
3 drops of essential oil of sandalwood
3 drops of essential oil of cedarwood
3 drops of essential oil of myrrh
1 tsp gum tragacanth powder
3–4 tbsp triple-strength rosewater

1 Mix the dry herbs and spices and add the oils, stirring gently.

2 Mix the gum tragacanth with 3 tablespoons of the rosewater and stir into the first mixture to form a paste. Add more rosewater if necessary.

3 Damp your hands with rosewater and roll the paste into beads. To increase their scent, use a darning needle dipped in essential oil to pierce the beads and thread onto strong oiled thread. Dry slowly. Paint with food dyes or ink.

Rose beads

Place finely chopped scented red and pink rose petals in a saucepan – a rusty pan will give a rich dark color. Barely cover with water and heat for 1 hour but keep below boiling point. Cool for 24 hours. Repeat four times. Damp your hands with rosewater, roll the pulp into beads, pressing hard, and then roll in powdered spices (cinnamon, cloves, nutmeg). Thread with a darning needle onto thick thread and dry in a warm place. Originally, rosaries were made with 165 rose petal beads.

Herbal dough toys

Combine 2 parts all-purpose white flour with one part salt and one part of strong herbal infusion. Knead for at least 5 minutes into a smooth pliable dough. Working on a piece of greaseproof paper, shape the dough into a flat-backed doll (use a cookie-cutter or a cut-out as a guide if it helps). Make some hair for the doll by pushing dough through a sieve or cutting thin strands, and shape an apron with a pocket, or form clasped hands to push dried herbs into. When joining the pieces of dough, moisten each end before pressing together. Transfer the paper, with dough, to a cookie sheet. Bake at 300 °F for 1 hour. Cool and apply paint sealer or thick acrylic paints. Dry thoroughly and varnish. Sprinkle essential oil onto the surface.

Alternatively, make a basket with a flat slab back and a shallow, curved, latticework front. Braid a handle and insert a wire in the back of the base as a hanging hook. Bake and finish as described above. Hang and fill with dried herbs.

Spiced apple granny doll

This may seem a slightly gruesome idea, but children seem to love it. Peel a firm cooking apple. Carve a face in the flesh, then soak and keep submerged in brine (5 percent salt by volume) overnight. Remove, drain, and mount on a wooden dowel. Add cloves for eyes and a cloth headscarf. Dress the dowel body and add an apron with pockets containing different spices such as cardamoms, coriander seed and nutmegs. As the apple face dries it wrinkles and "ages."

Lavender Bo-Peep mobile

This is a delightful idea for a mobile in a child's bedroom based on a nursery-rhyme character.

Make a small cloth doll and stuff the body with lavender; then make a few cloth sheep, and fill each with aromatic herbs. Make a circular hoop with wire and use nylon thread to hang the doll and sheep at different heights. The movement of the mobile will spread the soothing fragrance of herbs and lavender around the bedroom.

Toys

Aromatic stuffed toys and animal-shaped herb pillows delight children and bring comfort at night or during periods of illness.

Potpourri

The traditional way to capture the essence of a summer herb garden and bring it indoors is to make a potpourri, a mixture of fragrant, colorful flowers and leaves displayed in a bowl.

Potpourri has become a term for many aromatic mixtures, but the original French means "rotten pot," a moist mixture of pickled flowers and leaves. This older, "moist" method gives a longer-lasting perfume but it is more difficult to do and visually less attractive. The dry method is popular as it is easier and the colorful result can be displayed in bowls or potpourri balls, and used in herb pillows.

The basic ingredients fall into four categories: flowers for scent or color; aromatic leaves; spices and peel; and fixatives to preserve the blend. Many herbs are available as essential oils, a great asset to modern mixtures, but they must be used with discretion to avoid dominating subtler scents.

The leisurely activity of creating the mixture, focusing intently on scent and color, gives as much pleasure as the finished product. As you become familiar with your herbs and their seasons, you can preserve a few leaves here and a few blossoms there, slowly building up a store of aromatic ingredients. When you wish to create a mixture, assemble your aromas and consider how each will blend and harmonize with the others.

The recipes on p. 207 provide guidelines, but experience is the best teacher.

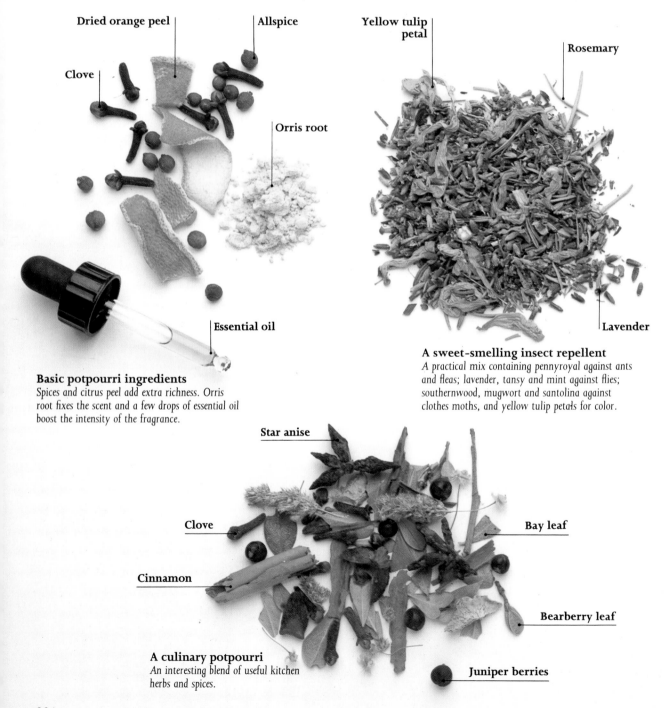

Dried orange peel | **Allspice**

Clove

Orris root

Essential oil

Basic potpourri ingredients
Spices and citrus peel add extra richness. Orris root fixes the scent and a few drops of essential oil boost the intensity of the fragrance.

Yellow tulip petal | **Rosemary**

Lavender

A sweet-smelling insect repellent
A practical mix containing pennyroyal against ants and fleas; lavender, tansy and mint against flies; southernwood, mugwort and santolina against clothes moths, and yellow tulip petals for color.

Star anise

Clove | **Bay leaf**

Cinnamon

Bearberry leaf

A culinary potpourri
An interesting blend of useful kitchen herbs and spices.

Juniper berries

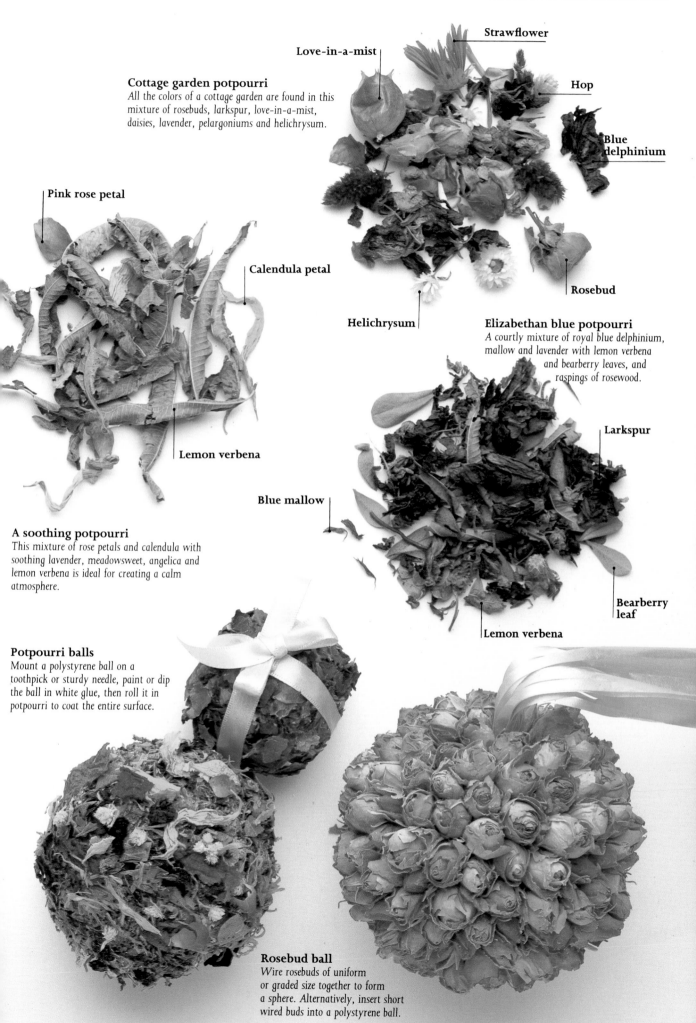

Strawflower

Love-in-a-mist

Hop

Blue delphinium

Cottage garden potpourri
All the colors of a cottage garden are found in this mixture of rosebuds, larkspur, love-in-a-mist, daisies, lavender, pelargoniums and helichrysum.

Pink rose petal

Calendula petal

Rosebud

Helichrysum

Elizabethan blue potpourri
A courtly mixture of royal blue delphinium, mallow and lavender with lemon verbena and bearberry leaves, and raspings of rosewood.

Larkspur

Lemon verbena

Blue mallow

A soothing potpourri
This mixture of rose petals and calendula with soothing lavender, meadowsweet, angelica and lemon verbena is ideal for creating a calm atmosphere.

Bearberry leaf

Lemon verbena

Potpourri balls
Mount a polystyrene ball on a toothpick or sturdy needle, paint or dip the ball in white glue, then roll it in potpourri to coat the entire surface.

Rosebud ball
Wire rosebuds of uniform or graded size together to form a sphere. Alternatively, insert short wired buds into a polystyrene ball.

205

Making potpourri

INGREDIENTS

To blend your own potpourri, select ingredients from each of the categories below. Use one of the recipes opposite as a guide for quantities.

Flowers for scent

Traditionally, flowers dominate any mixture, especially rose petals and lavender, as they retain their perfume the longest. For fragrance, select perfect, whole flowers just before they open fully. Dry by laying as flat as possible on stretched cheesecloth to allow air to circulate. Large-flowered roses and thick-petaled lilies and hyacinths should have their petals separated. Small rosebuds can be dried whole; they look exquisite but have little scent at this stage. Select from:

acacia, broom, carnation, elder, freesia, honeysuckle, hyacinth, jasmine, lavender, lilac, lily of the valley, linden, Madonna lily, meadowsweet, Mexican orange blossom, mignonette, mock orange, musk mallow, narcissus, nicotiana, orange blossom, rose, stock, sweet rocket, violet, wallflower.

Flowers for color

Choose from the following to include in display mixtures for extra color:

bergamot, borage, calendula, cornflowers, delphinium, endive, feverfew, forget-me-not, foxglove, larkspur, lawn daisy, poppy, sage, tansy, tulip, viper's bugloss, zinnias, and any of the small "everlasting" flowers.
Use pussy willow and sweet myrtle buds to give extra texture.

Aromatic leaves

These represent the second largest group in a potpourri mixture, and as their scent is often more powerful than that of flowers, select those that will harmonize. Dry leaves whole and then break or crush them in the blend to release their scent. Choose from:

balm of Gilead, balsam poplar buds, basil, bay, bergamot, costmary, lady's bedstraw, lemon balm, lemon verbena, melilot, mints, patchouli, scented pelargoniums, rosemary, sage, southernwood, sweetbrier, sweet cicely, sweet marjoram, sweet myrtle, sweet woodruff, tarragon, thymes, and wild strawberry.

Spices, peel, roots and wood chips

These have a strong aroma and are used sparingly; about 1 tablespoon to 4 cups of flowers and leaves. Selected spices are usually added in equal proportions. The best scent is obtained by freshly grinding whole spices in a pestle and mortar or pepper grinder; grate nutmeg. To make dried peel, take a thin layer of peel with a zester, grater or potato peeler, avoiding any white pith. Dip in orris root powder to intensify the scent. Dry slowly, then crush or mince if desired. Roots should be cleaned, carefully peeled, sliced and dried slowly. Then chop, crush, mince or powder them. Select from:

alexanders (seed), allspice, aniseed, cardamom, cinnamon, cloves, coriander, dill seed, ginger, juniper, nutmeg, star anise, vanilla pods; dried peel of citrus fruits; roots of angelica, cowslip, elecampane, sweet flag, valerian, vetiver; and shreds or raspings of cedarwood, sandalwood, cassia chips.

Fixatives

These are available as powders and are used to absorb and hold the other scents so they will last longer. Most have their own perfume, which enters into the aromatic equation. The most popular vegetable fixative is orris root, as its sweet violet scent doesn't affect a blend strongly: use 1 tablespoon per cup of flowers and leaves. Gum benzoin has a sweet vanilla scent; use about $\frac{1}{2}$ ounce to 4–6 cups of flowers and leaves. The tonka bean from *Dipteryx odorata* also has a strong vanilla scent; use one or two crushed beans per recipe.

Some fragrances act as fixatives, including oakmoss or chypre, sandalwood, sweet flag root, sweet violet root, and frankincense and myrrh. Use $\frac{1}{2}$ ounce to 4 cups of potpourri.

Essential oils

Many of the above are available as essential oils (see pp. 228–237). This is a great boon to present-day potpourri blenders for adding intensity and depth to a fragrant mixture. Oils are particularly good for reviving an old potpourri that has lost its scent; but only a few drops should be added to each mixture or you will overpower the blend.

METHODS
Moist potpourri

In traditional recipes, this is made from highly fragrant damask or cabbage rose petals, which are partly dried until leathery and halved in bulk: this takes about two days of dry weather. Then the petals are layered with dry, noniodized sea salt (half coarse and half fine), using 1 cup of salt to 3 packed cups of petals. Alternate every $\frac{1}{2}$ inch of petals with salt, in a bowl until it is two-thirds full. Stand it in a dark, dry, well-aired space for 10 days until caked together. If it froths, stir daily and allow another 10 days.

Break up the caked petals into small pieces, mix with the other ingredients and seal in an airtight container for six weeks to "ferment." Stir daily. Add dried flowers and essential oils and seal again for two weeks to complete blending. Transfer to a decorative opaque container with a lid, and cover when not in use. Moist potpourri will keep its fragrance for several years.

Dry potpourri

Select a theme for the scent – such as woodland or citrus – and assemble paper-dry flowers and leaves. Gently combine the flowers and leaves, then mix the fixative with the spices and blend in with your hands. Sprinkle on essential oils if desired, a drop at a time, stirring between each drop. Seal and store in a warm, dry, dark place for six weeks to "cure."

Place the mixture in open bowls for display. Choose a container with colors that harmonize with the potpourri, or use clear glass containers to show off the potpourri between layers of lavender or rose petals. A lid will prolong its scented life.

POTPOURRI RECIPES

Traditional rose and spice mixture

(moist method)

4 cups "fermented" rose petals	2 tbsp ground mace
1 tbsp crushed bay leaves	2 tbsp ground allspice
1 tbsp crushed orange peel	1 tbsp ground cloves
$\frac{1}{2}$ cup orris root powder	1 nutmeg, grated
	1 cinnamon stick, crushed
	1 cup dried rosebuds

Rondeletia potpourri

(moist method)

This is based on a nineteenth-century perfume.

4 cups "fermented" rose petals	$1\frac{1}{2}$ oz tonka bean, crushed
4 cups lavender flowers	7 drops bergamot oil
2 tbsp cloves	3 drops clary sage oil

Culinary potpourri

(dry method)

Crush half of each ingredient for scent, leaving the other half whole for texture and use.

2 cups sweet marjoram	2 tbsp sweet myrtle leaves
$\frac{1}{2}$ cup lemon thyme flowering tops	2 tbsp orange peel
$\frac{1}{2}$ cup basil	20 cardamom seeds
2 tbsp bearberry leaves	20 star anise pods
20 bay leaves	20 juniper berries
	2 tbsp cloves
	2 cinnamon sticks

Fresh citrus blend

(dry method)

2 cups lemon verbena	$\frac{1}{2}$ cup peppermint
1 cup lemon thyme	$\frac{1}{2}$ cup alecost (costmary) leaves
1 cup spearmint	$\frac{1}{2}$ cup thyme (pine-scented)
1 cup variegated applemint	$\frac{1}{2}$ cup calendula petals
1 cup young bergamot leaves	20 crushed juniper berries
$\frac{1}{2}$ cup basil	$\frac{1}{4}$ cup lemon peel
$\frac{1}{2}$ cup pelargonium (lemon and peppermint)	2 drops each lemon, orange and bergamot oil

Soothing potpourri

(dry method)

2 cups lemon verbena	1 cup meadowsweet florets
2 cups rose petals	1 cup chamomile flowers
1 cup lavender flowers	1 oz angelica root
1 cup calendula petals	4 tbsp orris root

Cottage garden potpourri

(dry method)

2 cups rose petals	1 cup pinks
1 cup rosebuds	1 cup larkspur flowers
2 cups lavender	$\frac{1}{4}$ cup daisies
1 cup mock orange flowers	8 love-in-a-mist seed capsules or hop flowers
1 cup scented pelargonium leaves	8 helichrysum flowers
1 cup bergamot leaves	5 tbsp orris root

Elizabethan mixture

(dry method)

2 cups lemon verbena	$\frac{1}{2}$ cup violets
2 cups lavender flowers	$\frac{1}{2}$ cup blue mallow flowers
1 cup bearberry leaves	$\frac{1}{2}$ cup crushed roseroot
1 cup sweet myrtle leaves	1 oz rosewood
1 cup delphiniums	4 tbsp orris root
	1 tbsp gum benzoin

Fly-away potpourri

(dry method)

Sweet-scented insect repellent.

2 cups lavender flowers	$\frac{1}{4}$ cup tansy
1 cup rosemary	$\frac{1}{4}$ cup mugwort
1 cup southernwood	$\frac{1}{4}$ cup cedarwood chips
$\frac{1}{2}$ cup spearmint	10 yellow tulips
$\frac{1}{2}$ cup santolina	3 tbsp orris root
$\frac{1}{4}$ cup pennyroyal	

Woodland blend

(dry method)

2 cups wild strawberry leaves	$\frac{1}{4}$ cup patchouli
1 cup pine needles	$\frac{1}{4}$ cup rosewood
$\frac{1}{2}$ cup violets	2 tbsp sweet violet root
$\frac{1}{2}$ cup rosemary	3 drops cypress oil
$\frac{1}{4}$ cup cedarwood chippings	2 drops pine oil
	1 oz oakmoss

Family heirloom

(dry method)

Begin with a simple blend of rose petals, lavender flowers, rosemary leaves, allspice and orris root. Whenever you have a special occasion involving flowers, dry the petals and add them to the potpourri. As the scent fades it can be revived with essential oils. The character of the potpourri will develop with your family history, and each petal will have a story to tell.

Herbal fragrance for the bedroom

Discover refreshing new ways of using herbs in the bedroom. All the pretty things shown on these pages are enhanced with herbal fragrances of different kinds. A scented sachet can be slipped under your pillow so that turning over in the night produces a soothing drift of bergamot. A lingerie drawer can be perfumed with the sweet scent of rose potpourri. Or a scented hanger can give a shirt the clean, fresh aroma of lemon verbena. See the following pages for more ideas.

Classic potpourri
Countless possibilities for recipes make concocting potpourri an absorbing art. A classic rose-scented mix has an intoxicating perfume.

Colorful potpourri
Tossing in a few vivid, dried flower heads for their color makes mixtures more decorative.

Lavender bundle
Pretty be-ribboned bundles of lavender make enchanting presents and are easy to slip into drawers and cupboards. Fresh-cut stalks of lavender are used, and pastel ribbon holds the flower heads in place.

Herb pillow
Especially treasured by those confined to bed, a herb pillow is easily constructed with a muslin inner slip. This holds the herbs, allowing the outer case to be laundered. A sleep pillow could include the heady-scented flowers of golden hop.

Country scent potpourri
This English garden mixture includes lavender, bergamot, rose petals, mock orange and eau de cologne mint. A hay-scented meadow mixture can be made from melilot, lady's bedstraw and sweet woodruff.

Lavender bags

Tiny and neat, handmade lavender bags have a peaceful fragrance. They can be stitched from fabric and lace scraps, or made up to match a scented hanger. Different shapes can be filled with dried lavender or a fragrant mixture of your choice.

Scented hanger

The floral fabric covering this padded coat hanger encloses a selection of fragrant dried herbs, caught beneath muslin strips wound around the hanger. Rose and lavender mixtures are suitable, or, for a man's hanger, a minty citrus blend of spearmint, costmary, lemon verbena and pine-scented thyme.

Pomander

This traditional aromatic pomander is made with an orange, some spicy cloves and a length of ribbon to hang it by.

Perfumed box

The old-fashioned fragrance of lavender can be used for a new idea. A pretty, fabric-covered box for keepsakes or handkerchiefs conceals a secret — padded, lavender-filled panels in the lid and base.

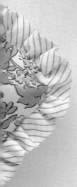

Herbal fragrance in the home

LIVING ROOM

Fresh, scented flowers and herbs arranged in a vase are one of the easiest ways to fill a room with scent. Other ways to freshen or perfume the air are listed below. All are based on simple ideas that have been practiced for centuries and are now enjoying something of a revival.

Herbal decorations Generous bunches of fresh herbs in vases or garlands will cool and perfume a room (see pp. 150–162). Herbs that sweeten the air include:

basil, bay, costmary, germander, hyssop, lavender, lemon balm, lemon verbena, mints, rosemary, roseroot, santolina, sweet myrtle, thyme, woodruff and wormwood.

Essential oils Add a few drops of lavender oil to a bowl of near-boiling water and place in the room. Alternatively, moisten a sponge with boiling water and add a few drops of an essential oil. Place the sponge in a dish in the room, and moisten it with boiling water twice a day, adding a few drops of oil twice a week (also see p. 235).

Chafing pan Use a heavy pan to burn aromatic herbs and spices over a low heat for fragrance and fumigation. Try angelica seed, dried angelica root, elecampane root, roseroot, sweet violet root, and cloves or mixed spices. When the dry ingredients begin to smolder, remove the pan from the heat and carry it around to freshen the air.

Scented water Mix $\frac{1}{2}$ cup triple-strength rosewater with 1 tablespoon powdered allspice or cloves. Store for a week to mature, then sprinkle a few drops on a hot pan or fire grate to scent a room.

Scented wood Keep any prunings of herbs like lavender and rosemary in a jar by the hearth, to sprinkle on the fire and scent the room. For special occasions burn scented wood such as apple, cedar, cherry, cypress, juniper, larch, lilac, pear or pine.

Lavender incense Soak dried lavender stems in 1 tablespoon saltpeter dissolved in 1 cup of warm water for 30 minutes. Dry out and light for a slow, smoldering scent.

Potpourri Try out the recipes on p. 207 and display in pretty bowls, inviting the potpourri to be touched so that the scent is released.

Lavender soother Put a dish of lavender by the telephone for its soothing fragrance.

Herb cushions Fill two rectangular muslin bags with favourite potpourri blends. Cover each with material to match your sofa or chair. Join the two bags with two strips of fabric and hang over the back of the sofa so the fragrance is released whenever anyone rests against them. Swap the bags around occasionally.

Scented books Put small sachets of lavender, southernwood, santolina or wormwood and cinnamon or cloves on your bookshelves to scent the books and protect them from pests.

Scented candles The easiest way to make candles is to buy a candle-making kit. Add small pieces of dried alecost, bergamot, germander, lavender heads, lemon thyme, mint, rosemary, sweet myrtle, or powdered cinnamon, or a few drops of essential oil to the melted wax, just before pouring it into the mold.

For decoration, apply aromatic leaves to the outside. Hold a candle by the wick and dip it in hot water for a few seconds to soften the outside; then roll it over dried herb leaves pressing gently. Alternatively, put the leaves around the edge of the mold. Salad burnet is a very pretty and delicate leaf to apply.

If you want to make a herbal wax, boil the leaves of bog myrtle (*Myrica gale*) or the pale gray berries (nutlets) of bayberry for about 15 minutes to extract their wax. Skim it off, remelt and strain. This wax burns with a mild spiciness.

HERBS FOR THE KITCHEN

Use herbs in the kitchen to freshen the air and disguise cooking fumes. Make decorative hangings (see pp. 156–7) and incorporate the herbs listed below that deter flies.

Kitchen potpourri Try the recipe on p. 207, or the following blend, to reduce kitchen smells and deter flies. Use 4 parts lemon verbena, 2 parts mints, 2 parts bay leaves, 1 part tansy leaves and flowers, 1 part lovage, a few crushed cloves and orris root. Handle the leaves as you pass by.

Fly-away posies Kitchen bouquets of chamomile, hemp agrimony, mugwort, pennyroyal, peppermint, rue, tansy or wormwood, or pot plants of basil and shoofly (*Nicandra physalodes*) should deter flies.

Potholders Sew rosemary, thyme or spices into the padding of potholders so they release their scent when warm.

Tea cozy Make pockets in a tea cozy and fill with lemon verbena, rose petals or jasmine; the warmth of the teapot will activate their perfume.

Scented oven Whenever baking, place a sprig of rosemary or any savory herb in the oven to scent the kitchen.

HERBS FOR THE BEDROOM

Fragrant herbs can help you sleep, sweeten the air and your clothes, and are particularly welcome in a bedroom where someone is ill.

Herb pillows Make a small muslin or cotton cover and fill with your favorite potpourri mixture. Keep it under your usual pillow. As you turn in the night, soothing wafts of herbal fragrance will aid your sleep. Fresh scents, not overly sweet, are best for the sickroom or a convalescent. Hops have sleep-inducing properties, but not everyone enjoys their beery scent; adding a little lavender, lemon verbena, mint or rosemary helps to counteract the aroma. Another sleep mixture includes 1 part chamomile (to dispel nightmares), 2 parts each rosemary and pine needles (both refreshing), 2 parts lavender (alleviates sadness) and a little sweet marjoram (a sedative) with crushed aniseed or dill, orris root and a few drops of bergamot oil.

Drawer bags (sweet bags) Use lavender, lemon verbena, mint or rose petals to fill individual sachets of lace, silk or cotton to lay among lingerie, sweaters, gloves and linen. Add a loop to hang sachets on hangers under dresses and shirts. Choose more robust materials for sachets to store herbs inside shoes, boots and suitcases so they stay sweetly scented. Tuck small sachets in the pockets or hems of winter coats in storage.

Perfumed boxes Make thin rectangular lavender pillows and tack them into the lid and base of a small box for storing jewelry or mementos.

Scented hangers Include herbs in the padding when making fabric-covered coat hangers.

Lavender bundles To make lavender bundles you need an odd number (13 or more) of long stems of lavender, freshly picked on a dry day, and about 3 feet of lavender or blue quarter-inch ribbon. Make a bunch of the lavender stems, lining up the base of the flower heads. Leave an 8 inch length of ribbon free at one end, then tie the stems together just below the heads. Gently bend back each stem until the flower heads are enclosed by the stems. Take the length of ribbon you saved and weave it under and over each stem, traveling around the bundle several times until the flower heads are covered with ribbon. Tuck in the short end of the ribbon and tie a bow with the other end. Trim the stalks and the ribbon.

Pomanders Press cloves into the skin of an orange, pricking the skin with a darning needle first if necessary. Either cover the whole orange with cloves, allowing a clove space between each to allow for shrinkage as the orange dries, or set them in patterns around the orange. Roll the finished orange in a mixture of orris root and spices – cinnamon or allspice. Tie a ribbon around it to suspend the pomander, which should hold its scent for a year or more.

Pomanders can also be made with apples, but they bruise and shrivel more than oranges. Select a large, firm cooking apple for the best results. A cidery clove scent eventually develops.

CLOTHING AND HOUSEHOLD LINEN
Scented bed linen and sweet-smelling clothes add a touch of luxury to your life at very little cost in time or money.

Sweet rinse waters Make a strong infusion of aromatic leaves or flowers by simmering them for 15 minutes in a covered pan. Strain and use the liquid as the final rinse for hand-washed articles, or add it to the washing machine's final rinse cycle.

Single herbs or mixtures can be used: rosemary with lavender is very refreshing. Choose from the following:
leaves of alecost (costmary), angelica, bay, bergamot, eau de cologne mint, lemon verbena, rosemary, sweet marjoram or sweet myrtle; powdered root of roseroot; or flowers of cottage pinks, lavender, rose petals or violets.

A small teaspoon of powdered orris root can be dissolved in the mixture to fix the scent. The solution can also be sprinkled on clothes before ironing. Alternatively, add a few drops of essential oil to the final rinse.

Herbs to protect and scent fabrics Make up small bags of your favorite aromatic herbs (see pp. 206–7). Alternatively, you can use individual herbs to lay among your clothes. Choose from:
sprigs of costmary, lavender, rosemary or southernwood; dried lemon peel; or root pieces of elecampane, orris, roseroot or sweet flag.

HERBS FOR SMOKERS
Mixtures of herb leaves and seeds have been smoked for centuries, long before the commercial domination of the tobacco plant. Indeed, in times past, herbal mixtures were smoked to relieve chest complaints.

Scented tobacco An aromatic mixture of aniseed, balsam, cinnamon, clove oil and gum benzoin can be made into peppercorn-sized balls and matured for a month. Add one piece to a pipeful of tobacco to perfume a room.

Herbal tobacco There has been a revival of interest in herbal tobacco, in response to the dangers inherent in smoking tobacco leaves. Most herbal tobaccos are based on coltsfoot, and can be bought from herbal suppliers. Other herbs added include arnica, betony, buckbean, annual chamomile, eyebright, lavender, mallow, mugwort, rosemary, thyme and yarrow. The final blends include licorice, salt, saltpeter and sugar.

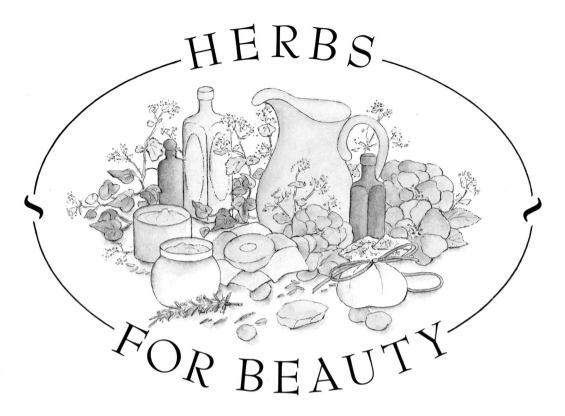

HERBS
FOR BEAUTY

The cosmetic use of plant material runs through all ancient cultures. Seven thousand years ago, the early tribes of the Nile Valley painted and anointed their dead, both to preserve the body and to make it more attractive for the world beyond. The Egyptians who followed assimilated their practices and developed them into an elaborate routine of beauty preparations for religious rituals and ceremonial occasions.

The ancient Greeks changed the focus of cosmetics from ceremonial to personal, developing a philosophy of all-around health and beauty akin to modern concepts. The famous physician Hippocrates formulated the study of dermatology and recommended diet, exercise, baths and massage for improving physical health and beauty. The Romans indulged further in aromatic rituals and body pampering. Citro, a Roman writer in the first century A.D., wrote four books on cosmetics with a range of recipes for bleaching, tinting and greasing hair, avoiding wrinkles, and dealing with body odors.

By the time of the Renaissance there was an awareness of skin care as separate from medicinal disorders. Recipes for soaps, creams, and herbal waters were collected and recorded in herbals and still-room books, which were handed down from mother to daughter for generations.

Commercial beauty products
During the nineteenth century, cosmetics became an organized industry in America. In 1846 Mr Theron T. Pond offered his "Pond's Extract" to the public and other manufacturers soon followed. The innovative use of preservatives and mass production created an unprecedented choice.

Today's commercial products are often expensive, having vast amounts of money spent on advertising, packaging, distribution and testing (which can involve cruelty to animals). Allergies have increased along with the use of chemical preservatives, synthetic perfumes and artificial colorings. As a result, demand has risen for natural ingredients, and since research has demonstrated the remarkable therapeutic properties of herbs, many firms are rushing to create their own ranges of herbal cosmetics.

Homemade herbal cosmetics
By making your own cosmetics, you can be sure of their contents. You select each ingredient and have control over its freshness and purity. The following recipes combine present-day knowledge with traditional ingredients and methods inherited from past ages, including the first face cream recipe recorded by Galen, a Roman doctor in the second century. This recipe used a formula of oil, water and wax and has formed the basis of day creams ever since. Some preparations take no longer than boiling a kettle, others require heating and blending but are no more complicated or time-consuming than preparing a simple sauce.

Note: *Before using any herbal preparations, you are advised to sample a small amount first, particularly if you have had allergic reactions in the past.*

USEFUL EQUIPMENT FOR HERBAL COSMETICS

This list is meant as a guide only, but do avoid using aluminum, copper and nonstick pans as their chemical contents can affect the ingredients' beneficial properties.

All containers and utensils must be scrupulously clean. Ideally they should be sterilized by being boiled or placed in a hot oven for 10 minutes. Have hot soapy water standing by to wash off wax before it hardens. Otherwise, stand bowls over boiling water to remelt traces of contents, and wash immediately.

Heatproof glassware or pottery cookware (to sit in or above pans of boiling water)
Enamel double boiler
Wire whisk or electric mixer
Measuring spoons
Measuring jug
Small glass measure
Small funnel
Nylon sieve
Pestle and mortar
Small weighing scale such as dieters use
Blender
Juice extractor

Glass dropper
Wooden spoons
Glass rods
Spatula
Clean dark glass bottles and jars with airtight lids
Labels
Indelible pen
A notebook for recording recipes

BASIC HERBAL PREPARATIONS

Most of the recipes in this section use one of these methods to extract the therapeutic properties from herbs.

Infusing Put one and a half handfuls of fresh herbs or 1 oz of dried into a heatproof container (not aluminum or copper). Bring 2½ cups distilled water to the boil. Pour over the herb immediately; cover with a lid to prevent the loss of any volatile elements through evaporation. Steep for at least 30 minutes. Strain and store in a refrigerator for up to three days.

Decocting This method is usually employed for the tougher parts of herbs — for example, roots, bark, stems and seeds. Put 1 oz of the herb, cut up if necessary, into a saucepan (not aluminum or copper). Add 2½ cups distilled water, bring to the boil and simmer for 30 minutes. By this time the liquid should have reduced by half. If more has evaporated, top up with water to make 1¼ cups. Cool, strain and bottle. Keep in the refrigerator and use within a few days.

Macerating Herbs likely to lose some of their therapeutic value if heated should be steeped in oil, vinegar or alcohol. Pack a glass jar with the crushed, fresh herb. Cover with vegetable oil, cider vinegar or pure alcohol. Seal and leave for two weeks, shaking the jar each day. Strain and top up with fresh herbs. Repeat until the liquid smells strongly herbal. Strain, seal and bottle. Keeps well.

Pulverizing Grind, bruise or mash plant fibers and seeds in a pestle and mortar or blender.

NONHERBAL INGREDIENTS

The following can be bought from any good pharmacist.

Agar agar Derived from seaweed. Used to make gels.

Alcohol A colorless, flavorless preservative and solvent. The best alcohol for perfumery, and least irritating to the skin, is ethyl alcohol. Isopropyl alcohol (rubbing alcohol) is second best but has a medicinal scent. Vodka can sometimes be used instead.

Beeswax Acts as an emulsifier for oil and water in creams. Usually sold in blocks. To make measuring easier, line egg box compartments with foil, melt the wax gently and put 1 teaspoon or 1 tablespoon in each compartment. When it has cooled and solidified, remove, wrap in foil and store until required.

Benzoin A preservative, astringent and antiseptic.

Borax A white, crystalline, mineral powder used as an emulsifier. May be omitted from recipes.

Bran Used in face masks, soaps and body scrubs as a cleanser.

Buttermilk Soothing and astringent.

Calamine lotion A soothing alkaline lotion useful for skin problems.

Castile soap A pure white soap with no added color or perfume. Makes a useful base for homemade soaps.

Cocoa butter A thick fat from the cocoa bean, which makes a rich emollient in creams.

Distilled water Only pure water is suitable for making cosmetics. Tap water and rainwater contain too many impurities.

Emulsifying wax A wax used to emulsify oil and water in creams.

Fuller's earth A fine gray powder derived from single-cell algae found on seabeds. Its absorbent properties and mineral richness make it an excellent face mask.

Gelatin A colorless, odorless, tasteless glue and a rich source of water-soluble protein, obtained by boiling animal bones. Used in eye ointments and nail-hardening lotions. Agar agar is a vegetable substitute.

Glycerin A thick, colorless, odorless syrup and byproduct of soap manufacture. It mixes with water, is soluble in alcohol and has softening properties.

Honey Softening, healing and binds other ingredients together.

Iodine Used as an antiseptic.

Kaolin The purest form of clay, useful in face masks.

Lanolin A thick, sticky fat obtained from sheep's wool. Softens and nourishes the skin.

Liquid paraffin A mineral oil that is not absorbed by the skin, making it useful in barrier creams.

Oatmeal See **Bran**

Oils See p. 230 for notes on essential oils and vegetable oils. Almond, avocado, wheatgerm, carrot, coconut and nut kernel oils are particularly skin-enriching. Castor oil disperses in water, making it a good vehicle for scented bath oils.

Oleic acid An emulsifying liquid that can rescue separated creams.

Petroleum jelly A pale yellow translucent mineral jelly insoluble in water. Does not turn rancid when exposed to air. Used in lip salves.

Vinegar Used in cosmetics to soften, cleanse and soothe the skin.

Vitamin capsules A convenient way of adding vitamins to skin creams.

Zinc oxide A white powder derived from zinc which has mild antiseptic and astringent qualities. Usually available as an ointment.

Knowing your skin

To appreciate how herbs can benefit your skin, it helps to know something about why skin deteriorates. Like eyes and hair, skin is a reflection of your general health, so diet and lifestyle are major contributors to its appearance. Its surface needs to be kept moist and clean to protect it from drying winds, the sun and environmental pollution. The first line of defense is to avoid as many of these factors as possible; the second is to clean and nourish your skin with care.

SKIN TYPES

To give your skin the correct treatment you need to ascertain your skin type. Test by cleaning your face thoroughly; rinse well and dry with a towel. Allow it to rest for two hours or overnight and then press a tissue onto your face. If the tissue comes away full of grease, you have oily skin; if there is grease on only parts of it (usually from around the forehead, nose and chin), you have combination skin. If the tissue comes away unmarked, wash your face with soap and water. If your skin feels supple and smooth afterwards, it's normal; if it feels taut, it's dry.

Normal skin is soft, smooth and springy with a translucent glow. Why it is called normal when it is the rarest form is a mystery. A simple care routine is sufficient.

Dry skin feels taut and dry and has no shine. All types of skin become drier and more sensitive to changes as they age. This type of skin requires moisturizer at an earlier age. It should be treated with mild cleansers and gentle care.

Oily skin has a definite shine and is supple. The pores are open and the skin may look coarse and sallow. An oily skin is less vulnerable to sun and winds, and a further benefit comes later in life as it appears supple for longer. It needs thorough cleansing as the greasy surface acts like a magnet for dirt and a breeding ground for acne, but cleansing must be gentle to avoid stimulating the sebaceous glands into further oil production.

Combination skin is the most common type, as the pores on the forehead, nose and chin are usually larger than those on the rest of the face. This "T" panel is oily, while the remainder of the face is dry. It is best treated as two types of skin, using different recipes for the appropriate areas.

Skin creams and lotions

All skin creams are based on a combination of melted waxes, oils and scented waters, which must all be at a similar temperature. The waxes are melted over a low heat, the oils are warmed and beaten into the waxes, then the heated waters are dribbled slowly into the blended wax and oil, and the mixture is stirred until cool. It is like making mayonnaise, only easier – a 10-minute operation.

The proportions of the ingredients govern a cream's consistency and are easy to adjust. To make a cream firmer, add more beeswax; to make it softer, add more oil. Adding more water will make it lighter and fluffier but also makes the ingredients more prone to separation. The addition of herbs such as marsh mallow and houseleek, which contain an emollient mucilage (a sticky substance in the roots, stems or leaves), will make a cream spongier. Add a few drops of essential oil for both the fragrance and its beneficial properties. Rose, geranium and lavender are particularly good for all skin types.

Spooning creams into small jars is an acquired skill. It's best to begin with a small spoon and to use a knife around the inside edge to remove any air pockets. Some lotions become firmer after a few hours, so until you are familiar with a recipe put your creams into wide-necked jars. What you pour into a bottle may become too thick to pour

out. (Gently reheat to remove if this does happen.)

Always label and date products immediately, keeping a record of each recipe and its success. As perishable ingredients are involved, refrigerate creams and use within a few weeks. To prevent the possibility of introducing bacteria, make sure your hands are clean before dipping into your creams, or use a small spatula.

ALLERGY

No cosmetics can claim to be nonallergenic, because every ingredient holds the possibility that someone might be allergic to it. One of the main benefits of making your own cosmetics is that if you do have an allergic reaction you know what ingredients you have used and can soon find the culprit. Test for a reaction by placing a spot of any ingredient on the inner, gauze area of a Band-aid and attaching this to your inner arm, between the wrist and elbow. Leave in place for 24 hours, by which time any reaction you may have will show.

Some essential oils can irritate sensitive skins, particularly on the face. Oils to watch out for are bay, bergamot, geranium, neroli, pennyroyal, peppermint, sage and spearmint.

For those with highly sensitive skins, the following ingredients can cause allergic reactions:

Agrimony	Glycerin	Lovage
Almond oil	Henna	Nettles
Cocoa butter	Ivy	Pennyroyal
Cowslips	Lanolin	Primrose
Cucumber	Lime blossom	Violet leaves

CLEANSING CREAMS

These are more efficient than soap and water at removing heavy dirt and makeup, which can lodge in skin crevices, aging the skin more quickly and making it seem dull and lifeless. Massage into the skin and then wipe off with absorbent cotton or tissue. Avoid dragging the skin; stroke lightly upward and across the face.

Glycerin and rosewater cleansing cream
(for dry and normal skins)

Most recipes for creams follow this procedure. Waxes are melted in one container while oils are warmed in another. All ingredients should be at about the same temperature when you mix them together or the mixture may curdle. You can substitute any suitable herbal infusion for the rosewater.

4 tbsp lanolin
2 fl oz almond oil
1 tbsp glycerin
⅛ tsp borax
3 tbsp rosewater
1 tsp zinc oxide ointment
6 drops essential oil of rose

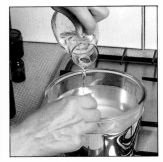

1 Melt the lanolin and gently heat the almond oil and glycerin together. Slowly pour the oil and glycerin mixture into the lanolin, beating constantly.

2 Dissolve the borax in the warmed rosewater and add gradually to the lanolin and oil mixture, beating all the time. Leave to cool.

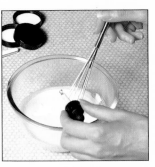

3 When cool and creamy, beat in the zinc oxide and rose oil. Spoon into prepared jars and label.

PLANTS TO USE IN CREAMS AND LOTIONS

Many plants and herbs have beneficial cosmetic uses. Those listed here are particularly effective in skin creams. Follow the preparation instructions on p. 213. For equivalent strengths, use half the quantity of dried herbs to fresh. Many of these herbs are also beneficial in face packs, baths and hair treatments and are listed in those sections of the chapter.

Aloe vera The sap from the leaves is soothing and healing.

Avocado An excellent skin food with high vitamin E and A content.

Borage Good for dry, sensitive skins.

Calendula A healing herb for rough, damaged and problem skin.

Chamomile A gentle, soothing herb that also softens and whitens skin.

Comfrey A healing and soothing herb that contains allantoin, a protein which speeds up cell renewal. Good for rough and damaged skin.

Cucumber A cleansing agent and toner. Soothing and healing.

Dandelion Contains a rich emollient useful in cleansing lotions for dry, mature and sallow skins.

Elderflower A good tonic for all skins, especially mature or sallow skins. Reputed to soften skin and smooth wrinkles, fade freckles and soothe sunburn.

Essential oils These are excellent additions to creams and lotions. See p. 236 for details of their properties.

Fennel Cleansing and soothing. Add crushed seeds to face packs.

Houseleek A healing, softening and soothing herb especially good for dry, sensitive skins.

Ivy Relieves sunburn; helps to disperse trapped fluids and toxins in the fight against cellulite.

Lady's mantle A healing herb for soothing dry, sensitive skin and rough hands; makes a good astringent for large pores.

Lavender A healing and gentle cleanser and tonic for all skin types.

Lemon An astringent that restores the skin's natural acid balance.

Linden blossom Soothes and softens the skin. Deep cleansing.

Lupine seed A cleanser and pore refiner for oily skin.

Marsh mallow A healing softener for dry skins, chapped hands and sunburn.

Nettle A deep cleanser, particularly good for oily skin.

Orange flower An excellent skin tonic, said to help restore the skin's acid barrier. Also treats dry skin and broken capillaries and stimulates cell replacement.

Parsley A conditioner for dry, sensitive and troubled skins.

Peppermint A stimulating astringent that clears the complexion.

Rose A soothing and gentle cleanser that has a refining and softening effect on the skin.

Rosemary An invigorating tonic and antiseptic which boosts circulation and deep skin cleansing.

Sage A cleansing, stimulating astringent which also tightens pores.

Thyme A stimulating but gentle antiseptic cleanser.

Violet A gentle, soothing astringent.

Watercress Expressed juice can help to clear blemishes.

Witch hazel Soothing and astringent. Distilled witch hazel contains 15 percent alcohol.

Yarrow A healing and cleansing astringent.

Chamomile cleansing milk
(for dry and sensitive skins)

Use elderflowers, sweet violets or lime blossom
in place of chamomile.

$\frac{1}{2}$ cup creamy milk   2 tbsp chamomile flowers,
fresh or dried

1 Heat together in a double boiler for 30 minutes. Do
not let the milk boil or form a skin.

2 Leave to infuse for 2 hours, then strain. Keep
refrigerated and use within 1 week. Apply with cotton
wool and remove excess with tissues.

Orange-flower cleansing cream
(for dry and normal skins)

Essential oil of neroli (extracted from the orange
flower) is used to stimulate the loss of old skin
cells and their replacement with new ones.

2 tbsp soy oil   2 tbsp orange-flower water
2 tbsp almond oil $\frac{1}{8}$ tsp borax
1 oz cocoa butter   5 drops essential oil of neroli
1 tbsp beeswax

1 Mix and warm the oils. Melt the cocoa butter and stir
it into the oils. Melt the beeswax, then beat it into the
oil mixture, a little at a time.

2 Warm the orange-flower water and dissolve the
borax in it. Beat this into the main mixture. Leave to
thicken and cool.

3 As the mixture starts to thicken, stir in the essential
oil. Once cool, spoon into prepared jars and label.

Cucumber and yarrow cleanser
(for oily skins)

Cucumber is an active cleanser while yarrow is
both cleansing and astringent.

1 tsp emulsifying wax   6 tbsp yarrow
4 tbsp soy oil   infusion
$\frac{1}{4}$ cucumber, puréed in blender   5 drops tincture of myrrh
and strained to make 2 tbsp

1 Melt the wax over a low heat. Warm the soy oil and
then slowly add the oil to the wax, beating well.

2 Heat the cucumber juice with the yarrow infusion
then blend into the oil and wax. Take off the heat and
beat until the mixture cools. Once cool, stir in the
myrrh. Spoon into jars and label.

Buttermilk and fennel cleansing milk
(for oily skins)

Fennel helps to remove impurities from oily skins
with a deep cleansing action.

$\frac{1}{2}$ cup buttermilk   2 tbsp fennel seed, crushed

1 Gently heat the milk and crushed seed together in a
double boiler for 30 minutes.

2 Leave to stand and infuse for a further 2 hours.
Strain, bottle, refrigerate and use within 1 week.

Lemon cleansing cream
(for oily skins)

Lemon has a reputation for clearing greasy skin
and smoothing wrinkles, as well as having a
mildly antiseptic quality.

1 tbsp beeswax   1 tbsp lemon juice,
$1\frac{1}{2}$ tbsp petroleum jelly   strained
3 tbsp mineral oil $\frac{1}{8}$ tsp borax
1 tbsp witch hazel   6 drops essential oil of lemon

1 Melt the beeswax and petroleum jelly together over a
low heat. Warm the mineral oil, then gradually add it
to the wax mixture, beating for 3–5 minutes.

2 Add the witch hazel to the lemon juice. Warm
gently, then stir in the borax until dissolved. Slowly
add this to the wax mixture, beating steadily until it is
creamy and cool.

3 Once cool, stir in the lemon oil. Spoon into clean
jars and label.

TONERS

Called variously astringents, refreshers and skin
tonics, these are important for removing any
remaining trace of cleansing cream. They also
tighten the pores and impart a clean, refreshing
feeling to the skin. Toners can also be used as a
pickup or quick cleanser during the day.

Elderflower water, lavender water, orange-
flower water and rosewater are four classic tonics
still valued today for all skin types. They can be
purchased as distilled waters, which will keep
(avoid synthetics), or made as a strong infusion to
be refrigerated and used within three days.

Rosewater toner
(for dry skins)

The soothing properties of rose make this a good
tonic for dry, sensitive and mature skins.

$\frac{3}{4}$ cup rosewater $\frac{2}{3}$ cup witch hazel
6 drops glycerin

Blend all the ingredients in a bottle and shake well
before use.

Sage astringent
(for oily skins)

4 tbsp dried sage $\frac{1}{4}$ tsp borax
4 tbsp ethyl alcohol   3 tbsp witch hazel
(or 6 tbsp vodka)   10 drops glycerin

1 Macerate the sage in the alcohol for 2 weeks and then
strain.

2 Dissolve the borax in the witch hazel. Stir into the
alcohol. Mix in the glycerin and decant into a bottle
with a tight-fitting lid. Shake before use.

*Clockwise from the top: Light rose moisturizer (p. 218); Ivy cellulite cream
(p. 218); Orange-flower cleansing cream; Comfrey and calendula cream
(p. 218); Avocado and nettle moisturizer (p. 218); Lemon cleansing cream.*

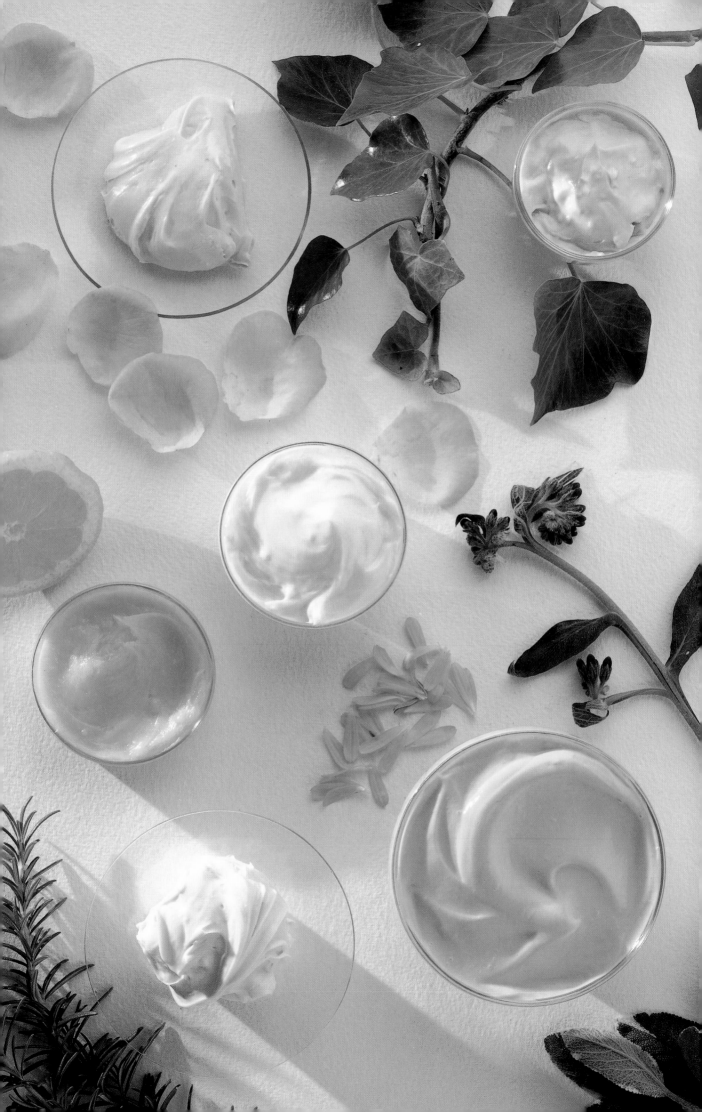

MOISTURIZING CREAMS

After the skin has been cleansed and toned it is ready for a protective film of moisturizer. The main function of a moisturizer is to maintain the skin's natural moisture level. It also protects from external dirt and drying atmospheres, and some formulations will add moisture to the epidermis (the skin's outside layer). Recent research has shown that massaging moisturizer into the skin regularly helps to speed the renewal of skin cells.

Light rose moisture cream
(for all skin types)

A pleasant light cream for daytime use.

1 tsp beeswax	3 tbsp rosewater,
1 tsp lanolin	warmed
1 tbsp almond oil	6 drops essential oil of rose,
$\frac{1}{2}$ tsp wheatgerm oil	or rose geranium
$\frac{1}{8}$ tsp borax	a few drops of red food
	coloring if desired

1 Melt the beeswax and lanolin together, stirring constantly.

2 Warm the oils gently and gradually beat them into the waxes. Dissolve the borax in the rosewater and slowly add to the oil and wax mixture, beating constantly until cool. Stir in the rose oil as the mixture begins to thicken.

3 Spoon into jars and label.

Rich moisturizing cream
(for dry skins)

Very penetrating if applied before a bath, as the steam will help the skin absorb the oils and moisture in the cream.

2 tsp beeswax	$\frac{1}{2}$ tsp glycerin
2 tsp emulsifying wax	4 tbsp rosewater
1 tbsp lanolin	$\frac{1}{4}$ tsp borax
$2\frac{1}{2}$ tsp avocado oil	6 drops essential oil of neroli
$\frac{1}{2}$ tsp wheatgerm oil	a few drops of red food
	coloring, if desired

1 Melt the beeswax, emulsifying wax and lanolin in a double boiler. Warm the avocado and wheatgerm oils with the glycerin and then gradually beat into the waxes until creamy. Remove from the heat.

2 Warm the rosewater and dissolve the borax in it. Dribble the rosewater into the cream, beating all the time. Keep stirring until the mixture cools and thickens. As it cools stir in the neroli oil.

3 Spoon into jars and label.

Avocado and nettle moisturizer
(for oily skins)

1 tsp beeswax	$\frac{1}{8}$ tsp borax
2 tsp emulsifying wax	2 tbsp strong nettle
8 tsp hazelnut oil	infusion, warm
4 tsp avocado oil	4 drops cedarwood
	essential oil

1 Melt the waxes together. Warm the oils and gradually beat them into the waxes.

2 Dissolve the borax in the warm infusion. Slowly beat this into the first mixture.

3 Allow to cool, then mix in the essential oil. Spoon into jars and label.

Comfrey and calendula cream
(nourishing cream for all skin types)

Especially good for rough, dry skin as these herbs are nourishing and healing. This also makes an excellent hand cream for sore, chapped hands. Comfrey contains a substance that helps cell renewal.

1 tbsp beeswax	$\frac{1}{4}$ tsp borax
1 tbsp lanolin	2 tbsp comfrey leaf
1 tbsp cocoa butter	infusion
$1\frac{1}{2}$ tbsp calendula oil	6 drops essential oil of
1 tsp glycerin	petitgrain

1 Melt the beeswax. Melt the lanolin and cocoa butter and gradually stir into the beeswax.

2 Warm the calendula oil and glycerin and slowly stir into the first mixture.

3 Dissolve the borax in the warm comfrey infusion and then add this to the main mixture, stirring well. Continue stirring until thick and cool, then mix in the essential oil.

4 Spoon into jars and label.

Ivy cellulite cream

Some doctors and scientists dispute the concept of cellulite; many women look at their skin and think otherwise. Whatever the outcome of this argument, the fatty "orange peel" deposits on the thighs and buttocks can benefit from extra attention. Massage into areas of cellulite.

2 tsp beeswax	4 tbsp double-strength
1 tsp emulsifying wax	ivy decoction
3 tsp almond oil	8 drops each essential oils of
1 tsp avocado oil	oregano, fennel, rosemary

1 Melt the waxes in a double boiler. Warm the oils and then stir them in well.

2 Beat in the ivy decoction and allow the mixture to cool before stirring in the essential oils.

3 Spoon into jars and label.

HERBAL SUN LOTIONS
Herbal sun products are suitable for skin that tans easily. Homemade products do not provide the heavy screening necessary for fair skin, young children, or protection against very hot sun.

Sesame suntan lotion
Bergamot improves the skin's ability to produce melanin, the substance that darkens the skin, but after a report suggesting it may have harmful effects, the research body for the world's perfumers recommended a maximum of 2 percent bergamot as a safe level.

1 tbsp lanolin	1 tsp cider vinegar
4 tbsp sesame oil	2 drops essential oil of
6 tbsp rosewater	bergamot

1 Melt the lanolin. Warm the oil, then gradually blend the two together.

2 Add the rosewater and vinegar, beating vigorously to create the lotion.

3 When cool, add the oil of bergamot. Bottle and label for use as required.

Lavender sunburn oil
Lavender oil is healing and soothing. Add a few drops more to lessen the pain (for serious burns consult a doctor).

| 6 tbsp olive oil | $\frac{1}{2}$ tsp iodine |
| 3 tbsp cider vinegar | 10 drops lavender oil |

Blend all the ingredients together and bottle. Apply very gently to relieve sunburn.

Herbal baths

Cleansing is the first and primary activity of external skin care, and an aromatic herbal bath is one of the most pleasurable and therapeutic ways of accomplishing this. You can add herbs to invigorate and stimulate circulation, or to relax and soothe muscles, unwinding the body for a peaceful night's rest (see p. 220). Select them for healing treatments to help a skin complaint, or simply for the pleasure of their aroma. Try to keep the water temperature around body heat. If it is too hot, the skin will perspire and will not absorb the therapeutic herbal properties. To get most benefit, relax in the water for at least 10 minutes.

Although it is a romantic idea to sprinkle scented leaves and flowers directly onto the water, it's not advisable – you will emerge from such a bath like a creature from the swamp, with plant bits clinging to every part of your body.

Herbal bath bags
The easiest way of adding herbs to a bath is to hang three or four herbal tea bags from the tap, or to place a small herb-filled tea infuser in the water. Alternatively, put a handful of herbs in the center of a piece of cheesecloth or fine gauze, gather up the corners to make a pouch and tie securely, adding a long loop to hang over the hot-water tap so the water will run through the bag. For a more permanent container, make simple drawstring bags from 4 × 3 in. squares of cheesecloth or gauze sewn together. Fill with your chosen herbs, fresh or dried, and suspend from the hot-water tap. Make the loop long enough to immerse the bag in the water so it continues to release its goodness. Use a single herb or mix up to four in one bath. For a body scrub, add a little fine oatmeal or bran

to the herb bag. Rub this over the body near the end of the bathing time. Herbal bath bags are reusable. Dry thoroughly after each bath and discard once the scent becomes faint.

Herbal bath infusions
Instead of adding the herb, you can extract its therapeutic properties by infusing 10 ounces of the dried herb or a large handful of fresh herbs in $2\frac{1}{2}$ cups of boiled water. Leave for at least 10 minutes, then strain and pour into the tub. Select from the list on p. 220.

Skin-soothing vinegar baths
A vinegar bath soothes itchiness and aching muscles and softens the skin. Add a cupful of the following mixture to your bath for its beneficial effects. Bring $2\frac{1}{2}$ cups of cider vinegar and a handful of fresh bath herbs slowly to the boil, then infuse overnight. Strain and bottle.

Skin-softening milk baths
Add 3 tablespoons of powdered milk (not skimmed, as it does not have the same healing qualities) to a fine gauze bag along with 2 ounces dried or 4 ounces fresh elderflowers, chamomile or linden blossom. Alternatively, infuse fresh flowers in 1 cup of cold milk for 2 hours, strain and add to the bath.

Therapeutic oil baths
The addition of 5–10 drops of essential oil to your bath allows you to lie in an envelope of fragrance and feel their beneficial power. Make your selection from the list on p. 236. Sprinkle the oil on hand-hot water after it has settled and gently swish around. Don't add oils under hot running

water or they will evaporate. The temperature of the water will affect you as well. A relaxing sedative bath should be just under blood heat. For a stimulating bath, use a temperature below 85 °F. If it is too low (below room temperature), the oils will not evaporate readily. A very hot bath is debilitating, even with relaxing oils, as well as aging for your skin.

● For dry skin, add the oils in a tablespoon of almond oil.
● For a more dispersible preparation, add the oil with a tablespoon of milk.
● For a bubble bath, add the oils with a tablespoon of mild liquid soap or baby shampoo.

Herbal saunas

Herbs rich in essential oils will release their properties in the heat of a sauna. Sprinkle in the water bucket a selection from basil, eucalyptus, lavender, lemon verbena, pine, rosemary, rose petals, sage, or thyme.

THERAPEUTIC BATH HERBS	
Relaxing bath herbs	
Chamomile	Linden flowers
Hops	Meadowsweet
Jasmine	Valerian
Stimulating bath herbs	
Basil	Mint
Bay	Pennyroyal
Eucalyptus	Pine
Fennel	Rosemary
Ivy	Sage
Lavender	Tansy
Lemon balm	Thyme
Lemon verbena	
Healing bath herbs	
Calendula	Lady's mantle
Comfrey	Spearmint
Houseleek	Yarrow
Spring tonic bath herbs	
Blackberry leaves	Lawn daisies
Dandelion	Nettle

Facial steams

A facial steam provides a thorough deep cleansing easily and inexpensively. The heat produces perspiration, which aids the elimination of toxins and stimulates circulation. The steam softens the skin and opens the pores, which helps the skin absorb the beneficial properties of the herbs.

Normal skin benefits from a weekly facial steam; oily skin from a steam two or three times a week, while those with dry skin should not have one more often than once every two weeks. Do not have a facial steam if you have thread veins, serious skin disorders, asthma or other breathing difficulties or heart problems.

To prepare a facial steam, assemble 2 handfuls of fresh herbs or 3 tablespoons of dried herbs. Tie back your hair, remove makeup and clean your face in your normal fashion. Place the herbs in a bowl or jug and pour over 6 cups of boiling water. Stir briefly with a wooden spoon or chopstick. Hold your face 12 inches away (or 18 inches if you have sensitive skin) and make a tent over your head and the bowl with a towel. Keep your eyes closed and maintain this position for 10 to 15 minutes.

Rinse with tepid to cool water and a few minutes later splash with cold water or witch hazel. A diluted herbal vinegar or an infusion of elderflower, peppermint, sage or yarrow dabbed on with absorbent cotton will tighten the pores. Avoid sudden changes of temperature, and don't go outdoors for an hour or so.

HERBS FOR FACIAL STEAMS	
Use leaves unless otherwise indicated.	
To remove impurities	
Fennel	Nettle
Linden blossom	
To boost circulation and aid deep cleansing	
Nettle	Rosemary
For soothing and gentle cleansing	
Applemint	Lemon balm
Chamomile	Rose petals
Chervil	Spearmint
Lavender	Thyme
For healing	
Comfrey (roots and leaves)	Fennel
For oily skin	
Calendula flowers	Crushed lupine seeds
Geranium (herb robert)	Sage
Horsetail	Yarrow
For dry, sensitive skins	
Borage	Parsley
Cornflower	Salad burnet
Houseleek	Sorrel
Lady's mantle	Sweet violet (flowers and
Marsh mallow (roots and leaves)	leaves)
For mature or sallow skins	
Dandelion	Red clover (flowers and
Elderflowers	leaves)
Lemon verbena	Tansy (flowers and leaves)

A selection of herbal bath products, including floral waters (p. 223); herbal bath bag (p. 219); face mask (p.222); aromatic bath oils (p. 219) and a facial steam.

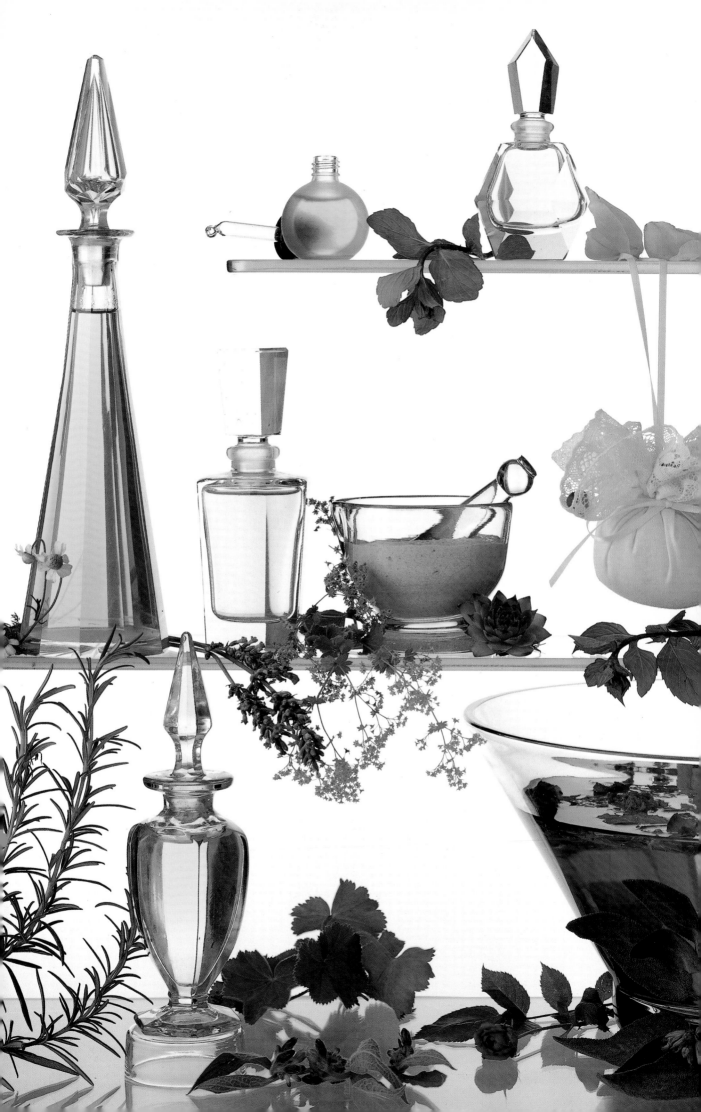

Face packs

A face pack or mask draws impurities to the skin's surface, stimulates the circulation and tightens the skin. It is doubly effective if applied after a facial steam before the pores have closed. Apply the mixture to slightly moist skin and then rest with your feet higher than your head so that gravity forces blood to the facial skin. Make cooling eye pads of cucumber or absorbent cotton soaked in a herbal infusion and place them against your eyelids to increase the absorption. Leave the mask on for 20 to 30 minutes before removing with warm water. Finish with a pore-closing infusion such as elderflower water, and then a moisturizer.

Do not apply a face mask just before preparing for a special occasion, as the drawing power of the mask, particularly one with a cereal or clay base, can flush the skin.

Green herbal mask
Any of the herbs recommended for a facial steam can be used to create a green mask. Take 2 handfuls of fresh leaves or 3 tablespoons of dried (softened by soaking in boiled water overnight). Add 2 tablespoons of distilled or mineral water and blend at high speed for a few seconds.

This makes a rather wet mixture, but if you are in a bath or lying on a towel it can be applied as it is. To thicken, add fuller's earth or ground almonds until it reaches the desired consistency.

Paste face packs
Ground oatmeal, ground almonds or fuller's earth used either singly or in combination form the basic carrier of a paste face pack. Each has the ability to draw impurities from the skin.

To 2 tablespoons of the basic carrier, add 2–3 tablespoons of a strong herbal infusion, or the juice of the herbs obtained using a juice extractor.

HERBS FOR FACE PACKS

For normal skin fennel, juniper berries, lady's mantle, linden flowers, mint, nettle

For dry and sensitive skin comfrey, houseleek, marsh mallow, pounded flax or quince seed (which contain a softening mucilage).

For oily skin sage, yarrow; 2 tablespoons of pounded fennel or lupine seed to refine pores.

NONHERBAL INGREDIENTS FOR FACE PACKS

● Milk products have softening and mild bleaching properties. Substitute 1 tablespoon of the herbal infusion for 1 tablespoon of creamy milk, or sour cream for dry skin, or yogurt or buttermilk for oily skin.

● Add 1 teaspoon honey for its healing properties.

● A few drops of lemon juice or cider vinegar help to restore the skin's acid mantle.

● Eggs are an excellent binding agent. Add an egg yolk for dry skin and a beaten egg white for oily skin.

● Mashed cucumber, strawberries, tomatoes, lemon juice and grapefruit juice are all good astringents. Avocado and ripe peach are rich moisturizers.

A deep pore cleansing mask
This recipe is based on an expensive face pack offered by a famous salon – so treat yourself!

1 tsp beeswax	3 tbsp rosewater
1 tbsp lanolin	1 tbsp fuller's earth

optional additions
1 tsp Irish moss or pounded quince or flax seed

1 Melt the wax and lanolin together over a gentle heat, stirring continuously.

2 Remove from the heat and add the rosewater, stirring until it has cooled.

3 Mix in the fuller's earth (and optional additions), stirring until you have a smooth paste.

Herbal soaps

Making soap from scratch involves the use of caustic soda – a dangerous ingredient to work with. It is much safer and easier to start with a bar of pure castile soap as a base.

Lemon and rosemary wash-balls
This recipe is based on the 16th-century method of soap making. Lemon is cleansing and toning, and rosemary is an astringent for all skin types.

5 oz bar of castile soap, grated	1 tsp dried, powdered lemon peel
3 tbsp lemon juice	6 drops essential oil of lemon
4 tbsp calendula infusion	4 drops essential oil of rosemary
1 tbsp rosemary leaves, pulverized	1 tbsp calendula infusion to moisten hands

1 Place the grated soap, lemon juice and calendula infusion in an enamel saucepan and heat gently until the soap has melted, stirring with a wooden spoon.

2 Leave to cool for 10 minutes, or until cool enough to touch, and knead with your hands to make a smooth paste. Add the rosemary leaves, lemon peel and oils.

3 Leave for 10 minutes, until it has begun to dry and is malleable. Form into approximately 6 plum-sized balls. Leave in a warm place for 2 hours, covered with plastic wrap so the outside does not crack. Then remove the plastic wrap, moisten your hands with the remaining calendula infusion and smooth the balls until shiny.

4 Cover with plastic wrap again and return them to a warm place to dry (approximately 24 hours). Wrap in tissue paper and store in a warm, dry place for a month before using.

Lavender and oatmeal soap

The healing and soothing qualities of lavender make it useful for many skin conditions, especially acne. The grittiness of the oatmeal removes dead skin cells; the coarser the oatmeal, the stronger the exfoliant action. For a whiter soap, substitute triple-strength rosewater for the lavender infusion and add either the lavender oil or a rose oil.

5 oz bar of castile soap, grated
1½ cups lavender infusion
⅓ cup ground oatmeal
a few drops of lavender oil

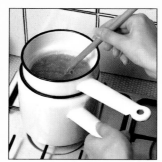

1 Put the grated soap flakes and the lavender infusion in an enamel saucepan and heat gently until the soap has melted. Stir occasionally.

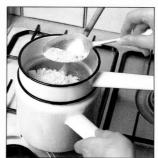

2 Remove from the heat and cool a little, then stir in the oatmeal and add the lavender oil.

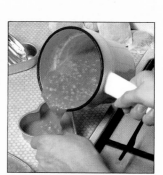

3 Pour into small oiled molds and allow to set. This can take from a few hours to a week. When dry, unmold, wrap in tissue and leave for a month in a dry cupboard.

Floral waters

Scent stirs the imagination as no other stimulus can, and aromatic leaves and flowers picked at perfection on a summer's day can be captured in a floral water (see right) to evoke pleasant memories throughout the year.

Herbs infused in water will not keep, so some form of alcohol or oil must be employed in order to preserve the scent. Use alcohol for a stronger scent. A floral water can be made with a strong infusion, adding 20 percent by volume of a 90° proof alcohol (ethyl alcohol) or 30 percent by volume of a 60° proof alcohol such as vodka.

Hungary water

Named after Queen Isabella of Hungary, who was said to have used this secret formula to restore her youth and beauty with such success that the King of Poland proposed marriage to her when she was 72. The original was made by distilling rosemary flowering tops, lemon verbena, rose and possibly sage.

2 fl oz ethyl alcohol mixed with the following essential oils:
30 drops of rosemary
12 drops of lemon
5 drops of rose
5 drops of neroli
2 drops of sage
2 drops of mint

Store in a screw-top bottle and shake before use.

Eau de cologne

2 fl oz ethyl alcohol mixed with the following essential oils:
44 drops of bergamot
15 drops of lemon
4 drops of neroli
1 drop of lavender
1 drop of rosemary

Store in a screw-top bottle and shake before use.

Floral waters

Suitable for use as a skin toner, scent or perfume.

1 cup lavender flowers, scented rose petals or orange blossom
¼ cup ethyl alcohol at room temperature

1 Steep for 6 days in a screw-top jar, shaking vigorously each day.

2 Strain and decant into a dark glass bottle.

Alternative method

If flowers are not available, use essential oils. Mix 25 drops of essential oil (traditionally lavender, rose or neroli) with 2 fl oz ethyl alcohol (or isopropyl or vodka). Shake them together in a screw-top bottle. Leave the mixture to settle for 2 days, then shake again. To store, decant into a dark bottle with a tight-fitting lid and leave almost no air space.

Roger's choice

This recipe was created in response to the challenge of a man who liked none of the scented products available for men. The basil makes it wonderful for clearing mental fatigue.

2 fl oz ethyl alcohol mixed with the following essential oils:
16 drops of basil
20 drops of bergamot
20 drops of frankincense
20 drops of lemon
20 drops of petitgrain
10 drops of coriander
5 drops of cloves
5 drops of black pepper
5 drops of patchouli
1 drop of sage
3 drops oil of benzoin

Store in a screw-top bottle and shake before use.

Aftershave

The above recipe made with witch hazel instead of ethyl alcohol makes a delicious aftershave.

Hands

The skin of our hands is subject to adverse weather conditions, hot water, detergents, polishes and garden soil. The best defense is to wear either cotton or rubber gloves, or gardening gloves, as appropriate, and to make lavish use of hand creams. Make up several bottles of your chosen recipe and leave them wherever you wash your hands. If you dislike wearing gloves or find that you keep removing them unconsciously, apply a barrier cream before doing any dirty work.

To make a particularly healing barrier cream, follow the recipe for comfrey and calendula nourishing cream on p. 218, and add 1 tablespoon warmed liquid paraffin to the wax mixture before adding the comfrey infusion. The recipe below is for a much stronger barrier cream.

Regular herbal hand treatments

To soften and soothe hands, soak them in an infusion of lady's mantle, fennel, comfrey, yarrow, or marsh mallow; an infusion of calendula or chamomile flowers is also effective.

Heavy-duty barrier cream

4 tbsp petroleum jelly	2 handfuls fresh elderflowers

1 Gently melt the petroleum jelly, then add the elderflowers.

2 Leave to macerate for 45 minutes, reheating the jelly each time it solidifies.

3 Warm to a liquid and strain through a sieve into a screw-top jar. Cool and then seal.

Glycerin and rosewater hand cream

A useful everyday skin softener.

4 tbsp glycerin	3 drops essential oil
1 cup rosewater	of rose
4 tbsp cornstarch	

1 Blend the glycerin, rosewater and cornstarch. Heat the mixture over a double boiler until it thickens.

2 Allow to cool, then add the rose oil, stirring well. Pour into screw-top jars and label.

Dill and horsetail nail bath

Both these herbs contain silicic acid, which helps to strengthen nails. Warm the mixture before using and soak your nails in it for 10 minutes every other day.

2 tbsp chopped horsetail	2 tbsp dill seed
	1 cup boiling water

1 Pour the water over the two herbs and steep for at least an hour.

2 Strain the liquid into a bottle.

Lady's mantle hand lotion

2 tbsp glycerin	10 drops essential oil of
2 tsp carrageen moss	lemon, rose, geranium or
melted in a little hot water	sandalwood
4 tbsp alcohol	2 tbsp strong infusion
	of lady's mantle

1 Stir the glycerin into the melted moss.

2 Add the essential oil to the alcohol, mixing well, and then blend the two mixtures. Stir in the herbal infusion, blending well.

3 Pour into a screw-top jar and label. Shake before use, if necessary.

Hand mask

Once a week treat your hands to this mask to whiten and soften the skin. Apply to the hands for 20 minutes, preferably just before going to bed. Wash off, then apply a rich moisturizing cream for the night (and wear cotton gloves while you sleep). Wash off the cream the following morning.

2 tbsp finely ground oatmeal	1 tsp avocado oil
1 tbsp calendula petals or lady's mantle infusion	1 tsp lemon juice
	1 tsp glycerin

Mix the ingredients together to form a smooth paste. Use as instructed above.

Feet

Any of the above treatments for hands can also be applied to feet. The enriching mask is particularly beneficial, but remember to wear cotton socks if you put moisturizer on your feet overnight.

Herbal foot baths

The traditional foot bath is one of the most therapeutic treatments.

To refresh tired feet choose from: bay, lavender, sage, sweet marjoram, thyme. Place a large handful of fresh or a quarter cup of dried herb and 1 tablespoon sea salt in a bowl of hot water. For convenience, these can be loose in the water.
● **To make a warming foot bath,** add 1 table-spoon black mustard seed, bruised, to the water. (Black mustard seed can be obtained at Indian or Pakistani grocery stores.)
● **To soothe itchy feet,** add 4 tablespoons cider vinegar to your foot bath.
● **To deodorize feet,** soak them in a strong decoction of sage or lovage.

Cold feet

Add 1 teaspoon cayenne to talcum powder or fuller's earth and sprinkle on your feet to get a quick warming sensation.

Hair care

Although most aspects of hair – its color, rate of growth, thickness and curliness – are hereditary, a wide range of herbal ingredients has been used through the ages to improve and enhance what nature provides.

Advertising agents have decided we all fall into one of four hair types: dry, greasy, normal or "problem" hair, but herbal trichologists state that all hair is normal for that person and problems should first be dealt with by looking holistically at a person: that is, looking at his or her lifestyle. Too many spicy foods, fats and sugars can be responsible for greasy hair, and synthetic shampoos can cause dry hair. There is also concern about the effects that medicated shampoos can have on the hair and scalp if used routinely. Stress, hormonal changes, lack of sleep, too much sun, chemical hair treatments, rinses and dyes all cause hair problems too.

HERBS USED IN HAIR CARE

To condition dry hair burdock root, comfrey, elderflowers, marsh mallow, parsley, sage, stinging nettle.

To condition greasy hair calendula, horsetail, lemon juice, lemon balm, lavender, mints, rosemary, southernwood, witch hazel and yarrow.

To prevent dandruff burdock root, chamomile, garlic and onion bulbs (powerful but unpleasantly scented), goosegrass, parsley, rosemary, southernwood, stinging nettle and thyme.

To soothe scalp irritation catmint (leaves and flowering tops), chamomile, comfrey.

To provide a hair tonic (giving body and luster) calendula, goosegrass, horsetail, linden flowers, nasturtium, parsley, rosemary, sage, southernwood, stinging nettles and watercress.

To dispel lice an infusion of quassia chips, poke root, or juniper berries with a tablespoon of cider vinegar. Apply at two-week intervals, three times.

Hair treatments

Dry hair, and any hair lacking luster, will benefit from a warm oil treatment before a shampoo.

Make a herbal oil using one of the above herbs and a polyunsaturated vegetable oil such as peach kernel, almond or sunflower. Alternatively, add 6 drops of essential oil to 2 tablespoons of almond oil or any vegetable oil. Warm the oil, pour a small amount into your palm and rub your hands together. Massage well into the scalp and along the hair strands. Repeat as necessary. Cover the head with foil and a plastic shower cap and wrap in a hot towel (wrung out in hot water), replacing the towel when it cools. Try to leave on for 20 to 30 minutes for greatest penetration, then wash off with a mild shampoo.

A quick herbal shampoo

Pour one application of a mild baby shampoo into a cup and add 2 tablespoons of a strong decoction of your selected herb, or 4 drops of essential oil. Mix together and use in the normal manner.

Soapwort shampoo

A very gentle cleansing shampoo which doesn't make much lather – but then lather does not equal cleaning power.

2 tbsp finely chopped soapwort root or a handful of leaves and stems	1 large handful of herb (see box) $2\frac{1}{2}$ cups boiling water

1 Pour the boiling water over the soapwort and herb and infuse for at least 30 minutes.

2 Strain and use when cool. About half a cup should be enough for average-length hair.

Soapbark shampoo

Good for greasy hair. Simmer 2 tablespoons soapbark chips (available from many health-food stores) in $2\frac{1}{2}$ cups water for 30 minutes.

Dry shampoo

2 tbsp powdered orris root	2 tbsp powdered arrowroot

Mix together. Part the hair in narrow regular bands and sprinkle the powder along each row. Leave on for 10 minutes to absorb any grease and then brush out vigorously and thoroughly until the hair is shiny.

Herbal hair rinses

Use these after your shampoo as the quickest and easiest way to improve hair shine. Prepare the herbal rinse before shampooing so it will have cooled when you are ready to use it.

1 tbsp selected herb 4 cups boiling water	1 tbsp cider vinegar (or lemon juice for fair hair)

1 Infuse the herb in water until cool. Strain well. Add the vinegar.

2 Pour through the hair, massaging the scalp. Catch the runoff in a bowl and repeat until either your patience or arms give out. If the final rinse is of cool rather than warm water, it makes all the outer cells on the hair strands lie flat, giving a smooth, shiny finish.

Rosewater pick-me-up

This is an excellent way to clean and revive your hair between shampoos. Orange-flower water can be used instead, or lavender water for greasy hair.

You will need a number of 4 inch squares of gauze dipped in rosewater. Force the gauze over a natural bristle brush and stroke through the hair in sections, removing dirt as you brush. Repeat with fresh gauze squares until the cloth picks up no more dirt. This treatment also gives a lovely fragrance to the hair.

Herbal hair colorants

Make your selection from the herbs listed in the box below. Unless otherwise stated, make a strong decoction, simmering 2 ounces herb in 4 cups of water for 20 minutes, keeping the lid on the pan. Cool, strain and pour through the hair, catching the rinse in a bowl. Repeat as many times as possible. Use an old towel to pat hair dry as some color will come off. These are progressive dyes, so the more you use them, the stronger the effect.

For a more intense color, make the rinse into a paste. Use only 1 cup of water for the decoction and 1 ounce of herb. Boil, strain and add kaolin powder to make a smooth paste. Apply to the hair roots wearing thin rubber gloves and gradually work down the hair strands. Cover the head with a small hot towel and a plastic bag to retain the heat. Leave on for 20 minutes, then rinse off. If further color is required, leave the paste on longer next time.

HERBS TO COLOR HAIR	
To lighten hair Chamomile: infuse 8 tablespoons and use regularly. Mullein flowers: make a decoction. Rhubarb root: make a decoction. Privet leaves: make a decoction. Hollyhock (blue-purple flowers): improves dingy yellow hair. Use as a decoction.	**To redden hair** Alkanet root: make a decoction. Calendula: make a decoction. Henna: follow product instructions carefully, as results are variable. Red hibiscus: make a decoction. Saffron: make a decoction.
To darken hair Sage: make a decoction. Sage and rosemary leaves: make a decoction. Sage and dried raspberry leaves: make a decoction. Green outer shells of unripe walnuts: crush in a pestle and mortar, add a pinch of salt, cover with water and soak for 3 days. Then add 3 cups water and simmer for 5 hours, adding more water as necessary to maintain at least 1 cup liquid. Strain and reduce to 1 cup by boiling. Ivy berries: make a decoction.	**For black hair** Elderberries: make a decoction. Indigo leaves and henna in equal quantities: make a decoction. **For gray hair** Hollyhock (blue-purple flowers): removes yellow tones. Use as a decoction. Betony: highlights yellow tones. Use as a decoction. Sage: darkens gray hair and adds luster. Use as a decoction.

Eye care

The best recipe for clear bright eyes is a good night's sleep. "Just enough regular and natural sleep is the great kindler of woman's most charming light," wrote a famous beauty of the nineteenth century. Failing that, eyes that are tired, irritated or bloodshot can often be soothed with a cooled herbal decoction. However, if you experience frequent or continuing eye irritation, it is advisable to consult a doctor.

When you are dealing with the delicate eye area, scrupulous cleanliness is vital. Sterilize all utensils and fabrics and use only absolutely fresh decoctions. Always boil herbs for an eyebath for 20 minutes to kill the greatest number of bacteria. Then filter the solution three times through a coffee filter paper to ensure no small bits remain to irritate the eye.

The most famous reputation for giving a brilliance and sparkle to the eyes goes to the modest little plant eyebright (*Euphrasia rostkoviana*). It is called *Augentrost* (consolation to the eyes) by the Germans, *luminella* (light for the eyes) by the Italians, and *casse-lunette* (discard your spectacles) by the French. It can relieve tiredness and soreness, and halt running eyes from a cold or hay fever.

Eyebright eyebath
Boil 2 tablespoons of the fresh plant or 2 teaspoons of the dried herb in 2 cups water for 20 minutes. Cool, strain and use immediately in an eyebath.

Agrimony eyebath
This herb is second to eyebright in its fame for adding luster to eyes. Boil a handful of fresh tops in $2\frac{1}{2}$ cups of water for 20 minutes. Cool, strain and use immediately.

Eye compresses
The following herbal teabag compress refreshes tired eyes at work.

Make 2 cups of chamomile or rosehip tea, using 2 teabags, and brew for 3 minutes. Remove the bags and cool. Place the teabags over your eyes for 15 minutes, put your feet up and rest. This can also be done with black teabags.

Eye gels
Lotions or gels for the delicate, thin skin around the eye must be light so that the application does not drag or pull the skin. The ingredients should treat only the surface of the skin. Rich penetrating oils can contribute to a puffy appearance around the eyes.

Eyebright or elderflower gel
Dissolve a strong decoction of eyebright or elderflower water in gelatin (following manufacturer's instructions) for a soothing and cooling eye gel.

Soothing eye gel
Use equal quantities of chamomile, calendula and cornflower flowers and mallow leaves to make a strong decoction.

6 tbsp decoction	pinch of sodium benzoate
2 tbsp witch hazel	if required to improve
$\frac{1}{4}$ tsp agar agar	keeping qualities

1 Heat the herbal decoction and witch hazel until just below boiling point. Stir in the agar (and benzoate) to dissolve. The agar agar must be thoroughly dissolved or it will feel grainy.

2 Leave to cool and thicken. If it forms a solid gel, put into a blender for a few seconds to thin. Store in screw-top jar in refrigerator.

HERBAL EYE REFRESHERS

Make a strong decoction of the herb. Strain, then soak sterilized squares of gauze in the solution and apply over closed eyes while resting.

Calendula Soothes sore or inflamed eyes
Chamomile Reduces inflammation and removes a "tired look"
Cornflower Soothes and helps reduce puffiness
Fennel seed Removes inflammation and gives sparkle
Horsetail Reduces redness and swollen eyelids and can be effective for styes. (Must boil for 30 minutes.)
Mallow Softens skin around eyes
Mint Minimizes dark circles under the eyes
Rose Softens and soothes skin around the eyes
Wormwood Reduces eye inflammation and redness; dab on a decoction with absorbent cotton.

For an extra-refreshing application, freeze any of the above strained decoctions in ice-cube trays and rub a cube over the eyelids and around the eyes.

Teeth

Most commercial toothpastes contain damaging abrasives, detergents and sweetening agents. Homemade products can achieve a better result without the harmful ingredients.

Instant tooth cleansers
● Rub a sage leaf over the teeth and gums to make them feel polished and clean.
● Peel a twig of flowering dogwood, chew the end to create a brush and rub on the teeth and gently on the gums.

Peppermint toothpaste
To make your own cleansing paste, take 1 teaspoon bicarbonate of soda, charcoal or powdered strawberry roots and 2 drops essential oil of peppermint. Add enough drops of water to create a paste. Mix and use.

Stain removers
Strawberry: rub half a strawberry (alpine is best) over the teeth.
Lemon peel: rub the wet side on the teeth. The blanching property of lemon is good for removing tea and other brown stains.

Mouthwashes
Commercial mouthwashes are often so powerful that they damage the proper balance of digestive juices and can irritate the lining of the mouth. Seek further help for persistent bad breath, as the digestive system may not be functioning properly. To sweeten the breath, chew fresh parsley, pulverized nettle leaves or watercress, which are all high in chlorophyll, the green plant pigment used in many commercial breath sweeteners. For a quick mouthwash, gargle with a peppermint infusion, rosewater, lavender water, or dilute witch hazel (1 part witch hazel to 6 parts water).

Toothache
To ease the pain, apply a drop of oil of cloves.

Mint and rosemary mouthwash
Both herbs sweeten the breath, and rosemary has antiseptic properties. If you wish to make up larger quantities, add 1 teaspoon tincture of myrrh for its preservative properties.

$2\frac{1}{2}$ cups distilled or	1 tsp rosemary leaves
mineral water	1 tsp aniseed
1 tsp fresh mint leaves	

1 Boil the water and infuse the mint, rosemary and aniseed for 20 minutes.

2 When cool, strain and use as a gargle.

Apricot and lemon lip balm
A delicious, protective and healing gloss, especially good for chapped lips.

1 tsp beeswax	a few drops essential oil of
1 tsp apricot kernel oil	lemon or orange
1 tsp calendula oil	

1 Melt the beeswax. Add the apricot and calendula oils, stirring constantly.

2 Remove from the heat while stirring, and when partly cooled add the essential oil. Store in a small pot.

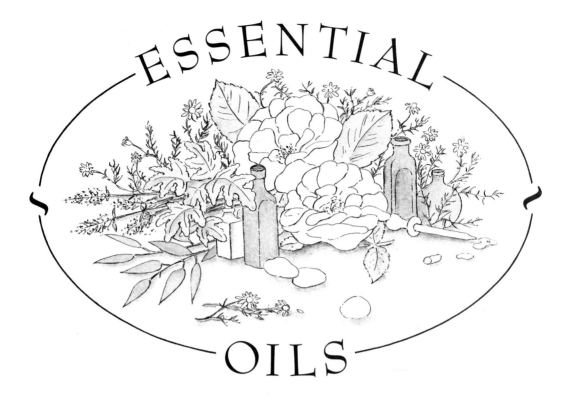

ESSENTIAL OILS

Essential oils are the concentrated vital essences of aromatic plants. They contain potent therapeutic properties and are much used in cosmetics, perfumes and flavorings, and in aromatherapy – a system of healing the body through massage, inhalation or bathing with blended essential oils. Although called "oils," they are more like water, being a liquid that readily evaporates.

Essential oils are found in minute glands in one or more parts of aromatic plants: in leaves (basil), flowers (rose), fruit (lemon), seed (coriander), wood (sandalwood), resin (frankincense), bark (cinnamon) and roots (calamus). Heat causes these essences to evaporate, creating a protective aura around the plant which seems to fight bacteria, fungi and pests, and also seems to act as a buffer against extremes of temperature.

Historical background
Aromatic oils have a long, rich history and were highly valued in ancient cultures in the Far and Middle East, including Egypt, China and India. *Ayur veda*, a system of traditional Indian medicine dating back to 1000 B.C., includes these oils in many healing and rejuvenating recipes.

Numerous papyri and temple reliefs show us that the Egyptians used them to perfume their clothes and bodies, to preserve and flavor food and drink, to heal, and most famously, to embalm. When the tomb of Tutankhamen was entered in 1922, the scent of herb oils was still perceptible.

Over two thousand years ago, the Greek physician Theophrastus wrote a study of scent and its healing effects entitled *Concerning Odors*. In this, he laid the early groundwork for some of our current understanding of aromatherapy. He described the effects of different flower essences and noted that an aromatic plant poultice applied to a leg could produce fragrant breath – its essences could permeate the skin and enter the circulatory system.

In Arabia, the technique of distillation was perfected centuries ago. This method of extracting plant essences by steaming is still the most useful in terms of preserving a plant's fragrance and healing properties. During the eleventh century A.D., Persian chemists distilled highly exotic and sophisticated essences, including the famous attar of roses. Crusaders learned these skills and brought them back to Europe.

For the past few centuries, the world's essential-oil industry has been centered in Grasse, in southern France. With the sixteenth-century fashion for scented gloves, local glovers were licensed to scent their own leather and sell perfumes, and their use of lavender oil appears to have rendered them immune to an outbreak of cholera.

Today essential oils have an enormous range of uses, in food, cosmetics and medicines. Most research is into their remarkable healing potential.

Healing properties
The revival of essential oils for healing in the West was instigated by a French chemist, Professor René-Maurice Gattefosse, who originated the term "aromatherapy." He conducted experiments with

essential oils on wounded soldiers during World War I. At this time, the most commonly used antiseptic was phenol, which was good for cleaning hospital floors but not very effective for healing wounds. The soldiers Gattefosse was treating had badly infected wounds, which often resulted in serious poisoning as the body reabsorbed harmful substances produced by decaying tissue. His work proved that essential oils, particularly lavender, are superior to chemical antiseptics in their ability to detoxify and speed up the elimination of these substances. Gattefosse was convinced of the power of lavender after he accidently burned his hand in his laboratory. The wound became gangrenous and he applied lavender oil. The pain went almost immediately and the skin soon healed, perfectly cured.

Another attractive feature of the antiseptic essential oils is that they do not appear to lose their effect with repeated applications.

More recent experiments have shown that essential oils are carried through the circulatory system to all the organs and eventually through the elimination system, the process taking anywhere from 30 minutes to 12 hours. To appreciate this, rub the sole of your foot with a slice of garlic, then smell your breath several hours later. It seems that each organ takes from the essential oils the components it needs.

Both directly in the pleasure they give and indirectly, essential oils are therapeutic. The sense of smell is our most ancient sense and yet the one we know least about. A scent travels from the olfactory nerves in the nose directly to the part of the brain concerned with intuition, emotions and creativity. It registers almost twice as fast as a pain sensation. Because the sense of smell is so immediate, substances administered by scent are likely to affect the body's chemical balance. For this reason, psychiatrists and psychologists are taking great interest in the safe mood-changing potential of essential oils.

Aromatherapy
Madame Maury, a biochemist and student of Gattefosse, recognized the potential of plant essences for skin care and developed the massage techniques and formulae now usually associated with aromatherapy.

Trained aromatherapists draw on several diagnostic and treatment systems. Their approach is usually holistic (looking at how all aspects of a person's life affects their well-being), and is based on the idea that the most effective way to prevent illness is to strengthen the body's own defence systems. Essential oils are applied mostly through massage but also through baths and inhalations.

These techniques are all easy to use at home as long as you follow the recommended number of drops for treatments. The oils are so concentrated that even a few drops too many can reverse their beneficial effects and provoke a bad reaction.

HOW ESSENTIAL OILS ARE PRODUCED AND SOLD
The extraction of oils is a highly complex and expensive business. Most oils are collected by distillation (steaming) or enfleurage (in grease). Both methods are time-consuming, labour-intensive and require expert use of complicated equipment and top quality materials. Huge amounts of plant stock are needed to distil minute quantities of oil: it takes about 250 pounds (115 kg) of rose petals to produce 1 fl oz (25 ml) of essential oil. For these reasons it is not worth attempting to extract essential oils at home.

Pure essential oils versus synthetic
Continuous attempts are being made to create synthetic essences as substitutes for essential oils. Some scents have been reproduced quite successfully, but it is only the scent. This is often acceptable to the food and cosmetic industries but it is of no use to anyone interested in the therapeutic value of an essential oil. Each essential oil is composed of many active and effective ingredients so that it can have many functions; one oil may soften the skin, act as a preservative, and deter insects. No synthetic substances can replicate all these aspects.

Buying essential oils
As the popularity of essential oils swells, so a wave of new firms has appeared each selling its own labelled oils. When you are buying oils, check that the supplier runs tests on them for purity, that staff are knowledgeable about their qualities and uses, and that they handle and store them correctly. Never buy oils that have been displayed in a hot sunny window or in clear glass. They must be stored in airtight, dark glass containers in a cool, dark place but not a refrigerator. The ideal storage temperature is about 65 °F (18 °C).

Many shops sell oils labelled "aromatherapy oils", a mixture of about two percent essential oil in a carrier oil (a lubricating vegetable oil), which is meant for massage. Once essential oils are added to carrier oils, their shelf life is reduced from years to a few months.

As a further guarantee of quality, get to know the price range of essential oils. At the time of writing, jasmine, neroli and rose are 150 to 175 times more expensive than camphor, sweet orange and eucalyptus, with most oils being in the range of two, three and four times the price of camphor. If a selection of essential oils is offered all at the same price, be suspicious.

Essential oils in massage

Massage is the primary method of application in aromatherapy. Essential oils are selected and blended with a carrier oil before the massage, as described in the box below. When undergoing a massage, you first notice the fragrance but soon become aware of the many other benefits. Essential oils penetrate the skin more effectively than vegetable oils, taking from 20 to 70 minutes to enter the bloodstream. However, their benefits to the body and emotions go on for far longer.

General benefits of aromatherapy massage

● Depending on the oils selected and the individual, the fragrance can have a relaxing or stimulating effect on the mind and spirits. The sense of smell is our most immediate sense – an unpleasant smell can cause nausea within seconds. It is closely linked to memory and emotional responses. Because of the fragrance alone, a massage can have considerable effect.
● The oils combined with the massage help to relieve stress and tension by their effect on the mind, the nerve endings, and the muscles.
● Many oils are antibacterial and work to relieve or heal certain internal conditions as well as skin problems (see the chart on p. 236).
● The combination of massage and oils improves blood circulation.
● The combination of oils and massage is thought to improve cell growth on the skin and give the surface a smooth appearance by speeding up the elimination of old skin cells.
● The oils combined with the massage help to accelerate the elimination of wastes through the body's lymphatic system, which cleanses and nourishes the blood.

Specific benefits

Here are some ideas for using oils to treat a number of common problems. For further ideas on the specific treatments and the relevant oils to use, see the recipes on the following page and the charts on p. 236 and p. 258.
● Use of the correct oils can normalize an oily or dry skin (for oily skins, try cedarwood, juniper, lemon, ylang-ylang; for dry skins, try chamomile, geranium, clary sage, jasmine, lavender, neroli).
● To soothe acne and other skin eruptions, try juniper, chamomile, cedarwood, eucalyptus, lavender, lemon grass.
● To increase the elasticity of the skin and promote the growth of new skin cells, try lavender, chamomile, calendula, jasmine, frankincense, myrrh.
● Cellulite seems to improve with aromatherapy massage (try cypress, fennel, geranium, juniper).
● To eradicate feelings of apathy, try jasmine or rosemary.
● To lift depression, try camphor, chamomile, jasmine, thyme, basil, bergamot, clary sage.

CARRIER OILS FOR MASSAGE

As essential oils are highly concentrated, they are used by the drop, and must be diluted in a carrier oil for skin applications. A carrier oil is a lubricating oil, used in massage to allow the hands to glide smoothly over skin. Aromatherapy uses only vegetable oils, mainly cold-pressed from seeds. These do not evaporate when warmed, unlike essential oils, but they become rancid on exposure to air and do so more quickly once mixed with essential oils.

A blend will be at its best for two or three months, so it is wise not to mix more oil than you may use in that time. Store it in an airtight bottle in a cool, dark place.

A good carrier oil has penetrative properties to assist the essential oils; is 100 percent pure; should have little or no smell, an attractive texture for massage and should benefit the skin. Select from the following:

Almond oil The most popular carrier oil, as it has little smell, is rich in protein and is emollient, nourishing and slow to become rancid.

Apricot kernel and peach kernel oils Both have the same properties as almond oil but are more expensive.

Grapeseed oil Very fine and clear; it gives a satin-smooth finish without a greasy touch.

Hazelnut oil Hazelnut penetrates the most easily and deeply. It stimulates the circulation and nourishes the skin.

Jojoba oil Keeps well and gives a satin-smooth feel to the skin. Treats acne.

Olive oil Calming, good for rheumatism and to relieve the itching of skin ailments. Unfortunately the scent of olives can overpower the fragrance of the essential oils.

Sesame oil Keeps well, but the rich color and odor can be off-putting. Used in Scandinavia to treat cases of dry eczema and psoriasis.

Corn, soy and sunflower oils Acceptable. Soy has a nice feel and doesn't become sticky with pressure. Sunflower has the least keeping qualities but contains vitamin F.

The following oils are often added in small quantities to a massage mix for their special qualities.

Avocado oil Nourishing and penetrating; useful for fatty areas and muscle preparations. Becomes sticky when massaged into a large area.

Calendula oil Macerated calendula petals. Beneficial in any cosmetic preparation for chapped and cracked skin.

Carrot oil Tonic and rejuvenating and particularly good for neck massage. Rich in many vitamins.

Evening primrose oil Useful for scaly skin and dandruff. Recent research has shown that oil extracted from borage seed has a similar composition.

Wheatgerm oil Nourishing, rich in vitamin E, but would be rather "oily" on its own. It is a natural antioxidant (preservative); a teaspoonful added to 2 fluid ounces massage oil will extend its keeping time.

MIXING ESSENTIAL OILS FOR MASSAGE

Most essential oils are sold in bottles measured in milliliters. One milliliter equals about 20 drops of essential oil. To a 2 ounce bottle of carrier oil, add between 15 and 30 drops of essential oil. The usual amount is 25 drops. Trial and error teaches that some problems and some people respond to more dilute solutions, while others require greater strength. Start with the average amount or less. Lower concentrations often give the best results for emotional problems, whereas higher concentrations are often more successful for helping physical problems.

One full body massage uses 2 to 4 teaspoons of a blend, which can be mixed in a small measuring cup. For a deluxe massage oil in a 2 fluid ounce bottle, add 1 teaspoon wheatgerm oil for keeping quality, 1 teaspoon avocado oil for greater penetration, then top up with your chosen carrier oil and drops of essential oil.

When you make up a blend, label and date the bottle, reminding yourself whom it was blended for and for what conditions.

Selecting the oils

Decide which conditions you want to treat and then refer to the chart on p. 236. Usually two or three oils are added, occasionally four. Each oil has different properties so select those that are most appropriate and appealing.

For example, if you have a dry, mature skin and wish to make a facial oil as a night treatment, you will find quite a bewildering choice of oils. Think about their additional properties and select scents that appeal to you.

You may also want to consider an oil's "note." Essential oils, like perfumes, are described as having a top, middle or base note. In aromatic terms, top notes are noticed first; they are stimulating and uplifting. Middle notes form the character of a perfume and last longer. Base notes are mainly sedative and calming, and are very long-lasting. You may prefer to select one oil from each group to make a balance, but it is not essential. When I made a massage oil for one son's aching muscles after an overexuberant day of sports, I assembled eucalyptus, juniper, lavender, marjoram, rosemary, sage and thyme (all good for muscular aches and pains) and invited him to choose three. He selected (by sniffing preference) eucalyptus, sage and thyme, which are all top notes, but which helped to clear his head cold at the same time as soothing his muscles.

The box (right) shows a suggested list of recipes for drops added to 2 fluid ounces of carrier oil. To make less, cut all ingredients proportionally.

THERAPEUTIC BLENDS	
TREATMENT	**FORMULA (in drops)**
Skin facial oils	
Normal skin	6 frankincense 6 geranium 3 jasmine 12 lavender
Dry skin	8 chamomile 8 rose 8 sandalwood
Oily skin	8 cedarwood 10 lemon 6 ylang-ylang
Massage oils	
Stretch marks	10 frankincense 15 lavender 5 neroli
Post-diet saggy skin	8 lemongrass 8 pine 8 sage
Cellulite (use hazelnut oil)	8 oregano 8 fennel 8 rosemary
Muscular cramp	10 basil 8 cypress 8 sweet marjoram
Muscular aches (use hazelnut oil)	8 bergamot 8 coriander 6 eucalyptus 8 rosemary
Arthritis	10 juniper 10 lemon 5 thyme
Arthritis (before sleep)	6 benzoin 6 chamomile 8 cypress 8 sage
Rheumatism, acute	9 ginger 9 pine 9 rosemary
Rheumatism, chronic	6 eucalyptus 8 juniper 8 rosemary 6 thyme
Colds and flu	7 cinnamon 7 eucalyptus 7 tea tree 7 pine
Bronchitis	10 eucalyptus 5 hyssop 10 niaouli 5 sandalwood
Asthma	4 hyssop 8 lavender 8 pine 8 rosemary
Eczema (dry)	10 calendula 5 chamomile 5 geranium 5 lavender
Eczema (weeping)	5 bergamot 10 calendula 10 juniper
High blood pressure	10 clary sage 10 lavender 10 ylang-ylang
Sinusitis	7 basil 7 eucalyptus 7 lavender 7 peppermint
Circulation, poor	12 black pepper 12 juniper 8 cypress
Nausea and diarrhea	9 lavender 9 peppermint 6 sandalwood
Menstrual pain	7 chamomile 7 clary sage 7 cypress 4 jasmine
Mosquito repellent	5 clove 10 eucalyptus 5 geranium 5 peppermint
Massage or inhalation (see p. 235)	
Cough and cold	3 benzoin 2 cypress 3 eucalyptus 2 hyssop
Head cold	3 basil 3 eucalyptus 3 ginger
Bronchitis	4 eucalyptus 4 niaouli 2 hyssop
Sinus	2 basil 2 eucalyptus 2 lavender 2 peppermint

GIVING A MASSAGE

With a friend, it is easy to enjoy and give a beneficial massage using therapeutic oils and basic massage strokes. A warm quiet room with soft lighting, no drafts or interruptions and perhaps the addition of some gentle meditation music (without sudden changes in tempo) will provide the atmosphere for a deeply relaxing experience.

Make sure your friend has plenty of space to lie comfortably full length on a firm surface. Professional masseurs use a massage table which is level with the upper thigh and 2 feet 6 inches wide. Ideally, the height should be level with the flat of your hand when holding your arm down at your side. You can use a long table with a padded covering; a narrow, very firm bed; a thin foam mattress or blankets on the floor as a substitute for a massage table. Protect whatever you use with a towel, as you will probably spill some oil. You'll also need somewhere less than an arm's length away to put the oil bottle between applications, to enable you to keep in continuous contact with your friend's skin, even if with your elbow.

The fewer clothes your friend wears, the easier you will find it to do long flowing strokes, but it's important that your friend feels comfortable. Cover any bare parts that you're not working on with a towel to keep them warm.

Before starting the massage, ensure that your hands are clean and warm. Rub them together for a second or two if they feel cold. A cold hand on the back is not a good way to start a massage.

WHEN MASSAGE IS INAPPROPRIATE

Although there are many benefits to an aromatherapy massage, the effects can be so far-reaching that sometimes it should be avoided.

● After a very hot bath, steam bath or sauna, the skin will be eliminating excess heat, toxins and surplus moisture for up to an hour. When the body is eliminating, it is not absorbing, so except for giving a pleasant fragrance, the therapeutic benefits of the oils would be wasted.

● Do not massage any area if it causes discomfort either to you or your friend.

● Do not massage if the person has a temperature, fever or viral disease, as this may spread the infection further via the lymphatic system. For the same reason, do not massage if cancer is suspected.

● Do not massage someone who has recently undergone a serious operation.

● Avoid areas where there are fractures, broken skin, sprains, bruises, swelling, rashes, torn muscles or ligaments, or varicose veins.

● Do not massage anyone who has heart trouble.

● Do not massage someone who has acute back pain.

● Do not massage the abdomen straight after a meal.

● If in doubt, don't massage.

MASSAGE STROKES

Aromatherapy massage employs a range of different strokes. Three of the easiest techniques to use are:

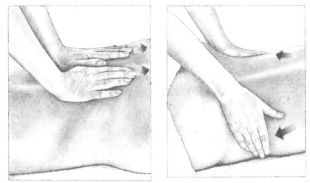

Effleurage This long stroking movement makes up most of aromatherapy massage. It helps movement in the veins and allows fresh blood to circulate more freely. The movement begins with a deep stroke made with pressure in the direction of the heart. The return journey is a light stroke moving away from the heart over a large area. The whole hand must be relaxed and molded to the shape of the body as it glides rhythmically over the skin.

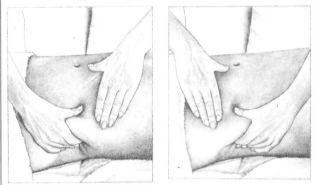

Kneading A vigorous movement, this stimulates muscle tissue, increases circulation and helps reduce fatigue by facilitating the removal of waste products. Pick up a handful of flesh and squeeze or roll it with one hand, then pass it to the other. Pick up the adjacent skin and repeat to make a rippling movement as if you were kneading dough. Do this slowly and rhythmically, after relaxing the area with effleurage.

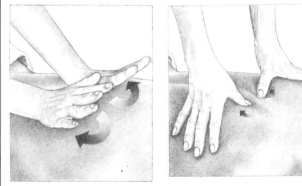

Frictions These movements stimulate circulation and help to remove excess fluid. Press the heel of the hand into the skin and move it in deep circles using a little pressure. After several circles, slide gently to the next area, always keeping in contact with the skin. On small areas of skin, use your thumbs instead of the heel of the hand.

Back massage

The back is a good area to start exploring the power of massage. It provides an expanse for your hands to experiment on and the opportunity to try out different massage strokes. It is also the area most people enjoy having massaged.

Have your friend lie on his or her front with arms comfortably positioned at the side or acting as a cushion under the forehead.

Start by placing one of your hands on the crown of your friend's head and the other at the base of the spine for a few seconds to establish contact. Breathe slowly and deeply, and relax. Take your selected oil and pour about a teaspoonful into one hand (it may be more fluid than you anticipate when you first pour). Take more later as you need it: 2 to 4 teaspoons should be sufficient for a back, depending on the dryness of the skin. Rub your hands together and cover the whole back with the oil.

The following is a suggestion of strokes for you to adapt or build on as you wish.

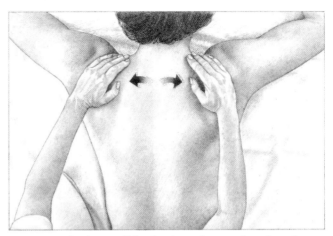

1 Start at the base of the back with your hands either side of the spine, fingers pointing upward. Move them up the center to the base of the neck, then slide them across the shoulders and bring them down lightly to your starting position. Repeat these long effleurage strokes until the back is oiled. Apply a series of dinner plate-size circular movements up both sides of the spine, then glide your hands slowly and rhythmically back down to the base of the spine.

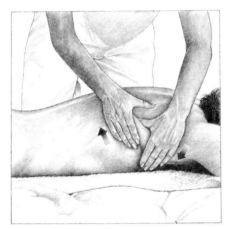

2 Move your hands to one side of the body and start to knead the flesh, working up the back and across the top of the shoulders. On the less fleshy areas knead more lightly, using just your thumb and fingers, not the whole of your hand. Be careful not to pinch. Repeat on the other side of the spine, then lightly slide your hands down, without dragging the skin.

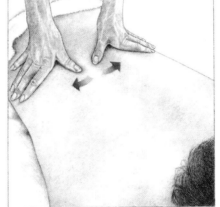

3 Starting again at the base of the spine, make small friction movements with your thumbs along either side of the backbone, working up to the neck and over the shoulder blades. Press into the muscles and outward, not into the bones, and work with both hands simultaneously. Return to the base of the spine, gliding your hands down the back in long, rhythmic strokes.

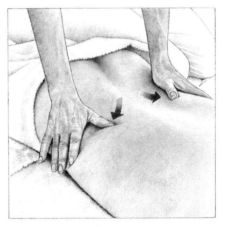

4 Make small friction movements with your thumbs, starting from the backbone at waist level and moving in an outward curve over the hip bone. Make three concentric curves. Complete the massage with a series of long, slow effleurage strokes, then finish by resting both hands lightly on the small of the back. Hold this position for a few seconds, then slowly lift your hands away.

Arm massage

Use a small drop of oil for each arm. Hold one hand in your hand and stroke from the wrist up the outside of the arm with your other hand. Repeat the stroke on the inside of the arm. Knead any areas of cellulite on the backs of the upper arms and make friction circles on any rheumatic areas. Knead into the shoulder muscles and finish with a few effleurage strokes up and down the arm, letting your hand trail off from the fingertips. Repeat the movements on the other arm.

Leg massage

Start on the backs of the legs so have your friend lie on his or her stomach. Put a drop of oil in one palm, rub your hands together lightly and place your palms over the soles of your friend's feet to establish contact. Now run your hands up the backs of the legs to the knees, pause and continue upward. Stroke firmly toward the tops of the legs and lightly back down several times until you have covered the legs in oil. Never apply pressure to the backs of the knees. Use kneading on any cellulite in the thighs followed by effleurage. Finish the backs of the legs by running your hands up to the tops of the thighs and sliding them off outward.

Turn your friend over, using the towels to keep him or her warm, and massage the front of each leg. Place your hands across the first leg, stroking sideways up to the top, one hand after the other. Go firmly upward, lightly downward. Repeat the treatment on the other leg. Make circular movements with the fingers (or lightly with the thumbs) around the ankles and the knees. Finish with relaxing effleurage strokes, working from the ankle up to the tops of the legs.

Foot massage

For a real treat, give yourself or a friend a foot massage. First bathe the feet to freshen them and then pat them dry. Pour about a teaspoonful of oil into your palm, rub your hands together and then take one foot in your hands. Place one hand under the sole of the foot and the other on top. Start to spread the oil by moving both hands up to the heel and down to the big toe. Work the oil well into the foot by repeating this stroke several times. Stroke each toe separately, running your fingers from the tip to the base. Work from the big toe to the little toe.

Repeat the routine with the other foot. Then take the tops of both feet in your fingers, and rest your thumbs on the heels. Slide your thumbs along from the heel to the toes and repeat several times, moving from the sides of the feet to the center of the soles. All movements on the feet should be done with confidence. If strokes are too light you will simply cause tickling.

Self face massage

Prepare by cleaning your face well, then pour 2 teaspoons of your oil mix into a saucer. Before oiling your hands, place them over your face, fingers on your forehead and palms over your cheeks and chin. Hold this for a few moments and then slowly draw your fingers out to your ears as if ironing out creases and tension from the forehead.

Now dip your fingers into the oil (very little is needed) and lightly rub your hands together. Always use gentle strokes on the face, particularly around the delicate eye skin. Start under the chin, glide up the face, then circle the eyes in the direction the eyebrows grow.

Add a little more oil and go very gently over the throat and up the face again. Place your fingers at the center of the forehead. Press lightly, then slide them apart toward the temples and off at the hairline. Repeat this movement, placing your fingers slightly higher up the forehead each time until you reach the hairline. Finish by pressing your fingers down harder in the center of your forehead for a few seconds. Repeat this movement along the brow bone until you reach the outer corner of the eyes.

Place your thumbs on your chin and pull them slowly along the jawline up to the ear. Repeat, moving slightly upward each time until you are just below the cheekbone. Then gently stroke the entire face with upward movements.

Work behind the ears, making small circular movements with your fingers. Then gently pinch the outer semicircle of the ear, starting at the top. Finish by pulling on the ear lobes three times.

Complete a face massage by "palming" the eyes. Press the base of your palms over your eyes to exclude the light for about 20 seconds. Do not lift away your hands immediately, let them slide down so they cover your face, hold them there for a few moments, then gently take them away.

Facial massage strokes

The drawings below show some of the basic facial massage strokes. To give yourself a soothing facial massage, follow the procedure described above.

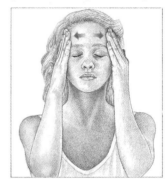

Ease away tension by stroking outward from the center of your forehead.

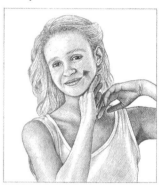

Lightly stroke up your neck and along your jawline to your ears.

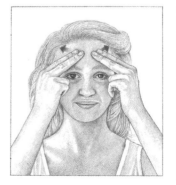

Smooth your fingers across your forehead, moving from the center outward along your hairline.

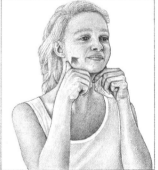

Draw your thumbs up along your jawbone, from your chin out to your ears. Repeat, moving upward.

OTHER WAYS OF USING ESSENTIAL OILS

You can experience the beneficial properties of essential oils by trying one of a number of other methods of application apart from massage. Use the chart on the following pages to select your oils.

Air purification
Essential oils have active antiseptic, antibacterial and even antiviral properties to differing degrees (see chart on p. 236). Some essential oil companies now sell various antiseptic oils in atomizers which are excellent for domestic use, especially in a sick room, and for use in hospitals and other public places.
● To make your own air purifier, half fill an atomizer with isopropyl alcohol and add 200 drops of essential oils per fluid ounce. Try 65 drops bergamot, 25 drops lemon, 25 drops lavender, 15 drops orange, 15 drops thyme, 15 drops clove, 10 drops juniper, 10 drops tea tree, 5 drops peppermint, 5 drops rosemary, 5 drops sandalwood, 5 drops eucalyptus. (If you don't have all these oils, any combination of them will be effective.) Top up with distilled water and spray as required.
   You can make up the mixture without the alcohol, but the oils will not disperse so you'll have to shake the atomizer before each spray, and the keeping qualities will be reduced.

Room fresheners
● Add a few drops of oil to a dish of warm water set on a radiator or in a sunny window. As it evaporates, its aroma will fill the room.
● Alternatively, place drops of one or more oils in a crucible over a small lamp, taking care that they don't burn, or the scent will spoil and the therapeutic qualities will be lost. Try thyme, lavender, pine or eucalyptus for their fresh fragrance.

Potpourri revitalizer
● A favourite use for essential oils is to top up the scent of fading potpourri. Lavender, rose, bergamot, pine, cedarwood, the citrus oils, and spice oils add intensity and freshness to other ingredients.

Car fresheners
● Sprinkle a few drops of an essential oil on a tissue and place it in an air vent inside the car. Use basil or peppermint to remain alert for long distances, or one of the citrus oils to refresh stale air.

Skin creams
● Many essential oils are particularly beneficial to the skin. Add a few drops to a fragrance-free commercial skin cream, or try making some of the basic cosmetic recipes in the previous chapter (see pp. 212–227).

Perfumes
Several essential oils smell beautiful on their own but from the range available you have enormous scope to make your own blends. Mixtures of alcohol and oil are necessary to preserve the scent of essential oils. Perfumes are 15–25 percent essences in pure alcohol. Eau de toilette is 12–15 percent essential oils blended with over 50 percent alcohol and some distilled water.
● See p. 223 for some recommended perfume recipes.

Baths
Aromatic baths using essential oils are highly therapeutic, particularly for muscular aches and pains, skin disorders, circulation problems, tension, fatigue and insomnia.
● Put 5 to 10 drops of oil into a bath of warm water after the water has settled. Mix it around in the water. Relax in the bath for about 10 minutes, with the door and windows closed so you get the full benefit of the aromatic vapors.

Saunas
● Two drops of pine or eucalyptus oil added to a ladle of water or 15 drops to a small bucket make a very pleasant and antiseptic fragrance for inhalation during a sauna.

Inhalants
Steam inhalation is an excellent method of application for everyone except asthmatics. It is particularly effective for treating problems of the respiratory system, such as colds, coughs and sinus, and relieving tension and headaches. The aroma goes straight to the brain while the therapeutic qualities of the oils breathed in pass from the lungs into the blood stream.
● Put 5 to 10 drops of oil in a bowl containing 2½ cups of hot water. Drape a towel over your head if you wish. Inhale the steam for 5 to 10 minutes about 9 inches above the water. Repeat no more than three times a day.
● Inhalation can also be accomplished by putting 5 to 8 drops of oil on a handkerchief or tissue and taking four deep breaths. A portable treatment when in bed, at work, or while traveling. When the tissue is not in use, place it against the breastbone where it will continue to work.

Compresses
These are excellent for treating local problems. Hot compresses soothe old injuries, sprains, muscular aches and pains, neuralgia, painful periods, cystitis and skin problems.
● Put up to 6 drops of chosen oil in enough hot water to soak a compress (an essential oil remains potent no matter how much it is diluted). Soak the compress and squeeze it until it stops dripping. Apply to the affected area and cover with plastic. Keep on for at least two hours. To help retain the heat, add a warmed towel and then place a blanket over the towel and the patient.
● Use a cold compress (made as above but with cold water and refrigerated for soothing coolness) on recent sprains, bruises or swellings and headaches.

Stress
Bathing in water with a few drops of essential oil added is one of the most effective ways to relieve stress.

Insomnia
To relieve insomnia, try putting a drop of basil, chamomile, clary sage, juniper or lavender on your pillow at night.

Studying
● When studying into the small hours of the night, add a drop of uplifting essential oil to a page in each book you are using. Try basil to clear your head; rose to lift your spirits; bergamot to bring freshness; cardamom to reduce mental fatigue.

Internal use
It is important to realize the strength and power of essential oils. One teaspoon of some essential oils taken internally could be lethal. For this reason they should only be taken under the direction of an aromatherapy doctor or herbalist trained in the use of essential oils.
● Teas can be flavored by adding 5 drops of, say, citrus oil to a packet of tea leaves. An alternative is to add one drop to a teabag and use this to make a whole pot of tea.

A GUIDE TO ESSENTIAL OILS

The oils listed below are commonly available and have many uses. The chart lists each oil's properties; conditions it treats; other oils it blends with, and any special points. Each oil is also described by its "note" (under the name).

In simple terms, this refers to its evaporation rate: top notes evaporate quickly; middle notes are mellow; base notes are lasting (see p. 231 for further explanation).

OIL	PROPERTIES	USE TO TREAT	BLEND WITH	SPECIAL NOTE
Basil top	Uplifting, energizing, antidepressant	Anxiety, concentration, digestion, headaches, respiratory problems	Bergamot, geranium, hyssop, neroli, marjoram, melissa, lavender	1 drop soothes wasp sting. More than 3 drops of oil may irritate some skins
Benzoin base	Penetrating, warming	Stimulates circulation; aids respiration; soothes irritated skin; reduces nervous tension	Cinnamon, coriander, cypress, jasmine, lemon, myrrh, rose, sandalwood	A useful fixative
Bergamot top	Fresh, uplifting, antiseptic	Anxiety, depression; stimulates appetite; aids digestion; soothes lung conditions; oily skin	Chamomile, coriander, cypress, geranium, jasmine, lavender, lemon, neroli, ylang-ylang	Do not use neat on exposed skin; may cause uneven pigmentation. Use only a $\frac{1}{2}$–1 percent concentration
Black pepper middle	Light, stimulating	Stimulates circulation, digestion; colds, coughs, muscular aches and pains	Cypress, frankincense, sandalwood, spice oils	
Camphor base	Cooling, highly stimulating	Depression, insomnia, shock, digestion, respiratory problems, oily skin, acne	Frankincense, neroli	Apply immediately in cold compress to reduce swelling of bruises and sprains
Cedarwood base	Sedative, antiseptic, insect repellent	Anxiety, cystitis, all lung conditions, acne, dandruff	Bergamot, cypress, jasmine, juniper, neroli, rosemary	Do not use in pregnancy
Chamomile middle	Refreshing, relaxing, pain reliever for dull aches	Depression, insomnia, digestive problems, menstrual problems, all skin conditions	Benzoin, bergamot, geranium, lavender, lemon, marjoram, neroli, rose, ylang-ylang	First choice for children
Cinnamon base	Warming, astringent, antiseptic	Exhaustion, digestion, coughs, circulation	Coriander, frankincense, citrus oils	
Clary sage top	Warming, soothing, nerve tonic	Depression, insomnia, sore throats, digestion, menstruation, dry skin, insect bites	Bergamot, cedarwood, citrus oils, cypress, geranium, jasmine, juniper, lavender, sandalwood	Small percentages may induce intoxication; large percentages induce headaches
Clove base	Warming, antiseptic, disinfectant, pain reliever, insect repellent	General debility, neuralgia, respiratory problems, toothache, mouth and skin sores	Basil, citrus and spice oils	A drop on a surface will kill ants. Use in air freshener
Coriander top	Sweet, uplifting	Nervous debility, digestion, rheumatic pain	Bergamot, lemon, neroli, orange, cypress, spice	
Cypress middle	Relaxing, refreshing, astringent	Circulation, influenza, laryngitis, muscular cramps, mature skin	Benzoin, bergamot, clary sage, juniper, lavender, lemon, orange, sandalwood	Useful for menopausal upsets
Eucalyptus top	Stimulating, antiseptic, antiviral, insect repellent	Diarrhea, colds and viruses, respiratory problems, aches and pains, cuts and wounds	Benzoin, hyssop, lavender, lemon, lemon grass, melissa, pine, rose	Aids formation of skin tissue. Massage into feet for deep sleep. Good air freshener
Fennel middle	Antitoxic, antispasmodic, diuretic	Digestion, constipation, nausea, oily skin, cellulite; menopause	Geranium, lavender, lemon, rose, sandalwood	Do not give to epileptics or children under 6.
Frankincense base	Warming, relaxing, tonic	Respiratory problems, aging skin, inflammation, wounds	All oils	Considered rejuvenating
Geranium (Pelargonium) middle	Refreshing, relaxing, astringent, insect repellent	Nervous system, digestion, liver and kidney disorders, menstrual problems; normalizes and cleanses skin	All oils	Most used oil in aromatherapy
Ginger base	Stimulating tonic	Digestion, loss of appetite, rheumatic pains, sore throat	Citrus and spice oils	Valuable bath oil to ward off colds
Hyssop middle	Sedative, decongestant	Anxiety, hypertension, normalizes circulation, digestion, respiratory problems, fades bruises	Clary sage, lavender, rosemary, sage, citrus oil	Do not give to epileptics. Can be toxic
Jasmine base	Relaxing, sedative	Depression, uterine pain, respiratory problems; tonic for sensitive skins	All oils	Expensive, but powerful fragrance

A GUIDE TO ESSENTIAL OILS

OIL	PROPERTIES	USE TO TREAT	BLEND WITH	SPECIAL NOTE
Juniper middle	Stimulating tonic, antiseptic, diuretic	Depression, respiratory problems, aching muscles, acne, skin sores, eczema	Bergamot, citrus oils, cypress, geranium, lavender, rosemary, sandalwood	Do not take during pregnancy
Lavender middle	Refreshing, soothing, antiseptic, insect repellent, relieves sharp pain	Insomnia, circulation, indigestion, headaches, infections, muscular pains, cell renewal; benefits all skin types	Most oils, especially citrus, chamomile, clary sage, geranium, pine, rosemary	Excellent first-aid remedy for insect bites and small burns. Low toxicity makes it good for children
Lemon top	Refreshing, invigorating, antiseptic, insect repellent	Circulation, respiratory problems, sore throats, oily skin, broken capillaries	Benzoin, chamomile, eucalyptus, fennel, frankincense, geranium, juniper, neroli, ylang-ylang	Whitens stained teeth; apply neat to insect bites. 2 percent solution in pure water stops small cuts bleeding
Lemon grass top	Toning, revitalizing, antiseptic	Circulation, digestion, muscle tone, acne, oily skin	Basil, geranium, jasmine, lavender	Excellent for post-diet saggy skin
Marjoram (Sweet) middle	Calming, warming	Tension, insomnia, high blood pressure, digestion, colds, headaches, muscular cramps, respiratory problems	Bergamot, chamomile, cypress, lavender, rosemary	
Melissa middle	Refreshing, antidepressant	Tension, neuralgia, digestion, fevers, painful menstruation, respiratory problems	Geranium, juniper, neroli, ylang-ylang	Good for the elderly
Myrrh base	Antiseptic, healing, anti-inflammatory, tonic	Digestion, loss of appetite, catarrh, bronchitis, skin inflammations	Camphor, lavender, spice oils	
Neroli top	Ambrosial, antiseptic	Anxiety, insomnia, diarrhea, rejuvenates skin	Most oils	Powerful scent. Expensive. Excellent for skin.
Niaouli top	Antiseptic, disinfectant, soothing	Respiratory problems, sore throats, colds, skin ulcers, rheumatism	Lavender, pine, mint	Used in many pharmaceutical products: toothpastes, cough drops
Patchouli base	Antiseptic, antidepressant, sedative	Anxiety, dry and mature skins	Basil, bergamot, geranium, juniper, lavender, myrrh, neroli, pine, rose	Small quantities are uplifting; larger doses are sedative
Peppermint top	Invigorating, antiseptic, pain reliever	Fatigue, shock, digestion, travel sickness, headaches, toothache, skin irritations	In small quantities with benzoin, black pepper, melissa, marjoram, spice oils	Use low concentration (1 percent) on inflamed or sensitive skin
Pine middle	Refreshing, antiseptic, disinfectant	Kidney problems, respiratory problems, asthma, sinus problems and flu	Cedarwood, eucalyptus, lavender, rosemary, sage, spice oils	Use in air freshener
Rose base	Relaxing, antidepressant, astringent, antiseptic	Stress, circulation, digestion, headaches; all skins, especially sensitive	Most oils	One of the least toxic oils. Good for children
Rosemary middle	Toning, invigorating, insect repellent	Fatigue, circulation, digestion, headaches, muscular pains, respiratory problems	Basil, cedarwood, frankincense, lavender, lemon, peppermint	Encourages hair growth
Sage top	Soothing, tonic, antiseptic, decongestant	Fatigue, low blood pressure, respiratory problems; clears sluggish skin, firms tissue	Bergamot, hyssop, lemon, lavender, melissa, peppermint, rosemary	Quite toxic. Use in moderation. Do not use if breast-feeding
Sandalwood base	Calming, antiseptic	Fatigue, diarrhea, nausea, respiratory problems; softens dry skin: mildly astringent for oily skin	Benzoin, black pepper, cypress, frankincense, jasmine, lemon, myrrh, neroli, ylang-ylang	
Tea tree top	Powerful antiseptic, fungicide	Respiratory problems, skin infections, wounds	Lavender, rosemary, citrus and spice oils	Highly disinfectant without being toxic
Thyme top	Stimulant, antiseptic, nerve tonic	Fatigue, depression, circulation, headaches, digestion, colds and respiratory problems, muscular pain	Bergamot, citrus oils, melissa, rosemary	In the presence of infectious diseases it is said to stimulate the production of white blood corpuscles
Ylang-Ylang base	Sedative, antiseptic, antidepressant	Anxiety, insomnia, frustration; regulates circulation	Most oils	Use sparingly. Too much may cause headaches

HERBS FOR HEALTH

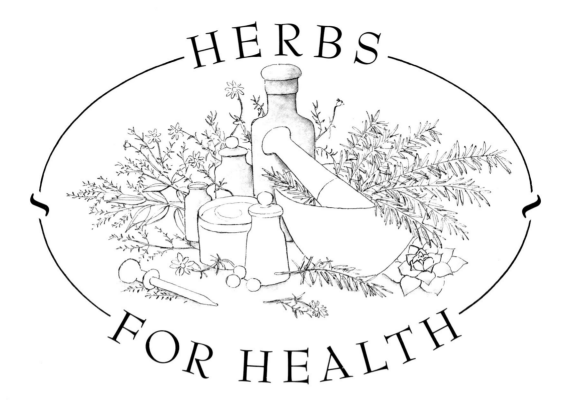

Since the beginning of time, people have turned to plants for healing help. It is rather ironic that this form of medicine, the oldest and still the most important in many parts of the world, should in some way be considered alternative, while the relatively new science of synthetic drugs in Western medicine should be called orthodox. What is important is that the best in every system should be valued and that proper attention should be paid to the dangers of any method. For emergencies, disasters and rapid infections, antibiotics, surgery and powerful drugs are vital to save lives; for minor or chronic ailments other forms of healing may have better results. In 1975 a Chief Medical Officer in Britain commented that "the number of admissions to hospital for treatment of adverse reactions to [medical] drugs now exceeds 100,000 a year."

But it must be recognized that plants too are potent drugs. Indeed, their active principles, isolated and synthesized, form the basis of many of today's drugs, from aspirin to morphine. Consequently, accurate dosage is vital: herbs should never be taken in excessive amounts.

Whenever you are in doubt or have a serious or recurring complaint, you should consult a trained herbalist. Most herbal practitioners follow the holistic approach to medicine. Holistic thinking has a way of spreading outward – like waves from a pebble dropped in water. Just as a whole plant is considered as being greater than the sum of its parts, a person's whole lifestyle and physical, mental and spiritual existence are examined before any treatment takes place. A herbalist will consider your diet, your work, general exercise, home life and environment, as well as the overall balance of your body's systems. Therefore what is prescribed for one patient may well differ from what is prescribed for another with the same symptoms.

Common ailments can be treated at home with a range of simple herbal remedies; follow the preparation instructions and advice in this chapter. You can also assist your health by including herbs in your daily diet. In times past it was the tradition to take herbal tonics in the spring to restore the body's vitality after a winter diet lacking in fresh green vegetables. Among the herbs used as tonics were yarrow, dandelion, sage, peppermint and rose hips, which helped to cleanse the system, and other herbs which were thought to strengthen the whole body, toning and invigorating its systems. Mint, for example, was taken for the digestive tract, and hawthorn berries were taken to improve the circulation system.

As research into the active constituents of herbs continues, increasing numbers of ancient treatments and tonics are becoming validated, revalued, and brought back into common use.

A history of herbal healing

For thousands of years early tribes accumulated a useful body of herbal knowledge through a process of trial and error. Women, with the restricted mobility of the childbearer, assumed the tasks of collecting and administering herbs, so that medicine was almost universally a female vocation in prescientific cultures. Early peoples also saw a link between health renewal and a woman's ability to create new life. The healing craft and plant knowledge were handed down from mother to daughter, and the efficiency of this system depended on both the accuracy of their observations and the nurturing qualities of the healer involved. To help their memories, nomadic tribes would select a visual attribute of each herb to remind them of its usage.

Difficulties in describing and remembering plants lessened with the advent of written language, and, by 3000 B.C., parallel cultures in China, Babylon, Egypt and India had begun to record their knowledge of medicinal plants.

Chinese herbalism
The country with the longest unbroken tradition in herbal medicine is China. By the time he died in 2698 B.C., the legendary Emperor Shen Nung had "tasted one hundred herbs." His Canon of Herbs deals with 252 plants, describing how to preserve and administer them, and many are still in use.

A hundred years later the Yellow Emperor, Huang Ti, formalized medical theory in the Nei Ching and displayed a sophisticated understanding of human disease for the time: "In treating illness, it is necessary to examine the entire context, scrutinize the symptoms, observe the emotions and attitudes. If one insists on the presence of ghosts and spirits, one cannot speak of therapeutics." It was an optimistic book, stating that, with the growth of knowledge, all kinds of disease would eventually be curable.

The Nei Ching was updated in the sixth century A.D. and again in the seventh century, when a certain Su Jing had a vision of a more complete herbal, and approached the Tang dynasty for sponsorship. The court responded with the provision of 20 experts and a command to each province to submit records and illustrations of the useful herbs in their area. After two years A Revised Canon of Herbs was published, describing the source, collection methods, flavor and therapeutic properties of 844 herbs. More than 800 years before the Western printing press was invented, the Tang government printed and distributed the revised herbal throughout China.

During the Ming dynasty, a world-famous Compendium of Materia Medica was compiled by Li Shizhen (1518–1593). From childhood he had always followed his father, collecting herbs and copying prescriptions, and he became aware of the real need for an accurate and comprehensive manual. His Materia Medica was completed in 1578 after 27 years of research: it is a thoroughly practical and scientific manual, listing 1,800 healing substances, mainly herbs, and 11,000 recipes or compounds. This process of updating and revising information has continued to the present day.

From the Far East to the Middle East
Clay tablets from 3000 B.C. record herbal imports into Babylon, and there is evidence of trade in ginseng between China and Babylon around 2000 B.C. The Babylonians had an enormous pharmacopoeia, with 1,400 plants; they used poppy as an anesthetic and fennel as a digestive. The Greek historian Herodotus noted that every Babylonian was an amateur physician since it was the custom to lay the sick in the street and solicit advice from anyone passing by.

The first known Egyptian physician was Imhotep (2980–2900 B.C.), a priest healer who also designed one of the earliest pyramids. He was greatly respected as a skilled and compassionate healer and was eventually deified.

The Ebers papyri of 1550 B.C. list many herbal remedies and accompanying incantations, and around this time a form of astrology was incorporated into Egyptian medicine. Egyptian physicians worked with around 900 herbs, and, through their embalming skills, had a superior understanding of the human organism.

At about the same time, Indian physicians were developing advanced surgical and diagnostic skills, and used hundreds of herbs in their treatments. Like the Chinese, they used all five senses when diagnosing, and developed a keen sensitivity when assessing breathing, pulse and skin odors.

Herbalism in the Ancient World
The Ancient Greeks acquired their knowledge of herbalism from India, Babylon, Egypt and even China. In the thirteenth century B.C. there lived in Greece a healer named Asclepius, skilled in the use of herbs. He designed a healing system whereby people would live through a series of experiences intended to transform them by changing old thinking patterns. Many miracles of healing were attributed to Asclepius and his daughter Hygieia. Eventually he was deified and healing temples sprang up across Greece. His system was practiced in Greece for several hundred years, and some of his ideas are still relevant in today's health centers.

In the sixth century B.C., the philosopher and mathematician Pythagoras set up a university to teach advanced knowledge. Herbs, particularly aromatic gardens, played an important part in the healing and restorative regime that preceded higher learning. Herbs were also used in the special high-energy food mixtures created for Pythagoras's long sojourns for contemplation.

Hippocrates (460–377 B.C.) brought Western medicine into a scientific framework of diagnosis and treatment. He dismissed the idea of disease as a punishment from the gods and considered food, occupation and climate important factors in illness. He believed that it was the individual's responsibility to aid self-healing through diet and plant medicines. He gave the medical profession a code of conduct that is still respected by doctors throughout the world.

Around 300 B.C., in the new cultural center of Alexandria, a famous medical school was established where herbal research was conducted. By 60 A.D. herbal knowledge had increased to such an extent that the physician Dioscorides was able to assemble a *Materia Médica* of 600 herbs, with their description, preparation and effect, and a new emphasis on botany. This became the standard herbal reference book for 1,500 years.

Soon afterwards, in 77 A.D., Pliny the Elder, the much-quoted writer from Ancient Rome, completed a listing of over 1,000 plants in his *Historia Naturalis*. Though full of curious information, it is not considered accurate.

More accurate was the herbal written by Galen (131–201 A.D.), a great physician and philosopher who traveled widely, making detailed plant observations. His enthusiasm for drugs and exotic compounds marks the beginning of several hundred years of a fashionable leaning toward complex drugs concocted mainly for the wealthy.

The Dark Ages

During the Dark Ages, Persia became the center of excellence in medicine. There the Nestorians (an Eastern Church not affiliated with Rome) established a famous school and hospital where Greek medical manuscripts were translated into Arabic. At about this time Avicenna (980–1037 A.D.), a gifted physician and scientist credited with inventing the process of distilling essential oils, wrote his *Canon Medicinae*, full of information on disease, remedies and medical philosophies.

In contemporary Europe medical progress was hampered by the authorities of the Christian church: scientific learning was not highly regarded, experiment was discouraged and originality considered a dangerous asset. Most significantly, the Church viewed disease as punishment for sin. However, plant medicine continued to be practiced by monks in the monasteries and by "herb women" in the villages.

The Renaissance

With the development in the fifteenth century of the Western printing press began a golden age of herbals. This was the beginning of the Renaissance, a time for re-examining old ideas, attempting to escape the limitations of old dogmas and giving rein to an eagerness for discovery. A new scientific attitude spread through medicine. The results of herbal remedies were observed more accurately, and the more bizarre drugs were dropped. Rather oddly, in this environment of growing reason, there occurred the cruelest witch hunts in history. Women were forbidden to study, while non-professional healers were pronounced heretics. Because of this, even today some people equate herbalism with superstition, quackery and magic.

Herbalism today

With the ascendancy of science in the nineteenth century came the ability to synthesize plant parts and concentrate doses. Herb usage probably reached an all-time low in the mid-twentieth century. But now, because of a greater concern about the side effects of drugs, an understanding of ecology and people's desire to take greater responsibility for their own health, herbal medicine is experiencing a remarkable revival. Research into plants such as feverfew, used to treat migraines; rosy periwinkle, which can control leukaemia; and *Rauvolfia serpentina*, which was used in tranquillizers, has highlighted the potential of herbal materials.

Pharmaceutical companies on the one hand recognize the value of herbs and are busy investigating worldwide herbal lore with unprecedented zeal, while on the other hand wish to maintain their lucrative near-monopoly on medicinal products. Some drug companies have tried to have herbs removed from the healing arena. One tactic has been to concentrate on finding and isolating a single toxic constituent in a herb. This happened in the case of sage some years ago, but attempts to quash its use failed after further research found that the other constituents in sage nullified any toxic element.

In order to use herbs safely, we need to find a sensible middle ground. One solution is a proposal on the statute books of Canada. This is to create a new class of "folk medicines." Each product would be labeled with botanical names, the plant parts used and the type of preparation. Ingredients would have to meet set standards of purity and concentration, and advertising would not make extravagant claims. Such a system would guarantee the safety of herbal medicines on the market and allow people to continue using these benevolent plants.

Herbal preparations

It is generally agreed that wild herbs or self-sown herbs, plants growing where Nature has decreed, have the most active ingredients, although, with home-grown plants, you are more certain of having the species you want when you want it. There is also less risk of mistaking one plant for another. The dangers of inaccurate identification cannot be stressed strongly enough. Some plants are dangerous under any circumstances, others are dangerous if taken inaccurately.

The quality of an herb is most important when it is to be used for healing. Pick perfect leaves, clean and unblemished, at their prime time, when most active constituents are present (see p. 269). Unless stated otherwise, leaves are at their prime just before flowers open; flowers are at their prime just as they open (coinciding with their moment of greatest beauty); fruit as it comes to ripeness, roots in the autumn, when goodness has passed from the leaves back into the roots; and bark after spring, when the sap has risen.

Use pruning shears or sharp scissors to remove parts cleanly, causing as little damage as possible to the plant. Do not pack tightly or allow to sweat before drying. Store carefully, label and date. Dried green herbs lose their medicinal potency after six or seven months; roots, seeds and bark after two or three years.

Remedy recipes and dosage

Generally a recipe can use either fresh or dried herb. Fresh herbs are likely to have the higher medicinal value, and the more recently picked, the higher it will be (unless it is an herb that changes chemically as it dries to give the active substance desired; see the Herbal Index). However, because dried herbs are available all year round, recipes are given in amounts of dried herb. On average, for infusions, or teas, and decoctions, one teaspoon of dried herb equals three teaspoons or one tablespoon of fresh.

To make a single dose use 1 teaspoon of herb to a cup of water. For a day's dosage add 1 ounce to $2\frac{1}{2}$ cups of liquid. For young children, the weak and very elderly the amount of herb (if using potent plants) should be halved.

The usual dosage is 7 fluid ounces of infusion, or a third of the reduced quantity for a decoction. As a guide, take this three times a day before meals for one or two days for a minor discomfort such as a mild sore throat, for several days for a cold, or for several weeks for chronic problems, such as migraine or constipation. Effectiveness also depends on lifestyle, general diet and fitness. With long-term problems, when conditions seem to be improving gradually, reduce the amount until you no longer need the remedy.

Although herbs do not have the side effects of drugs, they do affect major organic functions within the body and should not be taken unnecessarily. It is also important not to assume erroneously that, because herbs are "natural," any quantity or any combination can be taken. Herbal guidelines must be followed.

PREPARATION METHODS
Infusion or tea

Follow the quantities given below left for dosage. For a hot infusion, boil water, wait 30 seconds and then sprinkle the herb on the water to steep, stirring occasionally, for 10 minutes or until cool, or leave overnight. This method is preferable for leaves and flowers that easily give up their medicinal properties (especially vitamins and volatile ingredients) to the liquid, but remember to keep the container covered. Use a china, glass or enamel teapot or covered pan and use the purest water you can obtain, or bottled mineral water. Water with a high lime content (very hard water) can prevent plants from fully releasing their active principles. Strain the infusion into a cup and drink it lukewarm or cool as tea; but take it hot to break up a cold or cough. Drinks can be sweetened with honey or raw brown sugar to make them more palatable; or other herbs such as lemon verbena or spearmint can be added, as long as their own therapeutic effect is in sympathy with the desired result (see individual entries in the Herbal Index). Whenever possible, infusions should be made fresh each day and any unused portion kept refrigerated until needed, when it can be reheated in a glass or enamel pan.

A cold infusion is preferable for some plant parts with highly volatile ingredients. The text states when this is the case. Soak double quantities of these in cold water for 8–12 hours in a glass or enamel pan. Strain and drink. Make fresh daily.

Decoction

Follow the quantities given at left for dosage. Place the dried herb in an enamel or covered glass pan with cold water and slowly bring to the boil. Reduce the heat and simmer to reduce to a quarter of its original volume (10 minutes or longer); then steep with the lid on for 3 minutes or until cool. This method is used for hard materials such as roots, bark and seeds, which are bruised or crushed beforehand to release their active principles. It is also used for the green parts of plants, if mineral salts are required. Strain and take with honey or raw brown sugar if preferred. Make fresh daily when possible and keep any unused portion refrigerated. A decoction should keep for up to 3 days in this way.

Powder

Chop large dried plant parts, such as roots, bark or thick stems, into small pieces, then crush these or dried leaves and flowers with a pestle and mortar, or reduce them to powder in a coffee grinder. Powder can be added to drinks or soups, sprinkled on food, or put into gelatin capsules, which are obtainable from a pharmacist.

Pills

It is possible to make your own pills with a domestic press, although it is much easier (and safer) to buy them ready-made by a professional.

Syrup

Syrups are used to mask unpleasantly flavored herbs, especially for children, and to make cough medicine easier to take. Bring slowly to the boil $2\frac{1}{2}$ cups of selected infusion or decoction with 2–4 tablespoons honey until the mixture turns syrupy. Store in the refrigerator. This won't keep as long as a sugar-based syrup, but it is a healthier mixture.

To mix with a tincture, first heat $2\frac{1}{2}$ cups water with 4–6 tablespoons honey and stir until the mixture begins to boil. Remove from the heat. Mix 1 part tincture with 3 parts syrup. Store in the refrigerator.

Tincture

Put 4 ounces powdered herb or 8 ounces fresh chopped herb in a container with a tightly fitting lid. Add $2\frac{1}{2}$ cups alcohol, which must be at least 60° proof (e.g., brandy or vodka). Neither treated ethyl alcohol nor surgical spirit is suitable. Stand the mixture in a warm place and shake it twice daily for 2 weeks. Strain through double muslin, squeezing out as much liquid as possible, and store in a well-stoppered dark glass jar. Alcohol preparations will keep for a long time. The dosage is usually 5–15 drops, which can be taken directly or added to a cup of hot water. Homeopaths use very dilute tinctures in many of their preparations.

Essential oils

These are the concentrated essences of plants, usually extracted by steam distillation. It is possible to obtain minute amounts at home but more sensible to purchase them. It is important to find a source of pure, unadulterated essential oils to ensure that an oil contains all of a plant's active principles. Essential oils are excellent for making tinctures, adding to massage oils, ointments and other external applications. Infused or macerated oils are easy to make (see p. 188) and can be used as they are for massage or added to ointments.

Ointments and creams

Prepare and strain a strong decoction or infusion of the herb and add this to a quantity of pure, cold-pressed vegetable oil, such as sunflower. Boil until the liquid has evaporated (bubbles cease to appear) leaving the herbal principles in the oil. Alternatively use an infused oil (see p. 188). To stiffen as a cream, stir in melted beeswax – about 1 ounce should be enough for $2\frac{1}{4}$ cups of oil. You can make a cream by melting and blending 1 ounce beeswax, lanolin or cocoa butter with $\frac{1}{2}$ cup vegetable or herbal oil, following the method on p. 215. Add 1 ounce selected herb, simmer gently for 10 minutes, stirring frequently, sift through double muslin into a wide-necked container with a lid, label and date. A drop of tincture of benzoin or myrrh will extend its life. Do not use borax, as it can damage broken skin.

Petroleum jelly acts as a nonpenetrative base. Put $3\frac{1}{2}$ ounces petroleum jelly in an enamel pan or bowl over boiling water and melt. Leave to cool, then stir in a few drops of essential oil (say, eucalyptus for nasal relief), pour into a container, label and date.

Hot and cold compresses

A compress is useful for applying a herbal remedy externally to the skin. For a hot compress, soak a clean linen or cotton cloth in a hot decoction or infusion and apply it to the affected part as hot as can be tolerated. Cover the compress with plastic and a folded towel or blanket to maintain the heat. When the compress has cooled, either replace it with another one or apply a hot-water bottle over the plastic. Prepare a cold compress in the same way, but allow it to cool before applying.

Poultice

A poultice is similar to a compress except that plant parts are used rather than liquid extraction. Mash or crush fresh plant parts and either heat in a pan over boiling water or mix with a small amount of boiling water. Apply the pulp directly to the skin, as hot as can be tolerated, holding it in place with a gauze bandage. If using a dried herb, first powder it and make a paste with a little boiling water. If the paste is liable to irritate the skin, apply it between two layers of cloth.

Poultices are generally more active than compresses. They are used to stimulate circulation, soothe aches and pains or draw impurities out through the skin, depending on the herb chosen. Like massage with essential oils, a poultice will introduce the active parts of the herb into the body without stressing or being affected by the digestive tract before reaching its target area.

A-Z of herbal treatments

Here is a list of some common ailments and medical conditions that often respond to treatment with herbs at home. Do not attempt to treat more serious problems yourself and remember that many complaints are caused by incorrect diet, stress and other external factors.

Botanical names are supplied for the less common plants and for those where there may be confusion between species. Consult the Herbal Index for more detailed information. To be sure of getting the desired active principles, use the main species rather than varieties, cultivars or hybrids. You must be able to identify plants with complete confidence – many are easy to mistake for others and are highly poisonous.

It is always advisable to try a small quantity of any remedy before applying the full dosage. If you have an adverse reaction, or if a complaint seems to worsen or continue for a long time, seek professional advice from a qualified medical herbalist. For information on making up the recipes and on dosages, see p. 241.

Abrasions see **FIRST AID**

Acne
After washing, rinse the skin with an infusion of chamomile (*Chamaemelum nobile*), which is purifying, yarrow (*Achillea millefolium*), which helps eliminate toxins, catnip (*Nepeta cataria*), which is antiseptic, lavender (*Lavandula* spp), which is calming and antiseptic or thyme (*Thymus vulgaris*), which is a strong germkiller. Dab pimples with lemon juice to kill germs, cool inflammation and improve blood circulation. Apply a calendula ointment to reduce inflammation and improve local healing. Consider your diet and cut out sugars, fats and dairy products.

Appetite, lack of
Caraway (*Carum carvi*) and ginseng (*Panax pseudoginseng*) are good appetite stimulants, and a standard infusion of either can be drunk half an hour before a meal. Herbalists have had some success with both herbs in treating serious cases of anorexia nervosa. Horehound (*Marrubium vulgare*) tea, 1 cup taken three times a day, will stimulate the appetite after flu. Use with caution.

Arthritis see **Rheumatism and arthritis**

Asthma see **Coughs**

Bites, insect see **FIRST AID**

Boils and sores
To encourage boils to come to a head, apply neat lemon juice or secure over the boil half a warm baked onion (with the center layer removed to create a small dome). For boils and sores, apply a poultice of antiseptic catnip leaves (*Nepeta cataria*), antiseptic plantain leaves (*Plantago lanceolata*) or pulverized fenugreek seed to reduce inflammation and improve local healing. If there is any inflammation or fungal infection, calendula petal ointment is a safe treatment. If boils recur, seek professional advice.

Breastfeeding
To stimulate the flow of milk, a standard infusion of the leaves and seed of borage (*Borago officinalis*), dill seed, aniseed and fennel seed three times a day can help. A decoction of fenugreek seed is a strong stimulant. Simmer 1½ teaspoons seed in 1 cup water for 10 minutes and drink three times a day. A teaspoon of aniseed or honey will improve the taste. Another powerful stimulant is found in the flowering top of goat's rue (*Galega officinalis*): increases in milk flow of up to 50 percent have been recorded in tests with animals. Infuse 1 teaspoon dried leaves in 1 cup boiling water for 10 minutes and drink twice a day.

Bronchitis
For an effective bronchitis compound, combine equal parts of coltsfoot (*Tussilago farfara*), horehound (*Marrubium vulgare*) and aniseed. See also **Coughs.**

Bruises see **FIRST AID**

Burns, minor see **FIRST AID** and **Sunburn**

Chilblains and cold limbs
To warm hands and feet, massage gently with warmed macerated oil of honeysuckle flowers (*Lonicera caprifolium*). This will bring an increased flow of blood to the surface skin. For a foot bath to improve the circulation of cold feet and help chilblains, which are caused by poor circulation, use an infusion of 1 tablespoon freshly ground mustard seed to 2 quarts water. Cayenne seed powder is also a powerful stimulant to the circulatory system and helps blood flow to the extremities. In an ointment it can be used in moderation for unbroken chilblains.

Elder leaf (*Sambucus nigra*) ointment is useful for chilblains. Heat 1 part fresh leaves with 2 parts petroleum jelly until the leaves are crisp. Strain and label for storage.

To improve bad circulation, drink rose hip or horsetail (*Equisetum arvense*) or buckwheat (*Fagopyrum esculentum*) tea daily to strengthen small capillaries. Some spices and strongly flavored herbs, such as black pepper, cloves, cinnamon, coriander, cumin, freshly grated root ginger, garlic, marjoram, rosemary and thyme, improve circulation. Include them frequently in your diet, especially in the winter months.

Colds and fevers
To protect against colds, eat or take the juice of a raw clove of garlic three times a day. Essential oils are very efficient at destroying harmful bacteria and viruses. They can also be used in steam inhalants or as a room spray (see p. 235).

Rose hip tea, said to be high in vitamin C, can be used to build resistance to colds and other infections. Cayenne powder is also excellent at warding off colds as it strengthens and stimulates the circulatory and digestive system. Infuse ½–1 teaspoon cayenne powder in 1 cup boiling water for 10 minutes. Strain and take 1 tablespoon of this mixture topped up with hot water when needed or before each meal.

At the first sign of a cold, take a mixture of elderflower (*Sambucus nigra*), peppermint (*Mentha piperita*) and yarrow (*Achillea millefolium*).

Infuse ½ teaspoon of each together in 1 cup boiling water for 20 minutes. Strain, add 1 teaspoon honey and ¼ teaspoon cayenne pepper. This should decrease the intensity and the discomfort of a cold or flu. If the mixture benefits you, the herbs are worth storing as a dried blend for winter use. Another remedy to take at the earliest possible moment is 9 small horehound leaves (*Marrubium vulgare*) chopped finely and eaten raw with 1 tablespoon honey. Repeat as necessary.

To fight colds and flu, take hot lemon and honey as often as desired, as lemon has antibacterial properties. Take frequent hot drinks of elderflower (*Sambucus nigra*), peppermint (*Mentha piperita*) or yarrow (*Achillea millefolium*) tea to promote perspiration and to reduce temperature. Elderflower is also useful for reducing any nasal inflammation from catarrh. If this is accompanied by a penetrating chill, add grated ginger root or cayenne. Black pepper sprinkled over food also has a restorative effect, or you could take an infusion of mustard

seed, ¼ teaspoon powder infused for 5 minutes in 1 cup boiling water, three times a day, or add 2 quarts of mustard infusion to bathwater.

For catarrh and flu, golden rod (*Solidago virgaurea*) is good because it is antiseptic, expels catarrh and soothes inflammation. Infuse 2 teaspoons dried flowering stalks in 1 cup boiling water for 10 minutes and drink a cup three times a day. Licorice root (*Glycyrrhiza glabra*) is also excellent for its soothing and antiviral properties. Drink an infusion of ½–1 teaspoon of powdered root in 1 cup boiling water three times a day. Do not take if you suffer from heart or kidney problems. Take in moderation; in large amounts it can be harmful. You can also try a hot infusion of borage (*Borago officinalis*), coltsfoot (*Tussilago farfara*), comfrey (*Symphytum officinale*), or ground ivy (*Glechoma hederacea*) to relieve catarrh.

Relieve stuffiness by inhaling the vapors from a steam bath of chamomile flowers (*Matricaria recutita*) or eucalyptus leaves (*Eucalyptus globulus*) (see also p. 235 for additional inhalation ideas). A

pinch of basil taken as snuff can bring back your sense of smell. When your temperature has returned to normal, drink a warm infusion of cleavers (*Galium aparine*) three times a day to continue a mild perspiration action, help prevent gastric disturbance and promote restful sleep. Begin taking vegetable juices and progress to homemade vegetable soup, fresh fruit and salads. Reintroduce heavier foods slowly to avoid overloading the digestive system when it is still vulnerable.

Horehound tea restores an appetite that may need stimulating after flu. If lethargy or depression follow, take lemon balm (*Melissa officinalis*) or vervain (*Verbena officinalis*) tea. If this persists after a few days, seek professional advice.

Colic see CHILDREN'S PROBLEMS

Constipation
Long-term constipation, or any unusual changes in bowel habits, should be discussed with a medical herbalist or doctor. Roughage in the diet and regular exercise are

CHILDREN'S PROBLEMS

Colic
First choice for children is dill water (see p. 45). If you anticipate digestive discomfort, try giving the baby a teaspoonful before she or he feeds. Otherwise give a teaspoonful as required.

Diaper rash
If practicable, expose the baby's bottom to fresh air frequently. A cool compress of calendula or chamomile (*Matricaria recutita*) can be laid on sore areas for short periods. Use a lotion or ointment made with calendula, comfrey (*Symphytum officinale*) or marsh mallow (*Althaea officinalis*) to soothe the skin and promote rapid healing.

Diarrhea
Always seek the advice of a trained medical practitioner for persistent children's diarrhea. A standard agrimony (*Agrimonia eupatoria*) infusion is a specific herbal remedy for childhood diarrhea, as is a decoction of bistort root (*Polygonum bistorta*). Either can be drunk, 1 cup three times a day. An infusion of coriander also eases diarrhea safely for children. Use 1 teaspoon bruised seed infused

for 5 minutes and drink before meals or three times a day.

Head lice
Maggie Tisserand, in her book *Aromatherapy for Women*, has developed a recipe of essential oils which eliminates lice and leaves the hair lustrous and shining. Combine 25 drops of rosemary oil, 25 drops of lavender oil, 13 drops of geranium (*Pelargonium*) oil and 12 drops of eucalyptus oil in ⅓ cup vegetable oil. Divide the hair into small sections and saturate each section with the mixture down to the roots. Pile long hair on top of the head ensuring that every bit is oiled. Wrap plastic around the head and behind the ears to stop the oils from evaporating. Make sure that small children cannot move the plastic anywhere near the nose or mouth and restrict breathing. Leave it on for 2 hours. Remove the plastic, add shampoo and rub in well, rinse thoroughly and comb through with a fine nitcomb. Repeat three days later.

Sleep problems
Chamomile (*Matricaria recutita*) tea is a safe and gentle sedative for children and traditionally recommended for

those having nightmares. Give 1 cup of warm infusion half an hour before bedtime and remember to take the child to the toilet again just before bed. For small babies, put just 1 tablespoon in a sterilized feeding bottle. For older babies, use up to half a cup.

Teething
Chamomile tea calms some fractious children, as do homeopathic granules of chamomile (sold as chamomilla). Babies can be given a clean piece of marsh mallow (*Althaea officinalis*) root to chew on. Make sure that the baby cannot choke on the root.

Worms
As garlic kills intestinal parasites, make a garlic ointment and apply it around the anus nightly for two weeks. Pumpkin seeds (*Cucurbita maxima*) are among the most efficient remedies for killing intestinal parasites, including tapeworms, but a routine of fasting, cleansing the bowels and precise dosage must be followed, so it is wise to carry out the treatment under the supervision of a qualified medical herbalist.

important for healthy functioning bowels, while tension and emotional worries can contribute to constipation. Herbs can be used for short-term relief, but underlying causes should be addressed.

Syrup of figs is a valuable remedy, taken as required. An infusion of crushed flax seed (*Linum usitatissimum*) has a purgative action which brings relief: drink 1 cup morning and evening.

Licorice root (*Glycyrrhiza glabra*) is a mild and pleasant laxative. Chew root as desired, or make a decoction of 1 teaspoon root in 1 cup water and take three times a day. Stewed rhubarb in moderate doses is a gentle laxative for children; large doses cause a more powerful reaction. Rose hip tea is also a mild laxative. Use a decoction or infusion with halved hips, but strain through filter paper to remove the seeds and tiny hairs, which are an irritant to the body. Drink whenever necessary.

Coughs

To fight bronchial infections, eat raw garlic cloves for their strong antibiotic content. To help dispel fluid and mucus from the lungs and air passages, horehound (*Marrubium vulgare*) is the first choice. Drink a hot standard infusion three times a day. Another important herb in the treatment of lung problems, coughs and colds, and asthma is coltsfoot (*Tussilago farfara*). An infusion of the leaves and flowers will soothe the bronchi, encourage tissue healing and protect the delicate mucous membranes from further irritations.

To ease cough spasms and help expel mucus, make cowslip flower (*Primula veris*) syrup or decoct cowslip root, simmering for 5 minutes, and drink 1 cup three times a day. It can be combined with coltsfoot and aniseed (*Pimpinella anisum*). Aniseed has an expectorant action and can also help make cough mixture more palatable.

For an irritating bronchial cough with a great deal of catarrh, the expectorant, antiseptic action of elecampane root (*Inula helenium*) along with the soothing effect of its mucilage, makes it an excellent remedy, especially for children. Infuse 1 teaspoon of shredded root in 1 cup of cold water for 9 hours.

Drink it hot three times a day. An irritating cough can also be soothed by an infusion of powdered marsh mallow root (*Althaea officinalis*). It combines well with horehound (*Marrubium vulgare*) and licorice (*Glycyrrhiza glabra*). For dry coughs, combine coltsfoot with horehound and mullein (*Verbascum thapsus*).

To reduce catarrh in the lungs, apply a poultice of freshly ground mustard seed. Mix 4 ounces of seeds with warm water to make a thick paste. Apply the paste between two pieces of gauze with the bottom piece dampened so that is does not stick to the skin. Leave for one minute only. If skin is reddened, massage with an appropriate aromatherapy oil or any vegetable oil. Flax seed can be used with mustard to help reduce lung catarrh. A tea of plantain leaves (*Plantago major*) is a gentle expectorant; the herb is widely cultivated by Russian pharmaceutical companies. A standard infusion of star anise (*Illicium verum*) has expectorant and antibacterial properties. It mixes well with other cough remedies.

Cystitis

Drink a standard infusion of silver birch leaves (*Betula pendula*) against cystitis and other infections of the urinary tract, and to remove excess water from the system. It can be combined with bearberry (*Arctostaphylos uva-ursi*). A decoction of sweet Joe Pye root (*Eupatorium purpureum*), drunk three times a day, is helpful for urinary infections including cystitis. A standard infusion of yarrow (*Achillea millefolium*) is antiseptic to the urinary tract and assists recovery from cystitis.

Cuts *see* FIRST AID

Depression

A lavender flower infusion, taken three times a day, can be effective in clearing depression especially combined with rosemary (*Rosmarinus officinalis*) or skullcap (*Scutellaria lateriflora*). Rosemary is useful if your depression results from psychological tension or if you are feeling run-down after illness. Drink a standard infusion. It also combines well with skullcap.

Take a standard infusion of vervain (*Verbena officinalis*) to ease

depression and melancholy, which may follow flu. It also combines well with skullcap.

Diaper rash *see* CHILDREN'S PROBLEMS

Diarrhea

Sudden, painful diarrhea and chronic diarrhea need expert medical attention. Other cases are often the body's way of attempting to dump toxic material as fast as possible. Most herbal remedies attempt to assist this action while soothing the bowel and reducing inflammation.

Self-heal (*Prunella vulgaris*) has a gentle action which soothes inflamed mucous membranes. Drink an infusion three times daily. The same dose can be taken of agrimony (*Agrimonia eupatoria*) and coriander seed infusion (*see also* CHILDREN'S PROBLEMS).

Digestion

Most flavoring and seasoning herbs stimulate the flow of digestive juices in the stomach and intestine, and this increases the efficiency with which fats are broken down into fatty acids and nutrients are absorbed by the body. Classic herb partnerships reflect this benevolent fact: rosemary helps the digestion of fatty lamb, fennel assists the digestion of oily fish and horse-radish is thought to aid the digestion of beef.

Many of the aromatic seeds are useful digestives. Take 1 tablespoon ground aniseed boiled in 1 cup milk and drink this twice a day to improve the digestive system. Cardamom increases the flow of saliva and adds a pleasing aroma to digestive mixtures. Take 1 cup of infusion half an hour before each meal. Hot peppermint tea can be taken after a meal. A dish of digestive herbs including aniseed, caraway, dill and fennel seed is sometimes offered at the end of an Indian meal, and greatly assists the body in digesting rich foods.

If there is persistent or severe pain with digestion, consult a medical herbalist or doctor; if there are regular difficulties with indigestion not caused by disease, then rushed eating, an unbalanced diet or tension may be the cause, and it is sensible to consider solutions to these while taking herbs to alleviate the problem (*see also* **Stomachache**).

Earache
Eardrops made from a weak infusion of goldenseal (*Hydrastis canadensis*) soothe earache. Mullein (*Verbascum thapsus*) can be addded to the infusion. Where catarrh of the middle ear is causing tinnitus, an infusion of ground ivy (*Glechoma hederacea*) flowering stems is sometimes considered helpful.

Eczema, rashes and itchy skin
Make a weak infusion of goldenseal root (*Hydrastis canadensis*) and use externally as a wash or compress for eczema and itchy skin. Expressed juice of chickweed (*Stellaria media*) will soothe sores or itchy patches from eczema or psoriasis and will tone and invigorate the skin, while a poultice of crushed flax seed (*Linum usitatissimum*) brings relief to shingles and psoriasis.

For children's eczema and nervous eczema, nettle (*Urtica dioica*) is specifically recommended by herbalists. Drink an infusion three times a day.
For weeping eczema, drink an infusion of the flowering tops of heartsease (*Viola tricolor*) three times a day. It combines well with nettle and red clover (*Trifolium pratense*).

Comfrey oil (see recipe, p. 131) often brings relief from patches of itchy rough skin, and evening primrose oil can help.

Fevers *see* Colds and fevers

Flatulence
Seeds of aniseed, caraway or fennel are all effective at expelling wind but even more so in combination. Infuse crushed mixed seed and drink a cup slowly 30 minutes before each meal.

Many spice seeds help disperse wind; cloves or allspice can be chewed or infused as often as desired. Black pepper sprinkled on food removes wind. Infusions of root ginger, cardamom and coriander have pleasant aromas and relieve griping pains of wind. Star anise (*Illicium verum*) dispels wind and is often included with dill and fennel seed in colic preparations for young babies. Take a standard infusion three times a day.

Lemon balm (*Melissa officinalis*) relieves flatulent spasms, and a dose of $\frac{1}{4}-\frac{1}{2}$ teaspoon powdered angelica root (*Angelica archangelica*) will quickly expel gas from the stomach and bowel with a gentle action that is safe for children.

Hemorrhoids
A traditional choice for mild hemorrhoids is pilewort or lesser celandine (*Ranunculus ficaria*). It is said to shrink and soothe the swollen veins around the anus. Apply an ointment made with a strong infusion of the root. Do not take internally. For bleeding hemorrhoids, apply an ointment of self-heal (*Prunella vulgaris*).

FIRST AID

Bruises and sprains
Apply distilled witch hazel (purchased from a pharmacy) with sterile absorbent cotton promptly to small bumps and bruises. This will halt the swelling. Comfrey oil or ointment is good for messy scrapes, bruises and sprains. A poultice of comfrey leaves (*Symphytum officinale*) will reduce bruising and speed healing of sprains and fractures. It's best not used on deep wounds, as comfrey is such a powerful tissue healer that the surface skin may heal before the wound has healed deeper down. Comfrey also encourages good formation of scar tissue.

Both a lotion of St John's wort (*Hypericum perforatum*) and arnica (*Arnica montana*) ointment are excellent for sprains and bruises, especially if there is any pain or inflammation of the skin. **Caution:** Do not use arnica where the skin is broken.

An ointment of calendula petals, agrimony (*Agrimonia eupatoria*) or elder leaves (*Sambucus nigra*) is soothing and healing for bruises, sprains and other minor wounds.

Burns, minor
Immediately apply the cool inside surface of an *Aloe vera* leaf to reduce pain, speed healing and leave a protective seal against infection. Later, apply calendula as a cool compress or ointment to soothe and heal (*see also* **Sunburn**).

Major burns are an emergency: summon professional help at once. Cool the burn with cool (not ice-cold) water while waiting, and give the patient 6 drops Bach Flower Rescue Remedy and reassure him.

Cuts and abrasions
First clean the cut by soaking in witch hazel diluted with 4 parts water or an antiseptic herbal infusion; elder leaves (*Sambucus nigra*) are excellent. A speedy alternative is to add 3 drops thyme or rosemary oil or $\frac{1}{2}$ teaspoon tincture of calendula to 1 cup hand-hot, boiled water. The antiseptic wash can also be gently swabbed on with a series of sterile cottonwool balls. A dose of 4 drops Bach Flower Rescue Remedy has a calming effect, while an infusion of lady's mantle (*Alchemilla vulgaris*) can be applied as a compress to arrest bleeding.

For slow-healing wounds, apply a compress or poultice of comfrey (*Symphytum officinale*), self-heal (*Prunella vulgaris*) or yarrow (*Achillea millefolium*). Add plantain leaves (*Plantago major*) for their antibiotic properties. If applying a poultice to an open wound, dip leaves briefly in boiling water to sterilize them.

To continue treatment, a soft ointment of comfrey, calendula or agrimony (*Agrimonia eupatoria*) is soothing and healing.

Stings and insect bites
Wasp stings are alkaline: apply the inside surface of a houseleek leaf (*Sempervivum tectorum*), onion slices, or dab on vinegar (if possible, thyme vinegar). Bee stings and ant bites are acid: apply sodium bicarbonate dissolved in ice-cold water. Remember to remove the bee sting.
Reduce painful swelling with a drop of neat lavender or eucalyptus oil. To soothe lingering irritation, apply a cold compress of tincture of calendula or calendula ointment.
To soothe nettle stings, rub on crushed dock leaves (*Rumex obtusifolius*).

Travel sickness
Recent research confirms that the best treatment to settle the stomach and help prevent nausea is an infusion of ginger root. Take a bottle of tincture of ginger when traveling, and give 10 drops in half a cup of water for adults or 2–3 drops mixed in a little warm water for children.

Pick large leaves of fresh angelica (*Angelica archangelica*) and crush them on the journey; the scent allays nausea and refreshes stale air.

A herbalist may recommend an infusion of horse chestnut fruits (*Aesculus hippocastanum*) applied as a compress to tone and strengthen veins and help heal hemorrhoids (*see also* **Varicose veins**).

Hangover
Lemon in water or in orange juice for extra vitamin C, hot peppermint or wild thyme tea can alleviate the discomfort. A drink of yarrow (*Achillea millefolium*) and elderflower (*Sambucus nigra*) tea will help the body to eliminate toxins.

Hay fever
Sufferers from hay fever and other allergies may benefit from an infusion of golden rod (*Solidago virgaurea*). Take half a cup four times a day. The irritated mucous membranes are relieved and soothed by drinking a warm infusion of hyssop (*Hyssopus officinalis*), lavender (*Lavandula* species), marjoram (*Origanum majorana*) or thyme (*Thymus vulgaris*).

Apply cold compresses of witch hazel diluted in 4 parts boiled water to soothe the eyes. Hot mullein flower (*Verbascum thapsus*) tea and eyebright (*Euphrasia rostkoviana*) tea will help eliminate excess mucus, and eyebright will reduce redness around the eyes. Drink three times a day. Red and sore eyelids may result from other conditions. If symptoms persist, consult a qualified herbalist.

Headaches and migraines
Herbs may bring relief though they will not remove the cause. Fever-few leaf (*Tanacetum parthenium*) has justifiably become the primary remedy for migraine. A small to medium fresh or frozen leaf eaten between slices of bread (it can cause mouth ulcers in very sensitive people) three times a day has been found to reduce the intensity or frequency of 70 percent of migraines (usually in sufferers who gain relief from warmth applied to the head). Its action is cumulative and can take up to six months to show results. Do not take during pregnancy as it can stimulate the uterus. Alternatively take half a cup of leaf tea twice a day to reduce the pain of migraine.

Lavender (*Lavandula* species) is useful for stress-related headaches and combines well with valerian (*Valeriana officinalis*). Drink an infusion of lavender flowers three times a day. A standard infusion of valerian is useful in tension headaches, when it combines well with skullcap (*Scutellaria lateriflora*).

Head lice *see* CHILDREN'S PROBLEMS

High blood pressure
High blood pressure is a serious condition which must be monitored by a qualified medical practitioner. Ripe hawthorn berries (*Crataegus monogyna*) are a gentle yet powerful tonic for the heart and circulation, bringing both low and high blood pressure back to normal when used over a long period. Infuse 2 teaspoons berries for 20 minutes in 1 cup boiling water and drink up to three times a day for an extended period. For high blood pressure hawthorn combines well in an infusion with linden blossom (*Tilia cordata*) and yarrow (*Achillea millefolium*). Yarrow reduces high blood pressure by dilating peripheral blood vessels.

Chronic hypertension responds well to 1 cup dandelion leaves (*Taraxacum officinale*) infusion taken three times a day. Garlic is reliable, but it takes four weeks before there is any drop in blood pressure. Eat raw cloves up to six times a day. **Note:** *You must consult your own doctor first before trying any of these treatments.*

Insomnia
A cup of hop (*Humulus lupulus*) tea taken before retiring to bed is a useful sedative for insomnia except for anyone suffering from depression. It combines well with valerian (*Valeriana officinalis*) which reduces tension and anxiety, and passion flower leaves (*Passiflora incarnata*). Chamomile (*Chamaemelum nobile*) tea and catnip (*Nepeta cataria*) tea are traditional relaxing bedtime drinks that will reduce anxiety and promote restful sleep. Passion flower tea and orange blossom tea can also help insomniacs (*see also* **CHILDREN'S PROBLEMS**).

Itchy skin *see* **Eczema, rashes and itchy skin**

Joints, stiff *see* **Muscles and joints**

Kidney and liver complaints
Dandelion (*Taraxacum officinale*) is the ideal balanced diuretic as it supplies potassium, a substance lost during diuretic action. Decoct 1 tablespoon root in 1 cup water and drink three times a day.

Menstrual cycle
The best remedy for the dull headache, irritability, mild depression, fluid retention or breast discomfort experienced by many women just before their period is evening primrose oil. Tests at a London hospital indicated that 85 percent of those in the trial experienced improvement. The herb (*Oenothera biennis*) is easy to grow but extracting the oil from the seed is complex, so purchase capsules from a health shop. Those that also contain a marine oil are particularly recommended. Skullcap (*Scutellaria lateriflora*), chamomile (*Matricaria recutita*) and linden blossom (*Tilia cordata*) are safe teas to soothe and reduce discomfort of PMT (premenstrual tension). Take an infusion three times a day to relieve the symptoms.

For menstrual cramps drink an infusion of chamomile or valerian (*Valeriana officinalis*) three times a day, or half a cup of feverfew (*Tanacetum parthenium*) tea twice a day.

For cramps with a feeling of heaviness, a hot infusion of raspberry leaf (*Rubus idaeus*) tea is recommended.

To help reduce period pains and excessive bleeding, try lady's mantle leaves (*Alchemilla vulgaris*), taken in a double-strength infusion three times a day. This may also ease changes of the menopause.

To help relieve menopausal symptoms, try dried berries of the chaste tree (*Vitex agnus-castus*), which normalizes the activity of sex hormones. They are also of benefit in PMS and help to normalize the body's natural balance after taking contraceptive pills. Infuse 1 teaspoon berries for 15 minutes; drink 1 cup three times a day. Motherwort (*Leonurus cardiaca*) reduces the discomfort of the menopause. When symptoms include irritability and anxiety, St John's wort (*Hypericum perforatum*) is recommended. Drink a standard infusion of flowering tops three times a day.

Muscles and joints

Essential oil of fennel is one of several oils which, used in a massage oil, will ease muscular pains (see also p. 250). The moist inside surface of fresh silver birch bark (*Betula pendula*) applied over the area will ease painful muscles, while a poultice of mustard seed (see recipe, p. 60) stimulates circulation and relieves muscular and skeletal pain.

An ointment or poultice of wintergreen leaves (*Gaultheria procumbens*) has painkilling and anti-inflammatory properties that are excellent for chronic muscular problems. If you suffer from muscular cramps, a standard infusion of valerian (*Valeriana officinalis*) will bring relief.

Nausea

Freshly grated ginger or powdered cinnamon bark infused on their own or sprinkled in other teas can be taken whenever necessary to relieve nausea and vomiting. Cloves, as a flavoring in food or drunk as an infusion, will allay nausea and vomiting while stimulating the digestive system. Infuse about 10 cloves in 1 cup boiling water for 10 minutes and take as required, *see also* **Pregnancy and childbirth**.

Nervous tension

Unlike tranquillizers, herbs that work to relax nervous tension also counter stress by reviving and toning the central nervous system.

The two finest treatments are skullcap flowering top (*Scutellaria lateriflora*), which is suitable for a wide range of nervous complaints and valerian root (*Valeriana officinalis*), which is suitable for nervous spasms and tremors, phobias, insomnia and restlessness. Fortunately they work well together. Take an infusion individually or in combination. Take 1 cup infusion up to three times a day or half a cup every three hours in times of great stress, but not for long periods of time. A standard infusion of borage leaves (*Borago officinalis*) is a restorative tonic to the adrenal glands, which help the body to cope with stress. Borage flowers and leaves in wine have a traditional reputation for bolstering courage. The combination seems to cause a

significant rise in blood adrenalin level, and a wineglassful will relieve nervous tension during times of stress.

After a hectic day, try drinking a tea of ginseng (*Panax pseudoginseng*), linden blossom (*Tilia cordata*) or lavender (*Lavandula* species) to calm and tone the nervous system. Linden and lavender combine well to combat nervous exhaustion, while lemon balm (*Melissa officinalis*) relieves tension and stressful states with a mild antidepressant action. It combines well with lavender flowers and linden blossom. Take a cup of mixed teas morning, evening and when required.

Wood betony (*Stachys officinalis*) strengthens the central nervous system and is mildly sedative, being especially good for headaches and neuralgia of a nervous origin. Take 1 cup tea three times a day or combine it with skullcap.

For relaxants, try chamomile (*Chamaemelum nobile*), which can be drunk as desired, and cowslip (*Primula veris*), which is a relaxing sedative for stress-related tension. Make an infusion of the petals and drink 1 cup three times a day. It can be combined with linden blossom or skullcap.

To ease tension a standard infusion of St John's wort (*Hypericum perforatum*) has pain-reducing and sedative properties, making it useful for anxiety-related conditions, unless there is also depression. Rosemary, on the other hand, is a stimulant to the nervous system and is sometimes considered useful for treating psychological tension which is causing depression.

Pimples *see* Acne

Pregnancy and childbirth

Herbs with a strong action must be avoided during pregnancy, particularly those that stimulate the uterus, such as goldenseal (*Hydrastis canadensis*).

To prevent morning sickness, first try not to eat "junk" foods, which many herbalists feel contribute to this problem. Include plenty of fresh fruit and vegetables in your diet. Mild herbs that may help include meadowsweet flowering tops (*Filipendula ulmaria*), chamomile flowers (*Matricaria recutita*), linden blossom (*Tilia cordata*) and leaves of

peppermint (*Mentha piperita*). Drink a standard infusion on rising in the morning, at midday and in the evening. An infusion of powdered cinnamon bark and freshly grated ginger will allay nausea. These can be individually infused or sprinkled on the previously mentioned leaf and flower teas.

To tone and strengthen the tissue and muscle of the uterus, raspberry leaf (*Rubus idaeus*) tea has a deservedly high reputation. Take an infusion of 2 teaspoons with 1 cup boiling water and drink freely during the last few months of pregnancy. This is thought to tone the muscles to assist contractions and check bleeding in labor.

In the early stages of labor, a sponge wash with a sweet-scented floral water such as rosewater, lavender water or an infusion of rosemary has a pleasantly relaxing scent and mild antiseptic qualities.

Rash *see* **Eczema, rashes and itchy skin**

Rheumatism and arthritis

The causes of these ailments are complex, and a qualified herbalist should be consulted to discover which aspects of diet or lifestyle may be contributing to the problem. Devil's claw (*Harpagophytum procumbens*) has been found to be effective in many cases: it appears to detoxify the body and to stimulate the body's immune system. So far, no harmful side effects have been discovered, but it can be nauseous. Decoct $\frac{1}{2}$–1 teaspoon root in 1 cup water and boil for 15 minutes. Drink three times a day for at least a month to assess its effect.

To treat rheumatoid arthritis, try an infusion of celery seed, which helps to counter acid in the blood. Take 1 cup three times a day. It is said to work well combined with dandelion root (*Taraxacum officinale*) or devil's claw.

A standard infusion of valerian (*Valeriana officinalis*) will relieve the pain of rheumatism, and a double-strength infusion of chickweed (*Stellaria media*) steeped for 5 minutes has brought relief to some.

One of the beneficial side effects noticed by a significant number of patients using feverfew (*Tanacetum parthenium*) to treat migraine was a reduction in their pain from arthritis.

Try a dose of 1 leaf in a sandwich three times a day for up to six months (but not during pregnancy without seeking medical advice).

Essential oils such as rosemary, applied in a massage oil, can bring relief to rheumatic and arthritic pains (see p. 231). Wintergreen (*Gaultheria procumbens*) ointment contains useful painkilling and anti-inflammatory ingredients, arnica (*Arnica montana*) ointment reduces discomfort, and a compress of cayenne pepper infusion eases pain by increasing circulation.

Skin ulcers
The fruit of the fig tree has strong antiseptic and disinfectant properties. Apply a poultice of dried figs to chronic leg ulcers. A poultice of comfrey leaves (*Symphytum officinale*) has given remarkable results in many cases of chronic varicose ulcers, and is more beneficial if combined with the soothing properties of marsh mallow (*Althaea officinalis*). Calendula petals, applied either as a compress of the infusion or as an ointment, reduce inflammation and speed healing.

Sores *see* Boils and sores

Sprains *see* FIRST AID

Stings *see* FIRST AID

Stomachache
Sharp or prolonged pain in the stomach needs a professional medical diagnosis. For those who already know what is causing their ailment, herbs can be helpful as long as the condition is monitored carefully.
To soothe and heal the delicate mucous membranes in the stomach, drink chamomile (*Matricaria recutita*) tea for its anti-inflammatory effect or marsh mallow (*Althaea officinalis*) for its soothing properties, as desired.
For digestive disorders, slippery elm (*Ulmus rubra*) (purchased as a powder) is both a soothing remedy as well as a wholesome food for those unable to face solid food, and it is safe for children over 12 months. Make a paste with ½–1 tablespoon powdered bark and a little cold water. Stir in 1 cup of hot milk or water and sweeten with honey if desired.

For stomach cramps caused by indigestion, drink an infusion of antiseptic catnip (*Nepeta cataria*).
For stomach ulcers, chew licorice root (*Glycyrrhiza glabra*) as desired, or take a dose of ¼ teaspoon powdered root daily (strong doses are laxative). A calendula petal infusion, drunk three times a day, especially combined with marsh mallow root, soothes and aids the healing of stomach ulcers.
For gastric and duodenal ulcers, linden blossom (*Tilia cordata*) tea has useful anti-inflammatory properties, and the softening mucilage of comfrey (*Symphytum officinale*) makes it a soothing and healing treatment. Boil 1 teaspoon dried root in 1 cup water for 10 minutes.
For stomach ulcers and colitis: Half to 1 teaspoon of ground fenugreek seed (*Trigonella Foenum-graecum*), infused in 1 cup boiling water for 10 minutes is considered to be a tonic for all parts of the digestive tract. *See also* **Digestion.**

Sunburn
Aloe vera leaf juice is cooling and healing for sunburn and minor burns. Apply directly to the area of sunburn. A compress of sorrel (*Rumex acetosa*) also has a cooling effect. Sorrel tea is said to nullify the effects of sunstroke and exhaustion: take one cup three times a day.

A macerated oil of St John's wort (*Hypericum perforatum*) is excellent for minor burns once they have cooled.

Teething *see* CHILDREN'S PROBLEMS

Throat, sore
Purple sage (*Salvia officinalis* 'Purpurea') is an excellent treatment for sore throats. It is antiseptic and healing for inflammation of the mouth, throat and tonsils. Drink half a cup of infusion four times a day, and gargle with it as often as required. Do not drink it during pregnancy: it may cause abortion.

The bacterial qualities of lemon, another popular remedy, are increased if you take it in an infusion with a natural antiseptic such as eucalyptus (*Eucalyptus globulus*) and honey. Thyme (*Thymus vulgaris*) is a powerful disinfectant and excellent gargle for sore throats, laryngitis and tonsillitis.

Gargle with a standard tea of fenugreek seed, agrimony (*Agrimonia eupatorium*) or self-heal (*Prunella vulgaris*), or a decoction of bistort root (*Polygonum bistorta*) for relief of sore throats, inflammation of the mouth or tongue and laryngitis, or a cayenne infusion for laryngitis (see recipe, p. 243).

The anti-inflammatory and antiseptic properties of chamomile (*Matricaria recutita*) make it a useful gargle for sore throats and mouth infections such as **gingivitis.** Use a double-strength infusion of the flowers. The menthol in peppermint (*Mentha piperita*) makes it a pleasant antiseptic.
Soothe a sore throat by wrapping around it a hot compress of sage (*Salvia officinalis*) or thyme (*Thymus vulgaris*), kept warm and in place with a scarf. Chew licorice root (*Glycyrrhiza glabra*) as desired.

Toothache
Cloves are a powerful local antiseptic and mild pain reliever. Put a drop of oil of cloves (available from pharmacies and essential-oil suppliers) on the end of a cotton-wool bud and dab on or near the tooth; alternatively place a clove in the mouth near the tooth for as long as it is effective.

Travel sickness *see* FIRST AID

Ulcers, skin, *see* Skin ulcers

Ulcers, stomach *see* Stomachache

Varicose veins
Much can be done to prevent varicose veins. Tackle constipation; improve your diet, adding vitamins B, C and E; take more exercise; stop smoking; avoid hot baths and standing for hours.

Take spices that stimulate the circulation, such as ginger and cayenne, and an infusion of herbs that contain rutin, such as buckwheat (*Fagopyrum esculentum*), hawthorn berries (*Crataegus monogyna*) and horse chestnuts (*Aesculus hippocastanum*). Drink no more than three times a day, or use as a compress or lotion.

If your veins are inflamed or ache, a compress of calendula tincture or witch hazel will relieve the pain (*see also* **Hemorrhoids**).

THERAPEUTIC INDEX OF ESSENTIAL OILS

Essential oils are useful supplements for treating minor ailments, but for serious conditions, or if there is any uncertainty of diagnosis, be sure to consult a qualified practitioner. Apply the oils through massage, blended with a carrier oil, as described on pp. 230–4, or by one of the methods on p. 235. Do not take internally. Note that oils listed at the beginning of each group (out of alphabetical order) are considered most significant for that treatment. Use the oils in combination to treat your various symptoms. Refer to pp. 236–7 for ideas for blends.

Acne Cajuput, juniper, bergamot ($\frac{1}{2}$% concentration), chamomile, cedarwood, eucalyptus, lavender, lemon grass, sandalwood

Anxiety Jasmine, lavender, marjoram, neroli, basil, bergamot, camphor, chamomile, frankincense, geranium, juniper, melissa, rose, sandalwood

Apathy Jasmine, rosemary

Appetite, loss of Chamomile, bergamot, black pepper, coriander, fennel, ginger, hyssop, myrrh, sage

Arteriosclerosis Lemon, juniper

Arthritis Benzoin, chamomile, cypress, sage, juniper, lemon, thyme

Asthma Hyssop, lavender, pine, rosemary, basil, benzoin, cajuput

Athlete's foot Myrrh, lavender

Backache Chamomile, geranium

Blood pressure, high Clary sage, lavender, lemon, marjoram, melissa

Blood pressure, low Sage, hyssop, rosemary, thyme

Bronchitis, chronic Eucalyptus, hyssop, niaouli, cajuput, lavender

Bruises Hyssop, calendula, fennel

Burns and scalds (seek medical advice) Lavender, chamomile, eucalyptus, geranium, niaouli

Capillaries, broken Chamomile, cypress, rose, lavender, neroli

Catarrh Hyssop, basil, benzoin, black pepper, cedarwood, chamomile, eucalyptus, frankincense, jasmine, lavender, lemon, myrrh, thyme

Cellulite Cypress, fennel, oregano

Chilblains Lavender, lemon, camphor

Circulation, poor Black pepper, juniper, cypress, marjoram, lavender

Colds Lemon, pine, orange, tea tree

Constipation Fennel, marjoram, black pepper, rosemary, camphor

Coughs Cypress, eucalyptus, hyssop, thyme, benzoin, cedarwood

Cramp Basil, cypress, marjoram

Cystitis Pine, benzoin, bergamot, black pepper, cajuput, cedarwood, chamomile

Dandruff Chamomile, cedarwood, juniper, lavender, rosemary

Depression Camphor, chamomile, jasmine, thyme, basil, bergamot, clary sage, cypress, geranium

Diabetes Geranium, juniper

Diarrhea Lavender, black pepper, chamomile, cinnamon, clove, ginger, juniper, lemon, myrrh, neroli, peppermint, sandalwood

Earache Basil, chamomile, clove, hyssop, lavender, rose

Eczema, dry Chamomile, geranium, hyssop, lavender

Eczema, weeping Bergamot, juniper

Fevers Basil, black pepper, bergamot, camphor, chamomile, eucalyptus, hyssop, melissa, peppermint

Flatulence Coriander, fennel, peppermint

Flu Black pepper, eucalyptus, peppermint, rosemary, cypress

Fluid retention Cypress, eucalyptus, fennel, geranium, juniper, lavender

Food poisoning Black pepper, fennel

Hemorrhoids Cypress, frankincense, juniper, myrrh

Hair loss Lavender, rosemary, sage

Hay fever Chamomile, cypress, hyssop, lavender, lemon, pine, rose

Headache Chamomile, lavender, lemon, marjoram, peppermint, rose, rosemary

Herpes Geranium, lemon, myrrh, chamomile, eucalyptus, lavender

Indigestion Bergamot, chamomile, fennel, peppermint, rosemary, sage

Insect bites Lavender, basil, cinnamon, lemon, melissa, sage, thyme

Insomnia Basil, chamomile, clary sage, juniper, lavender, marjoram, neroli, rose, sandalwood, ylang-ylang

Itching skin Chamomile, cedarwood

Laryngitis Cypress, frankincense, lemon, sage, thyme, sandalwood

Lice Cinnamon, eucalyptus, clove, geranium, lavender, lemon grass

Liver, cirrhosis Juniper, rosemary

Lung disease Eucalyptus, tea tree, thyme, clove, pine

Malaria Eucalyptus, lemon

Menopause Cypress, sage

Menstruation, painful Cypress, peppermint, sage

Mental fatigue Rosemary, basil, peppermint

Mosquito repellent Eucalyptus, clove, geranium, peppermint

Muscular aches Eucalyptus, lavender, rosemary, black pepper

Muscle stiffness Rosemary, thyme

Muscle tone Lavender, lemon grass, rosemary, black pepper

Nausea Peppermint, basil, black pepper, fennel, lavender, rose

Nerves, panic Basil, bergamot, cedarwood, chamomile, geranium, juniper, lavender, marjoram, melissa, neroli, rose, thyme

Neuralgia, facial Chamomile, geranium, eucalyptus, peppermint

Overexertion Basil, lavender

Pimples Juniper, lavender, lemon

Premenstrual syndrome Benzoin, cedarwood, chamomile, cypress, frankincense, geranium, juniper

Psoriasis Bergamot, cajuput, lavender

Rheumatism Rosemary, ginger, oregano, pine, thyme

Sedatives Chamomile, lavender, lemon, marjoram, thyme

Shingles Eucalyptus, geranium, peppermint

Shock Camphor, melissa, neroli, peppermint

Sinusitis Basil, eucalyptus, lavender, lemon, niaouli, pine, thyme

Skin, chapped Benzoin, patchouli, chamomile, geranium, rose

Sore throat Tea tree, lemon, bergamot, clary sage, eucalyptus, geranium, ginger, sage, thyme

Sprains Eucalyptus, lavender

Stress Neroli, cedarwood, juniper

Sweating, offensive Cypress, pine

Tonsillitis Geranium, ginger, lemon

Toothache Clove, black pepper

Travel sickness Peppermint, ginger

Ulcers, skin Tea tree, bergamot, camphor, eucalyptus, frankincense

Ulcers, stomach Chamomile, geranium, lemon, peppermint, rose

Vomiting Basil, black pepper, chamomile, fennel, lavender, lemon, melissa, peppermint, rose

Warts and verrucas Lemon

Wounds (for serious bleeding get help immediately) Lemon on bandage to arrest bleeding; clean with lavender, eucalyptus, chamomile, geranium, hyssop, juniper

Wounds, infected Tea tree, chamomile, eucalyptus, lavender, myrrh, hyssop, thyme

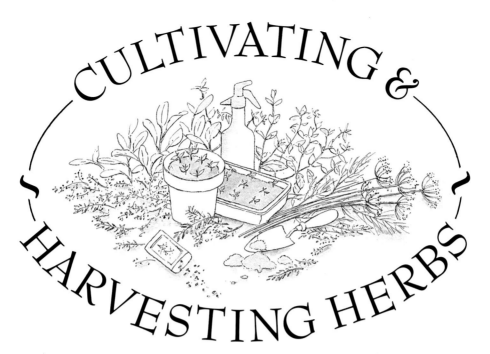

Herbs must be among the easiest plants to cultivate, being amenable to most conditions and rarely troubled by disease. The following pages provide information on growing herbs from seed and from cuttings; in the garden, in containers and indoors. There are practical ideas for making a variety of traditional herb garden features, notes on making herbal pesticides and fertilizers, and instructions on how to harvest and preserve different plant parts.

Soil preparation

Many herbs can survive on poor, stony ground, but few can cope with water-logged soil. Ideally, they prefer a light, open soil which is well aerated yet able to retain moisture and nutrients. To help them thrive, prepare the soil in early spring before sowing or plant-ing. Dig deeply and create a fine tilth, then rake to a smooth level surface. Allow the soil to settle at least one week before planting seed. Pot-grown plants can be planted almost immedi-ately in prepared soil.

Improving drainage
To increase air spaces and drainage in heavy soils, first dig over in early winter, as the presence of frost helps to break down solid clods of earth. In early spring, mix coarse grit, horticul-tural sand or vermiculite into the top 18 inches. Add compost to supply a more fibrous texture and nutrients. All these create space for extra oxygen, which means an increase in bacterial activity. This in turn results in more available plant food. They also make the soil more attractive to earthworms, whose presence enriches and lightens any soil.

When planting one of the Mediter-ranean herbs such as rosemary, sage, thyme, lavender or savory, incorporate a child's bucket of grit into each cubic foot of planting space to help the drainage.

If soil is very waterlogged, you can improve it for a few years by building a rubble drain. Dig an 18 inch–2 foot deep ditch angled toward an already

existing ditch or drainage facility. Half fill with coarse rubble and cover with a 3 inch layer of gravel, clinker or ash, replacing the topsoil. For a more permanent solution, make the ditch 2 feet 6 inches–3 feet deep, with plastic drainage pipes along the bottom leading to a soak-away, and proceed as before. Alternatively, if soil tends to be waterlogged, consider making raised beds (see p. 261).

Eliminating weeds
While preparing the soil for planting, get rid of persistent weeds such as bindweed (*Convolvulus arvensis*), couch grass (*Agropyron repens*) and ground elder (*Aegopodium podagraria*), which can quickly take over an herb bed. Dig up weeds with taproots, taking care not to break off any of the root or it will sprout. Fork out longer straggling roots over a period of about a month. Dig through the soil at weekly intervals. Don't throw uprooted weeds on the compost heap; you'll transplant them.

Enriching soil
A light, free-draining sandy soil does not hold moisture and is usually low in nutrients. Although the Mediterranean herbs can thrive on such a soil, others, such as mint and chives, may benefit from the addition of compost, or a well-rotted straw-based manure, to help retain moisture and supply nutrients. These are best worked in after winter rains so most of the nutrients will be available for spring growth. Peat helps to retain moisture, but it does not

contribute nutrients and may make the soil too acid if used in large quantities.

Most herbs are like vegetables in their preference for a slightly alkaline soil. If your soil is acidic, add a sprink-ling of lime, not as a plant food but as a catalyst to help the plants take up the nutrients present. Use the lowest amount recommended. Ashes from wood fires are also beneficial as they contribute lime and potash.

Avoid using artificial fertilizers as these can make growth too lush, which will result in a plant with poor flavor. However, if you know your soil is poor or lacking in minerals, try one of the herbal fertilizers listed on p. 267.

Mulching
Once herbs are established they will benefit from a mulch, a covering of organic matter spread over the soil. The mulch helps to stop the soil drying out and provides nutrients. Applied during the growing season, it boosts lush growth in salad herbs such as sorrel and purslane, and in shade- and moisture-loving herbs such as mint, angelica and sweet cicely. It can also protect plant roots from frosts.

Mulching is usually most beneficial after a heavy rain. Spread light, organic matter over the soil and around plants in a layer up to 3 inches deep. The Mediterranean herbs such as rosemary, thyme, sage and lavender may benefit more from a layer of gravel or clinkers if the soil is very moist. Mulching also helps to control weed growth by blocking out light.

Propagation

Many herbs will grow from seed and readily self-seed once established. A large proportion can also be grown from cuttings and division.

Sowing seed on site

Annual plants of the Umbelliferae family (anise, chervil, dill, coriander and cumin, and the biennial parsley) are best sown on site, where you wish them to grow, as any root disturbance in transplanting can make them run to seed before they have produced a useful crop of leaves, Parsley seed is exceptionally slow to germinate, so do be patient.

As a rule, sow seed in mid- to late spring after the soil has been prepared and warmed up. One of the most reliable signs is the emergence of new weed seedlings in the ground. Remove weeds and sow seeds thinly in shallow drills (see below).

If the soil feels heavy and lumpy, spread a layer of fine sand along the drill to give seeds a better start. Barely cover seeds with a fine sprinkling of soil and tap down gently. Water with a fine spray. Mark each row with the name of the herb and date of sowing.

Covering with cloches gives seeds a head start and provides protection from late frosts and hungry wildlife. Lay the cloches in position a few weeks before you sow so the soil warms up.

Thin out the seedlings when they have reached a height of 2–4 inches. Water the soil the day before you remove them. Use a trowel or your fingers to lift them from the soil and handle very carefully when replanting. See the Herbal Index or seed packet for planting distances.

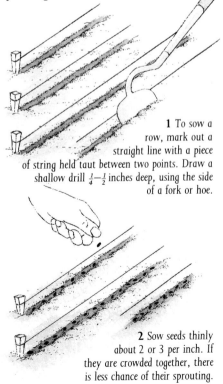

1 To sow a row, mark out a straight line with a piece of string held taut between two points. Draw a shallow drill $\frac{1}{4}$–$\frac{1}{2}$ inches deep, using the side of a fork or hoe.

2 Sow seeds thinly about 2 or 3 per inch. If they are crowded together, there is less chance of their sprouting.

Growing seed indoors

It is better to grow expensive, rare or unfamiliar seeds in seed trays indoors, where all conditions can be controlled. Sowing seeds indoors also allows you to start the plants off before the soil has warmed up.

Buy a proprietary loamless seed-growing mixture or mix your own with two parts sterilized loam, one part fine peat, one part coarse sand and a dash of fertilizer. Blend well and pass through a $\frac{3}{8}$ inch sieve.

A shallow seed tray 2 inches deep is the best size for sowing small seeds. Small pots can also be used and are better if you only wish to sow a few seeds. If using deeper containers, fill the lower section with clean drainage material – a layer of gravel, perlite or broken pottery. Add growing mixture to within $\frac{1}{4}$ inch of the top. Give the tray or pot a sharp downward tap, then press the soil surface gently with a flat board. If the mixture is very dry,

Preparing pots and trays

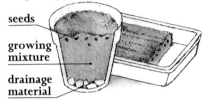

seeds
growing mixture
drainage material

water and leave it to drain. Sow seeds thinly, mixing fine seeds with sand so they spread out evenly. Sprinkle over a fine layer of potting mixture to hold the seeds in place. Cover larger seed with a layer as deep as the seed.

Water with a fine rose, beginning the flow off the tray and ending off the tray. Label, date and cover with a layer of glass and a layer of newspaper.

Seeds germinate faster in the warmth of a greenhouse or indoors (preferably

in a place with a constant, warm temperature), and need to be watched daily. If further watering proves necessary, set the pots in water until the top appears damp.

When sprouting begins, move the trays into the light. Lift the covering at one edge for two days. Then take off the cover, but shade the seedlings from bright sun for several days.

Transplanting seedlings

As soon as plants are large enough to handle, thin them out or transplant them to a larger box or a pot to prevent overcrowding. Wait, though, until the first pair of true leaves has formed, after the cotyledons – two seed leaves which are a completely different shape.

Handle young seedlings by a leaf rather than by their stems and take them carefully out of the soil to avoid breaking or bruising their tiny new roots and stems. Make a hole in the soil then insert the seedling. Firm the compost, water it and site the plants in a light location out of direct sunlight. Daily attention is important at this stage, as overcrowded seedlings or those not in good light can become weak and leggy within two days. If this happens, repot them at a lower depth, by burying half the elongated stem.

Once seedlings are growing well, remove any feebler ones and leave the strongest to grow on. Transfer to larger pots with potting-grade compost (see p. 264) or plant out.

Firm in a seedling after careful transplanting.

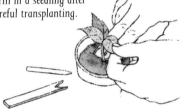

HERBS WORTH GROWING FROM SEED		
An enormous number of herbs, common and rare, can be grown from seed but the group listed below		is generally the easiest. If you require only one plant, it is often cheaper and quicker to buy one.
All the annuals		
anise	chervil	nasturtium
arugula	coriander	orach
basil	cumin	purslane
borage	dill	summer savory
calendula	mustard	sweet marjoram
chamomile, annual		
Biennials		
angelica	parsley, curled and broad	wild celery (smallage)
caraway	leaf	woad
Perennials		
catnip	lovage	salad burnet
chamomile, flowering	marjoram, French	sorrel
chives	marsh mallow	sweet cicely
fennel, green and bronze	onion, Welsh	thyme, common
feverfew	oregano	winter savory
good King Henry	rue	wormwood
hyssop	sage	

Planting out

All plants hate shocks; they need to get acclimatized to new conditions. Plants propagated indoors should move outdoors gradually. Set them out in a sheltered position during the day, and take them in at night. After several days, leave them out at night as well. Plant out after about a week.

Do not plant out half-hardy plants until you are sure spring frosts are over. Avoid planting out on hot or rainy days. The best days are calm and warm; early evening is often ideal, as the soil is warm and the sun low.

Water the soil beforehand, if it isn't already moist. Make a hole the size of the root, insert the plant, handling the root area very carefully; fill the hole with soil and firm the plant in.

OTHER FORMS OF PROPAGATION

Herbs can also be grown easily using vegetative means of propagation: cuttings, dividing and layering. With these methods, you can be more certain of the resulting flower and leaf shapes and colors on the new plant, whereas plants grown from seeds are often more variable. These methods of propagation are also beneficial to the parent plants, which might otherwise become overcrowded and straggly.

Propagating from cuttings

There are three main types of stem cuttings that are suitable for herbs: softwood, from new shoots which have not yet hardened; semihardwood, from new growth when it has started to firm up at the base; and hardwood, from woody shrubs and trees.

Softwood cuttings are taken in late spring from strong new growth, or in late summer after flowering. Semi-hardwood cuttings are usually taken from midsummer to mid-autumn, from shrubby herbs such as rosemary and myrtle. Hardwood cuttings are taken in mid- to late autumn. If you are propagating a variegated or colored leaf plant, choose the most highly colored pieces for your cuttings.

Planting cuttings

To plant cuttings in open ground, choose a warm sheltered spot out of direct sunlight. For softwood and semi-hardwood cuttings, a soil temperature of 55–64 °F is adequate. Dig in extra sand and peat to create a loose open soil, which will encourage quick root formation. An even easier method is to place a few cuttings under the mother plant, but remember to water them for the first few days and in dry weather. Softwood cuttings soon wilt, so plant them out promptly. Spray leaves lightly, and frequently during dry weather.

Planting cuttings in containers gives greater flexibility for positioning and for supplying bottom heat to speed root formation. Insert cuttings to a third of their depth in potting compost or garden soil lightened with sand and peat. Firm in no more than necessary to hold them upright; the looser the soil, the easier it is for roots to grow. Place several cuttings of the same species around the edge of a pot, add three tall sticks and cover with a clear plastic bag to retain moisture and warmth. Open the bag every few days to change the air and prevent mold building up. As soon as cuttings show signs of growth, place them in a sheltered sunny position and provide with some plant nutrients. Ensure that the plants don't get too much strong sunlight early on.

Softwood and semihardwood cuttings usually root in about six weeks (four for sages and pelargoniums).

Plant cuttings to one third of their depth in cutting compost.

Plant several cuttings from one species in a pot and cover with a plastic bag, raised so it doesn't touch the leaves.

Hardwood cuttings gradually develop roots over the winter. Transplant the following year to a permanent location.

Most herbs root easily without a hormone rooting compound. If you do use one, shake off any excess as too much can be worse than none at all.

PLANTS FOR CUTTINGS

The following grow well from cuttings taken from a healthy parent plant.

curry plant	rue varieties
hyssop varieties	sage varieties
lavender varieties	santolinas
lemon verbena	tarragon, French
marjorams	thyme varieties
myrtle	winter savory
pelargoniums	wormwood
rosemary varieties	varieties

HOW TO TAKE A CUTTING

Follow the same method for all three types of cutting. For softwood cuttings, take sturdy pieces 2–4 inches long with plenty of leaves; for semihardwood cuttings, you should take pieces 4–6 inches long; for hardwood cuttings, you need pieces 6–15 inches long.

Take cuttings from just below a leaf node; the collection of cells at leaf junctions encourages growth. Choose healthy, vigorous shoots without flower buds. Use a sharp knife or pruning shears for a clean cut without ragged edges. If the cutting is torn from the main stem, trim the heel,

leaving a neat sliver of the main stem wood, as the larger the cut surface the greater the chance of infection.

Strip the lower third of leaves away, taking care not to tear the stem, before planting.

For hardwood cuttings, trim the cuttings just below the lowest bud.

Softwood cutting

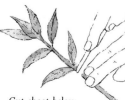

Cut shoot below a leaf node, leaving a short length of stem.

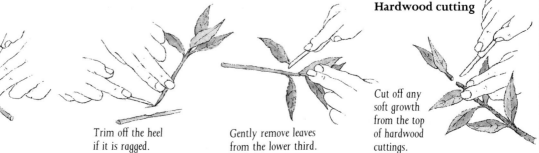

Hardwood cutting

Trim off the heel if it is ragged.

Gently remove leaves from the lower third.

Cut off any soft growth from the top of hardwood cuttings.

Plant division

Several herbs benefit from being divided. This method checks their spread and keeps them hardier. Dig up the plant, preferably in autumn or early spring, when it is dormant. Remove old flower stems and carefully separate the plant, into individual sections, each having a growing point and some roots. Replant, nurture and water these sections until the roots have reestablished themselves and there are signs of new growth.

Bulbous plants such as chives and everlasting onion are pulled apart in the same manner and replanted.

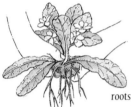

Divide young plants by hand, ensuring that roots have new growth.

HERBS SUITABLE FOR PLANT DIVISION	
alecost (costmary)	meadowsweet
bistort	primrose
chives	skirret
cowslip	sorrel
elecampane	sweet Joe Pye
good King Henry	sweet violet
lawn chamomile	tansy
lemon balm	tarragon
lovage	thymes
lungwort	wall germander
marjorams	wormwood

Root sections

This is the easiest form of propagation. Dig up the plant in spring or autumn and carefully take 2–4 inch pieces of roots, each with growing buds; plant these pieces approximately 1 inch deep in a pot of compost. Use longer pieces if planting straight into the ground. This method is most suitable for spreading plants with creeping roots: bergamot, dwarf comfrey, mints, soapwort and sweet woodruff.

Root cuttings

A few herbs, such as horseradish, comfrey and skirret, can be propagated from thick pieces of root cut 2–3 inches long. Insert the cuttings vertically into potting compost with a $\frac{1}{4}$ inch covering of sand (see below).

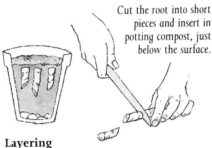

Cut the root into short pieces and insert in potting compost, just below the surface.

Layering

If cuttings are difficult to root, you can try layering. With this method, you encourage new sections of a plant to root while still attached to the parent plant. This is how many shrubby plants like thyme spread in the wild.

Peg a stem to the ground so its underside is in contact with the soil.

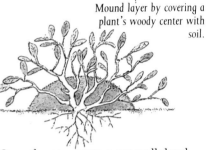

Layer by pegging down a stem against the soil.

Mound layer by covering a plant's woody center with soil.

Once the new roots seem well developed, separate the new shoot from its parent. If the soil is heavy, add some sand or peat before you start.

Another similar method is **mound layering**, which not only creates new growth but also improves the appearance of old plants, particularly sages and thymes, which can go woody in the center. In spring, pile soil (mixed with peat and sand when necessary) over the woody center until only the young shoots show. By late summer, roots will have formed on many of the shoots, and these shoots can be taken from the parent plant and planted in a new location.

Maintaining and creating plant shapes

Herbs are basically wild plants and have vigorous survival instincts to cope with poor or crowded conditions. When herbs are planted in rich garden soil, their growth is exuberant and often needs curtailing.

Controlling growth

Tenacious spreaders, such as the mint family, should have their roots contained in a sunken 14 inch pot, a black polythene bag with drainage holes or an 18 inch deep tube of drainpipe. Bottomless restraining barriers such as a pipe must be at least 18 inches deep, otherwise the roots will spread back up along the surface. Other vigorous-growing herbs, such as soapwort, dwarf comfrey and sweet woodruff, need to have spreading roots removed regularly.

For sorrel, lemon balm and the annual salad herbs, remove the flowering stems as soon as they sprout to ensure the production of more succulent leaves. Others, such as good King Henry and marjoram, can be cut

back hard just after flowering in time to grow a fresh young crop of leaves before autumn.

Depending on your priorities, you can harvest seed heads or leave them on the plant as winter food for the birds, cutting back hard early in the spring. Other late-flowering stalks can be left on over the winter if their dead leaves provide some wind and frost protection for themselves or their neighbors. Avoid leaving tall or thick stems standing if your soil is very light and the herbs are liable to be rocked about by winter winds. This can create pockets of frost around the stems and lead to rot.

Pruning

Lightly prune aromatic shrubby perennials such as lavender, hyssop, santolinas, southernwood and curry plant by cutting off their dried flower stalks in autumn; then cut them right back the following spring to encourage new growth. In general, cut back to about 9 inches, or to the previous year's

growth, as long as you can see some green shoots below this level. Sage needs more care as stems often refuse to break lower down. You may be better off replacing some sages and lavenders every four or five years.

It is preferable to do a regular gentle pruning each year. Many people leave shrubby herbs two or three years, then discover a tangled mass with leggy stems. The solutions are to cut back as far as green can be seen, to propagate cuttings for replacement plants or to dig up the entire plant and replant at a lower level, burying the long stems. Do make sure that the soil is well drained below the new depth, or the plant will rot.

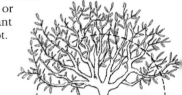

Prune shrubby herbs in autumn, cutting back to the previous year's growth.

All aromatic herbs are antiseptic, so you can use prunings in several ways: lay wormwood in the vegetable garden as an insect repellent or dry the leaves and hang them indoors to deter moths infuse thyme and rosemary to make disinfectant waters; burn any of the aromatic herbs on a fire to scent and purify the air.

Picking herbs

The way you pick leaves for use can make a plant grow bushier. Basil, tarragon, marjoram, oregano and the evergreens maintain a bushier shape if the growing tip is pinched out first. Then pick the larger side leaves. In general, do not remove more than a fifth of the total leaves of a herb before allowing the plant time to regrow.

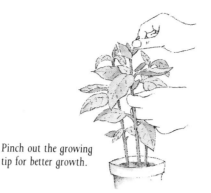

Pinch out the growing tip for better growth.

Mint produces small side leaves if the top is snipped off, but it's better to cut off a whole stem as the plant responds with more succulent growth.

Pick the outer leaves of parsley, sorrel, lovage and salad burnet to encourage continuing growth. If one of these plants produces a strong central stem as a prelude to flowering, remove it immediately. Parsley is a biennial and produces the best leaves in its first season. When replacing a parsley plant, add the old roots to a bouquet garni.

Small sprigs of rosemary, thyme, sage and winter savory can be picked on an aesthetic basis: remove pieces that spoil the look of the herb.

Chives and Welsh onion can be cut down to 1½ inches and then allowed to regrow. Less is wasted if you cut a few blades of chives down to 1½ inches instead of nipping a layer off the top of the whole plant, because each blade yellows for a further inch or two after being cut.

Winter protection for herbs

Many herbs will not survive a cold winter if left outdoors, but by being brought indoors in pots, annuals can have their lives extended by some months, and less hardy perennials often benefit too (see p. 264 for potting and pp. 266–7 for growing herbs indoors). At the first sign of crisp autumn air, basil should be brought indoors. Pale, mottled or otherwise unhappy leaves may be signaling the plant's displeasure at cold evenings. Before a heavy frost, pineapple sage (*Salvia elegans*), fringed lavender (*L. dentata*), pelargoniums, balm of Gilead (*Cedronella canariensis*) and Crete dittany (*Origanum dictamnus*) need to be brought indoors. All will reward your effort with aromatic leaves and occasionally with winter blossoms.

In colder climates with longer periods of frost and snow, rosemary, sage, winter savory, curry plant, lavender and the more delicate thymes should be brought indoors to survive the winter. Protect mature plants that winter outside by layering soil, straw or compost around their roots.

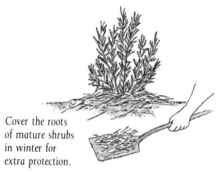

Cover the roots of mature shrubs in winter for extra protection.

If you grow herbs in pots all year (see pp. 264–5), plunged in soil in summer, it's easier to bring them indoors. Trim any roots which may have grown through the base, or repot if the maximum pot size has not been reached. Try to make the transfer while outdoor and indoor temperatures are similar. If that is not possible, go through an intermediate stage using an unheated greenhouse for a few days, or a cool garage for a few nights, to ease the transition.

Some herbs, such as chives, have an intimate relationship with the seasons and feel strongly that autumn onward is rest time. Practice a little deception: repot them in early autumn, water and cut back the growth as necessary. Put them in a warm, humid place, out of direct sun, for a week or two, to encourage root growth into the new soil. Then put them into a cooler location for a few weeks, while you still have other chives growing outside. When the other chives die back, bring the potted ones indoors to start their "spring" growth, with additional artificial light if possible.

Much less trouble to bring in is the Welsh onion, which has a larger onion leaf than chives and maintains some green throughout the winter, even outdoors. Chervil and winter purslane do well indoors as they prefer growing at this time of the year, while summer-sown parsley and tarragon will tolerate being moved indoors. Don't bother transplanting whole mint stems; pot 3–4 inch healthy cuttings with plump leaf buds. Within six weeks you should have fresh new mint leaves available for harvesting.

Enclosures

An important aspect of a traditional herb garden, an enclosure reduces wind damage, raises the overall average temperature, creates privacy and retains the perfume of aromatic herbs. It can be as permanent or as temporary as you require. Upkeep and expenditure vary from type to type.

HEDGING

Once established, this is the easiest form of tall, long-term enclosure, and gives further opportunities for using herbal and aromatic plants around the

Informal hedging

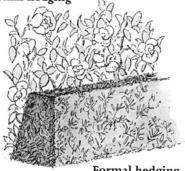

Formal hedging

garden, as many shrubby herbs are evergreen and clip well. Hedging can be neat and formal or soft and wild in effect, depending on the plants you select and how you trim them. However, it cannot be immediate. All hedging plants take some years to reach a good height.

Yew (*Taxus* species) is a classic hedging plant, for good reasons. Its dark green leaves are the perfect size and color as a backdrop to all shades of green, gold, bronze, silver and gray as well as any flower color, and it clips well. Yew has a reputation for being slow, but it rewards good cultivation. Enrich the ground with bonemeal and compost, and water yew plants well in their first season to help speed up their growth. Start with 18 inch plants and plant them at 2 foot intervals. To shape, prune in mid-spring and again in late summer. Following this procedure, our yew hedge reached waist-height in three growing seasons and head height in six years.

Box (*Buxus sempervirens*) is another traditional hedging plant. Although quite slow-growing, it has neat, small, glossy leaves which suit being clipped into tight, formal shapes. Plant at 18 inch intervals.

Sweetbrier rose (*Rosa eglanteria*) is often associated with herb gardens for the lovely apple scent of its leaves. It is large, untidy and prickly but can be trained into a natural-style hedge. Plant at 3 foot intervals.

Arbor vitae, the *Thuja* family of conifers, has aromatic foliage of a pleasant, fruity, almost pineapple scent, and T. *plicata* and T. *occidentalis* are excellent plants for tall hedges. Both appreciate clipping and are tolerant of shade and shallow soils. An annual pruning or pinching back is best in late summer to allow any new growth to ripen before the first frosts. Plant at 2–3 foot intervals.

The giant fir, *Abies grandis*, makes a good windbreak on all but very exposed sites, but it should not be clipped. Its foliage releases a refreshing orange-grapefruit scent when crushed. Plant at 6–12 foot intervals.

Low hedging

Low hedging is a feature of many herb gardens. It is used to separate species and beds as well as for ornament, as seen in knot gardens. In order of hardiness, dwarf box (*B.s.* 'Suffruti-cosa'), lavender, santolina and rosemary are the most popular plants for low hedges. When making your choice, it is important to know whether the species will survive the regular winter conditions in your area. Single plants can be replaced in the occasional severe winter but to have a hedge killed just as it reaches full glory can be a heartbreaking experience.

Rosemary can reach a height of 6 feet in sheltered areas, though 3 feet is more the norm. *Rosmarinus officinalis* 'Miss Jessup's Upright' provides the least sprawling form. A new form called *R.o.* 'Sawyer's Selection,' culti-vated at Suffolk Herbs, has reached 8 feet in four years and appears to have the same degree of hardiness as common rosemary, as well as a vigorous habit.

Next in size are the large lavenders at 3–4 feet, Old English lavender

(*L. angustifolia*), with 'Grappenhall' and 'Hidcote Giant' the two largest named cultivars. The intermediate-sized lavenders include white, pink, blue and purple flowering varieties, so you can grow an interesting hedge with a range of colors and flowering times. Clip the hedge after harvesting the flowers.

Santolina chamaecyparissus creates an intensely silver hedge that will grow about 2 feet high. Clipped regularly, it can make an attractive, dense shape, though you won't get the little yellow flowers.

Curry plant (*Helichrysum angustifolium*), hyssops in different colors, southern-wood, upright wall germander, rue, winter savory, shrubby thymes and the herbaceous chives and wormwood can all be planted and clipped to make good low hedges.

Planting and maintaining a hedge

It's easiest to grow a hedge from purchased container-grown specimens or cuttings, which can be set directly into position. As a rough guide, allow a space of two-thirds the eventual height of the plant between hedging specimens: for a 3 foot lavender hedge, set the plants 2 feet apart; for an 18 inch rock hyssop hedge, set the plants 12 inches apart.

To keep the growth healthy and dense, clip the hedge regularly along the top to encourage bushy side growth. Spread a well-rotted compost around the roots each spring and water well during periods of hot weather, as a thick hedge can prevent the roots from receiving much rainwater.

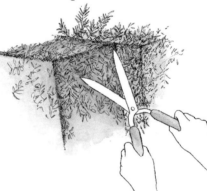

Trim the hedge so that the sides slope a little, making it broader at the base than the top. This will make the hedge grow sturdier and more able to cope with a weighty layer of snow.

KNOT GARDENS

Knot gardens were first recorded in the fifteenth century and are one of the most traditional syles of herb garden planting. This delightful skill of using clipped edging plants to create "rib-bons" (and hence "knots") of color is now enjoying a revival, albeit on a more intimate scale than in the grand

gardens of the past. It is a highly attractive method for separating plants and displaying color.

Try your hand by marking out a bed not less than 6 feet square (it is difficult to achieve any weaving of lines if the outside dimensions are less than this), following the method below. Plan it as a feature on its own or as the centerpiece of your herb garden. Well kept, it will make an entire garden appear mature and cared for.

Choose to plant a square or rec-tangle, as contained geometric patterns suit this style of planting. Carefully plan out your design on grid paper with the thickness of the hedging cor-rectly drawn. For inspiration, look at knot patterns featured in old herbals or turn to the art of ancient cultures which used geometric designs; Indian, Arabic and Chinese materials are a par-ticularly rich source of ideas.

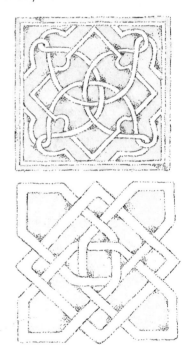

Two ornate knot-garden designs based on ideas from a 17th-century gardening book.

The interest in a knot garden comes from contrasting the foliage colors of different evergreen herbs. Choose from light green dwarf box (*Buxus sempervirens* 'Suffruticosa'), rock hyssop (*Hyssopus officinalis* 'Aristata'), the green *Santolina virens*; the dark green of upright wall germander, winter savory or rosemary; the silver of *Santolina chamaecyparissus* 'Nana' and the dwarf lavenders; the willow green of *Santolina* 'Lemon Queen.' In fact, by using just the three santolinas, you can make a highly satisfying pattern, with different colors of foliage and uniform growth and leaf size.

Traditionally, the space between the plants was covered with colored sand

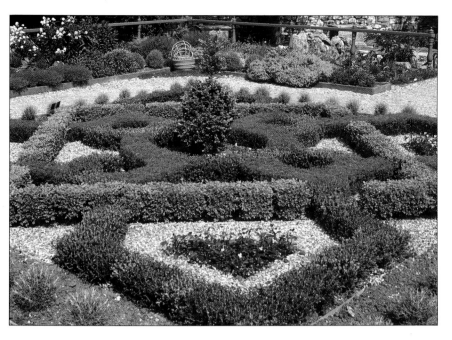

A reconstruction of an Elizabethan knot garden at the Tudor House Museum, Southampton.

or gravel, but this is difficult to obtain and maintain. Dark peat shows off the colored plants very well, or, as nature always rushes to fill a space, ground-hugging evergreens like creeping thymes can be used. Thymes range in leaf color from the dark green T. *herba barona* to the light green T. *caespititius*, and the gold variegated varieties. In high summer, their colorful flowers can add an extra dimension to your design.

Making and maintaining a knot garden
Before planting out the herbs, clear the ground of all weeds and cultivate it well, digging in additional coarse sand or grit to ensure good drainage.

After working out your design on grid paper, mark it out with lime, sand or string, using a card template for any small, repeated shapes.

Plant selected perennial evergreen herbs 9 inches apart for 9 inch high ribbons. Lower, 6 inch ribbons work with dwarf box, but any other plants in the ribbon will spend most of the season denuded from being constantly cut back. Plant the corner herbs first to ensure even spacing. With pot-grown plants, the first pruning can begin as soon as they are in the ground. Clip the top and sides so each plant is neat.

Cut back in late spring to encourage new growth. When pruning the shape, give extra flow and movement to the design by emphasizing any crossover of two ribbons by height. If a silver ribbon crosses a green ribbon, clip it to make a gentle hump-back curve, and make the ribbon passing "underneath" curve down as it nears the join.

Make your last cutting in late summer so the plants have some leaf protection during the winter.

An instant knot garden
A light-hearted and inexpensive way of trying out a knot garden or even creating a temporary pattern, perhaps for a special occasion, is to lay out a design with cuttings. Prepare the bed as described above, adding more peat and sand. Select one or two large plants of your chosen ribbon herbs to take cuttings from. Place 6 inch cuttings at 4 inch intervals to mark out the design. Water daily for the first two weeks and shade with a net curtain on twigs in high summer until rooted. Plant a few extra cuttings on the sidelines to replace any that die.

WALLS
A solid walled garden can give the equivalent in increased warmth to moving about 200 miles nearer to the equator. It also gives a feeling of privacy and solitude. High walls are expensive and require skilled construction. However, even a small wall provides shelter and a boundary.

When constructing a wall, choose materials that are sympathetic in texture and color with those of your house and of any other hard surfaces, such as a terrace or paths. Use local stone, hollow concrete blocks or bricks. If selecting bricks from a large range, take accurate color samples of materials from your house and paved areas to check compatibility. If pink is a predominant color in your garden, take along a few blooms, as these often clash with the colors of brick.

Limit yourself to constructing low walls about 2 feet high, as shown right. Drystone walls (those built without

mortar), retaining walls and low brick walls, with a double thickness of brick, can all be constructed in this way, so they contain pockets of soil which will accommodate a wide range of herbs. When constructing a double-thickness wall, set a good layer of rubble or stones in the center and then top up with a layer of soil.

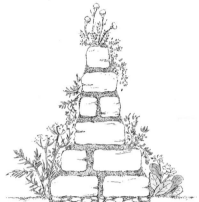

Making a stone wall
Dig a shallow trench the proposed width of the wall. Put a layer of rubble or stones in the base of the trench to hold the first layer of stones in position. Start with a broad base about two stones wide, and narrow to a stone's width at the top. Use soil between the stones as mortar and slot in plants as you go. Place long stones across the width of the wall at intervals as extra anchorage.

HERBS FOR WALLS
Any herbs accustomed to rocky hillsides will revel in a sun-facing wall. The following trailing plants are attractive for planting in crevices or on top of a sunny wall:

creeping thymes	low-growing
prostrate winter	artemisias
savory	maiden's pink
rosemary	alpine lady's
catmint	mantle
	prostrate sage

The following shrubby evergreen herbs add color and height if planted along the top of a wall:

lavender	juniper
hyssop	santolina

Herbs with the word "wall" in their name are obviously well suited to this situation:

wallflowers	wall germander
pellitory-of-the-wall	wall pennywort

Herbs that enjoy dry locations grow well on a wall:

perennial	houseleek
chamomile	

Moisture often collects along the base of a wall, making a good location on the shady side for:

primroses	mints
violets	meadowsweet
sweet cicely	angelica

FENCES

For those without the time or space to grow a hedge or build a wall, an interesting range of fencing materials is available. These give wind protection and privacy, and provide an instant screen around such utilitarian areas as a compost heap. Select materials such as timber, bamboo, sturdy wattle or trellis, which will harmonize in color and texture with the natural softness of herbs. Solid paneling gives the greatest privacy, but many climbing plants benefit from the extra light and ventilation that open fencing provides.

All fencing needs maintenance and eventually replacing, so choose the best-quality materials you can afford. As a rule, the cheaper the material, the shorter its lifespan.

Fencing posts must be solid and secure. If you use a lightweight open fence or trellis, support it with sturdy posts: a trellis is easy to replace, but the posts involve much harder work. Concrete posts set into concrete form the most solid support, but they are not the most attractive. Timber is more sympathetic but must be treated with a preservative. Remember that if you use creosote you cannot grow plants against it for a season. Timber posts set directly into the earth will rot relatively quickly. When possible, fix timber posts at ground level to a metal collar that is fixed into the earth, or set them in a concrete base partly filled with stone and rubble.

Use low fences to define boundaries and edges between beds. White picket fences are a charming feature of many

Wattle-fencing in the medieval style.

Traditional white picket fencing.

American herb gardens. They show off the plants, look trim and provide a tidy sense of order.

To give a more rustic feel around a small bed, you can renew a medieval tradition by making low-level sections of wattle fencing. These are woven using flexible, green branches of hazel, willow or dogwood approximately $\frac{1}{4}$ inch diameter. Select sturdy pieces as vertical supports, $\frac{1}{2}-\frac{3}{4}$ inch in diameter and about 12 inches long. Push them into the soil at 9 inch intervals, leaving about 5 inches above ground. Then weave the hazel strips between the verticals, pushing each one down firmly as you proceed.

Screens

To provide a visual barrier without heavy shade, create an open screen. Posts with garlands of rope or chain, along which climbing roses, honeysuckle, hops or ivies have been trained, often look effective. The idea can be developed further with a crisscross of

diagonal ropes stretched between posts. Train a climbing plant such as ivy along the ropes and clip in the spaces to keep the "windows" open. For a temporary screen lasting a few seasons, bamboo canes can be inserted at 6–9 inch intervals, wired together for support and planted with a lightweight climber such as nasturtium, sweet pea, or a climbing bean with attractive flowers or foliage.

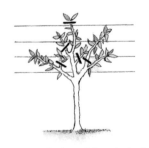

A fence of wire and canes covered in quick-growing nasturtiums.

A crisscross trellis covered in sweet-smelling honeysuckle.

Trellis

Treillage or trellis work, a combination of plant support and screen, is fast developing into an art form of its own. Available in a variety of patterns on different scales, trellis is bought in panels, which come in a range of widths, 6 feet high. It is a delightful way of adding lightness and decorative richness to large surfaces such as house walls or flat fences and dark corners. Select climbing plants from the list on p. 259, or grow tall herbaceous herbs

---

PLEACHING TREES

In this technique of training trees, young branches are braided together to form one flat wall of greenery with the lower section left open. All low branches are removed and eventually the trunks assume the stature of pillars. Early versions were a favorite in medieval herbaries, designed to form a green gallery or covered walk around the herb garden. Charming examples can be seen at the Queen's Garden, Kew, London, and in the National Trust gardens at Sissinghurst, Kent, and Hidcote, Gloucestershire.

Pleached trees create shelter and define areas without causing the claustrophobic feeling a tall hedge can give in a small space. They can frame features, block out tall eyesores, hint at vistas beyond and make a suitable architectural link between two styles of gardening; say between formal beds and an informal herb garden, or a formal herb garden and an informal swimming pool area. If they are grown as a single row, a

parallel hedge planted one path's width away will make a windbreak.

Hornbeam and lime are the two most frequently trained species, but willows, privet, whitethorn, sycamore, chestnut and the dogwood *Cornus mas* can all be used. Plan the desired size and shape carefully, testing out the heights with canes in the garden. Check the vista from every direction and from windows in the house.

Start with young trees which have straight stems. Prepare the ground well, mixing in additional bonemeal and good compost. If you're aiming for a slender wall of greenery, the trees will need a support system of posts and horizontal wires (similar to those used for espaliered fruit trees). Plant the trees at 4–8 foot intervals and prune as described at right. Each autumn, prune and train until a dense network of twigs is built up. Thereafter, just clip the foliage to keep its shape.

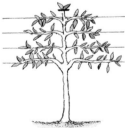

1 *Remove any side shoots below the level desired. Remove any branches not growing in the desired direction.*

2 *Prune upright branches or twigs above a set of buds and encourage this new growth along the wires.*

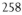

in the screen's shelter. For woody climbers, such as honeysuckle and jasmine, choose more permanent materials, because it is difficult to remove damaged trellis or wattle from a tangle of branches. With some ingenuity, pieces can be combined to create structures such as an arbor (see p. 262) or a pergola (see below).

PERGOLAS

A pergola consists of a series of rectangular or curved "arches" joined horizontally and covered with climbing plants to create a semicovered walkway. It is one of the quickest ways of bringing mystery and interest to a small, bland garden or flat landscape.

A pergola can also be built with vertical supports and horizontal beams extending from the house, creating a successful architectural link between house and garden and a delightful outdoor room. It can mask unsightly views, provide a strong, identifiable entrance into the herb garden or be used to emphasize a route.

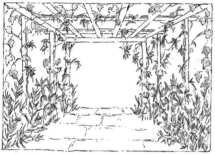

A traditional pergola makes an airy covered walkway or shelter.

When building a pergola, there is a difficult balance to draw between genuine rural charm and fairy-tale sweetness. Simple structures of metal arches, or rectangular frames of posts and rails, are usually the most successful. Plant climbers at each support post. If you are growing climbing roses, try to ensure that no thorns brush against those walking along the path.

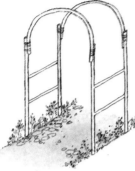

To make a double arch, position four stout poles at the required intervals and wire flexible branches, such as green hazel, between them. Add horizontal rails for rigidity.

A double arch makes an effective entrance as shown above. It can also be used at the crossroads of two paths, as in the illustration above opposite. The garden design on p. 31 features a pergola created from espaliered fruit trees.

For structures of timber, hardwood always lasts many years longer than softwood but is considerably more expensive. Treat all wood with a preservative that is safe for plants. For square posts, consider purchasing a metal collar with an extended pointed piece which you hammer into the ground. This supports the post just above ground level and prolongs its life by keeping it out of damp soil.

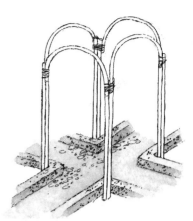

For arches at the crossroads of two paths, omit the side rails and add two extra arches at right angles to the first pair.

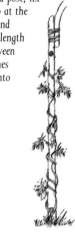

To train stems up a post, fix a screw eye or loop at the top and the base, and loosely spiral up a length of plastic wire between the two. As branches grow, tuck them into the wire.

CLIMBING PLANTS FOR THE HERB GARDEN

Roses This list includes only scented and continuous or repeat flowering roses, which have the soft colors and graceful growth of the old-fashioned species.
'Albéric Barbier': yellow buds to creamy white flowers.
'Bloomfield Abundance': miniature pink blooms in profusion, as the name suggests.
'Gloire de Dijon': buff yellow, early flowering. Will grow on a shady wall.
'Guinée': rich velvet scarlet, perfect buds to dry for potpourri.
'New Dawn': silver blush pink; fruity fragrance.
'Zephirine Drouhin': cerise pink.
'Blush Noisette': lilac pink; rich clove scent.
'Cécile Brunner': tiny blush blooms.
'Constance Spry': luminous pink; myrrh fragrance.
'Leverkusen': lemon-yellow flowers with lemon fragrance.
'Mme Alfred Carrière': blush white globes, very fragrant and hardy.
'Marigold': bronze yellow; strong fragrance, prickly.

Other scented climbers
Jasmine is easily grown in fertile soils and prefers a sunny position. Its heady fragrance can fill an arbor.
Jasminum officinale: clusters of tiny white fragrant flowers in summer.
J. beesianum: small deep red flowers in late spring.
J. x stephanense: small fragrant pale pink clusters in summer.

Honeysuckle grows well in most soil and enjoys half shade.
Woodbine *Lonicera periclymenum* A traditional cottage garden climber, vigorous and the most fragrant form.
L. japonica repens: flowers, leaves and shoots are flushed purple.
Akebia (*Akebia quinata*): grows 27–36 feet high and is an unusual and hardy semievergreen climber with delicate whorls of leaves. It produces tiny, scented, purple-red flowers in spring and small edible fruits if the summer has been a hot one.
A. trifoliata: 27 feet high, a similar elegant climber with dark purple flowers and pale lilac fruit.

Hops are easy to grow in most soils.
Humulus lupulus: 9 to 18 feet, large, deeply lobed leaves.
H. lupulus 'Aureus' is a golden form with soft yellow leaves. It prefers sun.

Unscented climbers
Ivies *Hedera helix:* There are 29 cultivars with silver, gold, variegated, large, tiny or crinkled leaves.

Clematis The prolific small-flowered varieties are most sympathetic to the intimate scale of a herb garden:
Clematis macropetala 'Snowbird' has tiny flowers.
C. montana 'Elizabeth' is scented.

Grapevines Probably the most ancient climber to be planted in gardens, these are vigorous plants with large, handsome leaves. Vines are easy to grow, but require a long, hot summer and skilled attention for a good crop of fruit.
Vitis vinifera 'Apiifolia' has divided leaves.
V. vinifera 'Purpurea' has rich red leaves later turning to wine color. Stunning next to silver herbs.

Herb lawns

"But those which Perfume the Aire most delightfully, not passed by as the rest, but being Troden upon and Crushed, are Three: That is Burnet, Wilde-Time, and Water-Mints. Therefore, you are to set whole Allies of them, to have the Pleasure, when you walke to tread."

Francis Bacon
An Essay of Gardens (1625)

A fragrant lawn carpet can be laid with several different perennial herbs. It is best to begin with a small area as all herb lawns involve a lot of weeding, although generally they don't need mowing. Start by creating a welcoming mat as you enter the herb garden or a "hearth rug" in front of a garden seat, so swinging legs will gently brush the surface and release a herbal aroma.

Planting a herb lawn
To prepare the ground, weed thoroughly to remove every trace of perennial weeds, then rake the soil to a smooth surface. In a lightly shaded or cool patch, add rich compost to hold moisture, and plant either pungent peppermint-scented pennyroyal at 9 inch intervals or the tiny-leaved *Mentha requienii* with its crème-de-menthe scent at 4 inch intervals. The water mint suggested by Bacon requires moist soil and would probably leave numerous gaps, but it could be tried with pennyroyal or lawn grass.

If the area is in sun, incorporate a sandy compost and plant Roman or perennial chamomile with its apple-scented leaves at 4 inch intervals.

'Treneague' is a nonflowering clone, which is convenient, as it saves having to remove flower heads, but the ordinary Roman chamomile can be started from seed, which is much less expensive. Prepare the soil and then broadcast the seed. Cover with a thin layer of soil and keep moist (not wet). Once seedlings appear and have at least two sets of leaves, thin them out to about 3 inches apart. Don't walk on them until they're beginning to bind together. Remove most flowerheads as they appear, to ensure leaf vigor, but allow occasional flowers to remain, as they form part of the lawn's charm. Avoid having a chamomile lawn bordering on a grass or wild garden area as creeping weeds will soon invade the lawn, and uprooting them will also mean disturbing the shallow-rooted chamomile plants. A surround of stone, brick or paving slabs is ideal.

A popular alternative to a lawn is to plant creeping thymes at 9 inch intervals or sow them in groups following the same procedure as for chamomile. Select thymes according to their leaf color (gold, variegated, gray, light and dark green) or leaf scent (thyme, lemon, pine, caraway) and flower color (see p. 142). In midsummer, the flowers (white, pink, mauve or cochineal) provide the possibility of a kaleidoscope of color and scent. Wait until spring before removing flowering stems as they supply some protection to the herb during winter.

Corn mint (*Mentha arvensis*), the farmer's nightmare, tolerates dry conditions and could be tried on its own or grown with grass. Several mints will grow amid grass if it is not mown low too often, or you can incorporate them into little-used paths as an aromatic treat.

The only suggestion of Bacon's I haven't tried is the salad burnet. It is a robust plant with a cucumber scent and could form part of a lawn.

Although all these lawns will take some traffic, they are not suitable for continuous heavy footfalls. Where necessary, paving stones or slices of redwood or elm should be used as stepping stones. Certain areas, often the center, receive rougher treatment, while lush vigorous plants around the edges continue to flourish. If this is the case, you can always transplant rooted pieces from the outside to the center.

LAWN HERBS
Chamomile
Chamaemelum nobile 'Treneague': apple-scented, nonflowering variety. Tolerant of dry conditions.
Mints
Corsican mint (*Mentha requienii*): tiny leaves, strong scent. Likes moisture. Pennyroyal (*M. pulegium*): bright green, pungent peppermint scent. Corn mint (*M. arvensis*)
Thymes
All the creeping varieties (*Thymus serpyllum*, *T. praecox*, *T. pseudolanuginosus*) are suitable for cultivation in lawns. Prefer dry, sandy soil.

Paths

Access to plants is essential in a herb garden to enable you to pick leaves, flowers and seeds whenever you wish, and to ease the task of maintaining the garden. A path can be as narrow as 18 inches or as wide as 6 feet, depending on the size and style of the herb garden and surrounding area.

Grass
A grass path is the simplest form of path, especially if you are cutting your herb garden out of existing lawn. Any of the lawn herbs listed above can also be used. The path must be at least the width of your lawnmower or else have an edging of flat bricks to take the weight of any wheels. Laid end-on between the path and the herb bed, a row of bricks gives space for plants to tumble forward without restricting traffic. In the absence of a hard edge, make a sharp cut, 3 inches deep, down each edge of the path, to stop the grass

spreading into the soil and to create a clear edge for maintenance.

The main drawback of a grass or herb path is that it won't stand a lot of heavy traffic. One way round this is to insert round cuts of timber at intervals as stepping stones – aromatic woods such as cedar are ideal. Alternatively, use pavers or bricks as stepping stones.

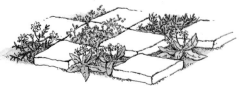

A checkerboard pattern of stone slabs interplanted with low-growing plants.

Gravel paths
Gravel or pea shingle is an attractive material for paths. Gravel differs in color depending on the stone from which it is broken. Use lighter shades

to brighten a dark area and darker shades to heighten distance or space. Gravel paths require regular rolling to maintain a level surface, and regular weeding. You may need to add a layer of gravel occasionally if the path has a lot of traffic. Planks of wood can also be embedded in gravel.

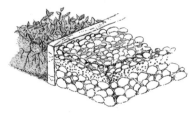

Making a gravel path
First lay a 4 inch layer of hardcore, then a thin layer of sand, and top with a 2 inch layer of gravel. For paths longer than 15 feet it is advisable to make a slope so puddles do not form during periods of heavy rain.

Stone and brick paths

Hard surfaces are preferable on well-used paths and for comfortable access in all weather conditions, ease of maintenance and durability.

Whatever material you choose, take care to select colors and textures which harmonize with the soft naturalness of herbs. Paving bricks and brick-sized concrete units are now produced in subtle colors. If selecting reconstructed stone or concrete blocks, look for irregular textures and changes in color. Any uniform coloring looks bland and lacks depth.

Old bricks are another classic paving material, suitable for almost every site. They are highly versatile for creating patterns. Running in the direction of the path, they make its extent seem longer; placed horizontally or in patterns, they make a path appear wider and shorter. Bricks can be set in many patterns: herringbone, fans, or mixed schemes of horizontally and vertically laid bricks as in the stretcher bond scheme shown below.

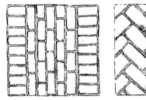

Stretcher bond   **Diagonal herringbone**

Particularly attractive is a narrow gauge $2\frac{7}{8}$ inch brick paver, which is especially suitable for the intimate scale of many herb gardens. The contemporary pavers require a hardcore of 4 inches and a 1 inch layer of mortar if the path will be in constant use. Otherwise, make the path wide enough to fit the brick layout plus edge retainers (see right). You should also aim to make a slight gradient to avoid puddles forming.

Making a brick path

Construct a traditional brick path to add character and permanence to a herb garden. Follow the steps below.

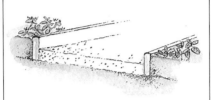

1 Dig out the whole area to a depth of 4 inches and insert metal or timber edging (see below right). Spread a 2 inch layer of sharp sand over the base and dampen slightly.

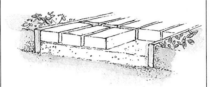

2 Lay the bricks on top, leaving $\frac{1}{8}$–$\frac{1}{4}$ inch gaps between, and bang them into place using a mallet and board, or a hired plate vibrator.

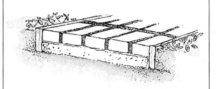

3 Spread the joints with a mix of fine, dry sand and cement (a mix of 1:4) and brush it in. The mixture will gradually absorb moisture from the atmosphere, so in time it will secure the bricks in place.

Concrete paths

Laying your own concrete path is a neglected opportunity for creative endeavor. You can make a highly individual path by adding mosaic-sized pieces of china or glass, seashells, iron-work, pebbles or bricks, or you can even use herb leaves to imprint their shapes on the concrete. Plan your ideas carefully on paper first. Follow these ground rules: to achieve unity there must be constants; either the same material used to create the patterns, or the same pattern repeated with different colors or different materials, or, most successful, the same pattern and material repeated with very slight variations. The Chinese use curved tiles laid edge to edge to create many shapes, and then infill the sections with oval colored pebbles.

Design the path in sections; a square at a time based on the path's width is easiest. Within each square assemble your chosen materials. Before laying, check that no sharp edges protrude and that colors harmonize. When positioning small pieces such as pebbles, make sure the space between them is less than the size of the pebble. If you are short of pebbles, don't spread them evenly; group them in tight patterns with larger spaces between the groups. Make sure all your materials are ready beforehand; once poured, concrete waits for no one.

Edge retainers

These help to hold bricks in place.

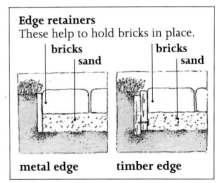

metal edge   **timber edge**

Raised beds

If your soil is poorly drained, and particularly if it's heavy clay, it would be advisable to grow your herbs in raised beds. In these beds the surface of the soil is higher than the surrounding area, thus improving drainage. Often depicted in medieval woodcuts, raised beds also help to define areas, stop trespassing feet and make weeding and harvesting easier. They are accessible for people in wheelchairs.

If drainage is not a problem, you can make a raised bed simply by piling soil higher than the surrounding area, flattening it and giving the area a slight slope on the edges. For more permanence, and better drainage, make a bed

Cross section of a raised bed

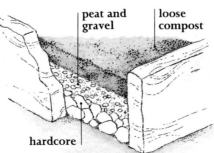

peat and gravel   loose compost

hardcore

with a layer of hardcore below, a layer of rough peat and gravel above that and a topping of loose compost, all contained by a timber or brick wall.

The best height for a raised bed is somewhere between 1 and 3 feet. Any higher and you will need solid foundations for the retaining wall so it can support the weight of the soil. Keep the width under 5 feet so you can weed and harvest the center.

For those in a wheelchair, a bed can be raised on concrete supports, like a large sink with drainage holes, and should be made at least 6 inches deep (deeper if there are strong winds). Most herbs can grow in such a bed, but the moisture-lovers, such as mint and sweet cicely, will need frequent watering. If possible, confine them to a bed near to the water supply.

Sloping banks

A good way to grow less hardy, sun-loving plants, especially if you live in a cool region, is to plant them on a sun-facing bank or slope. Not only does a bank increase the area of growing space available, but it can act as a windbreak or be created as part of a raised bed. It is also a useful device if you have surplus rubble to hide after building work. Arrange the rubble as a base for the bank, keeping the slope at a gradient less than 45°. Cover with topsoil and hold in place with netting pegged into the earth until the plants are established.

The top will drain very quickly — so plants in the upper sections should be drought-resistant — whereas the base will receive moisture. If you build a new bank, take particular care in the first two seasons to prevent erosion, either by covering the bank with netting or building a small retaining wall at the base. Thereafter the plant roots should bind the soil together; but on steeper slopes, it's best to have a low wall holding back the soil.

> "I know a bank whereon the wild
> thyme blows,
> Where oxlips and the nodding
> violet grows."

Shakespeare's choice of plants would make a colorful and sweet-smelling bank. The herbs listed on p. 257 for growing on a wall will enjoy the situation of a sunny bank. Marjorams, mugwort, alexanders, cowslips, calamint, Jacob's ladder, columbine and horehound are particularly suited.

Spreading herbs suitable for banks include dwarf comfrey, lady's bedstraw, bugles and lamiums, and in a shady area, sweet woodruff, periwinkle, bugles (the darker-leaved forms) and the wild or alpine strawberry.

For a damp bank such as the side of a ditch, the Tibetan cowslip (*Primula florindae*) is a spectacular addition, with its giant honey-scented flowers, which appear in midsummer.

Seats

Often considered as an afterthought, and sometimes not at all, a seat is most important in developing a relationship with herbs. For every gardener, there are always more jobs than hours in the day but with practice, the art of sitting and watching can be cultivated alongside the art of gardening.

Choose the site for your seat with care. Select a sheltered location, with the most attractive vista according to the time of day you are most likely to use the seat and whether you want to catch the sun early or late in the day.

Choosing a seat
The color and character of stone or reconstituted stone looks very attractive with the silver, gray and muted flower colors of many herbs; try, too, to choose a stone that is compatible with the style of your house. Stone seats are beautiful but rather uncomfortable for any length of time. Keep cushions handy for summer use.

Classic timber garden seats in hardwood are still firm favorites. Teak weathers to a silver gray and will last 70 years or a lifetime. There are also many interesting pieces of garden furniture available in wood made by a new generation of designers. Remember to renew preservative treatment on wood from time to time.

For further pleasure, plant sweet-smelling mints, lemon balm and pelargoniums around the seat, or site them in pots nearby.

ARBORS
A seat encourages one to take time to contemplate the delights of a herb garden, and the experience is bettered by a seat in a protective enclosure of aromatic plants called an arbor. You can buy metal or timber frames or construct a simple arch over a seat by fixing four stout timber poles into the ground and binding two flexible branches, such as green hazel, to form two arches. Add two crosspieces at shoulder height for extra rigidity.

Another simple but rectangular form can be made very easily using four 3 × 3 inch supporting corner posts and trellis sides, back and top. Choose the sturdiest trellis (usually with square rather than diagonal panels) and secure it to the posts. Although trellis is a lightweight material, I have found that the right angles of the structure provide sufficient rigidity. Climbing plants bind it together further, but you need substantial corner posts to prevent the whole structure leaning.

Check the sizes of materials available and plan the shape accordingly. For example, if panels are available 8 feet high in 3 foot and 4 foot widths, you could make each side of the arbor 3 × 8 feet, use two panels 4 × 8 feet for the back and a 3 × 8 foot piece for the top. You would have room for a 5–6 foot seat inside. An extra vertical support would be needed where the back panels join. A 6 foot height and width and 2 foot depth will just work, but more care is needed to stop plants infringing on the seat area. For an even less expensive enclosure, use plastic horticultural netting and train climbing plants over it.

Check the list of climbing plants on p. 259 and select a mixture to give

---

MAKING AN HERB BENCH

Attractive to look at and pleasant to sit on, an herb bench is a cross between a wall, a seat and a lawn. It's easy to make a comfortable solid bench as a brick box planted with scented thymes or chamomile.

Dig out the base to a depth of 14 inches. Put in a 4 inch layer of hardcore and then a 2 inch layer of sand. This leaves space for two layers of brick up to ground level. Five layers of brick above ground make a comfortable seat height with a further two layers as arm and back rests. Set the bricks with mortar, leaving some drainage holes, to ensure the seat is solid and safe. Instead of having a row of bricks along the top at the front, which would be uncomfortable to sit on, use an equal thickness of treated wood.

Fill with rubble to 6 inches below the seat and then infill with good compost. Plant perennial chamomile at 6 inch or thyme at 9 inch intervals. Alternatively, put 6 inch wide slats across the top at 3 inch intervals and plant herbs between them. To help maintain the herbs, add a thin layer of compost each spring to replace soil and to provide a surface for new runners.

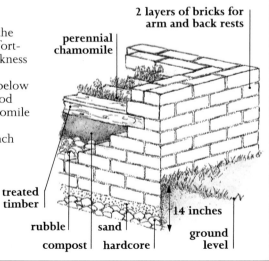

2 layers of bricks for arm and back rests

perennial chamomile

treated timber

rubble   sand

compost   hardcore

14 inches

ground level

fragrance over a long season and if possible, fruits to nibble. Choose one or two with evergreen leaves for the garden in winter and look for a contrast of leaf shapes and sizes so you can enjoy the special magic of looking up to see sparkling sunlight filtered through large and decorative leaves.

The frequent advice to plant climbers 6 feet apart is necessary only if you wish to have a 6 foot run of wall displaying a single plant. If you are happy for climbers to mingle, they can be planted as close together as

2–3 feet. Alternatively, a single vigorous climber such as honeysuckle can cover an entire arbor in just a few seasons.

Arbors can also be shaped out of hedges. In the 1st century A.D., Pliny the Elder commented on the Romans' invention of the *romora tonsilis*, the clipped arbor. In this practice, one enormous Mediterranean cypress was clipped into a protective shelter open at the front with a seat inside. The idea can be transferred successfully to a yew hedge in colder climates.

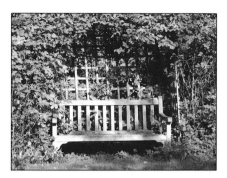

A fragrant arbor in the author's garden.

Focal points

Being a place of contemplation, an herb garden often incorporates a focal point. Traditionally, this is positioned as a centerpiece or set at the end of a path to draw people along its length. It may take the form of a piece of topiary such as a ball bay (see below). Or it may be associated with the wildlife which is drawn to herb gardens – a beehive, or a feeding table or water area for birds. A wide shallow bowl or a pond is appealing, as the water reflects the sky, and can be used to float flowers. An attractively planted urn or other large container also draws the eye. A sundial has long been a favorite centerpiece, often inscribed with philosophical meditations, such as Plato's advice that turning from the shadow to the sun is the mind's supreme activity. Statues of St Fiacre, the patron saint of gardeners, or Kwan Yin, the Chinese goddess of mercy, are both classical, tall, slender shapes with pleasing proportions. Representations of the mythical piper, Pan, are also enjoyable and light-hearted garden sculptures.

TOPIARY

Many of the evergreen herbs are suitable for this ancient form of sculpture. It is a way to bring order and architecture to a garden, an enjoyable contrast to the voluptuous disorder of many herbs. The Mediterranean cypress (*C. sempervirens*) has long been popular for making into shaped forms, as have the hardier yew and box. Bay, santolina, savory, sweet myrtle and upright germander can all be shaped, as can rosemary, which was much clipped as hedging in Shakespeare's time.

A good eye is needed for judging shapes, especially where curves are involved. Simple geometric shapes like the sphere and cone are most successful, although a little eccentricity can make a garden memorable.

For small-leaved plants like dwarf box, start clipping them once they have reached the desired height. To maintain a topiary shape or a formal

geometric hedge, two clippings a year are needed: one in late spring or early summer, after new shoots have formed, and a second in late summer, allowing time for subsequent new shoots to ripen before winter frosts. This keeps the plant clothed in fresh new shoots for most of the year.

TRAINED SHAPES

Medieval gardeners used several ingenious ways of training climbing plants into ornamental shapes, some based on designs originally developed to support grapevines. One form often seen in medieval illumination is that of a tiered structure with one central pole supporting three or four circular wire trays. Sometimes these "estrades" had climbing plants trained into the tiers (see right) and sometimes the trays were used to hold pots of plants hung with decorative colored balls.

You can make a simpler version of this idea with just one circular wire frame fixed atop a central pole. Train a quick-growing climber round this shape by allowing two of its stems to twist up the central pole, cutting back

any side shoots, and twisting its branches into the wire frame so that it eventually forms a disk of foliage.

A stunning focal point can be created within two years using a tripod or single vertical post as support for a vigorous climber such as scented honeysuckle, grapevine, golden hop, decorative ivies or *Akebia quinata*.

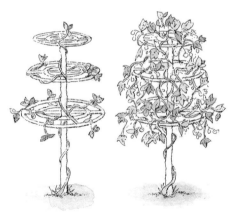

A three-tiered "estrade" with hops trained up it becomes an eye-catching shape in a few seasons.

MAKING A BAY TREE BALL

Plan the shape you want on paper, especially if the bay is to be container grown, so the proportions of sphere,

stem height and container are right. Generally, the taller the stem, the bigger the sphere should be.

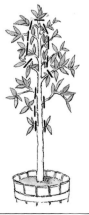

1 Grow the tree 6 inches higher than the desired finished height. Then clip back the tip, remove the side shoots below where you want the ball to begin and trim the side shoots in the sphere down to two or three leaves.

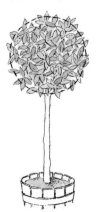

2 When the side shoots have formed four or five leaves, clip back again to two or three, and repeat with all shoots until you have a ball shape. Thereafter prune with shears in early and late summer to maintain its appearance.

Growing herbs in containers

Most herbs are willing to grow in pots, so town dwellers with a balcony, roof garden or outdoor window sill can enjoy them. Herbs in containers look pleasing in groups and benefit from the microclimate that grouping creates. The flexibility of containers means they can be repositioned to catch the sun, rearranged to make a focal point or used to fill seasonal gaps. The plants are easy to monitor.

Before planting out containers on a balcony or roof garden, check the strength of the structure, as the combination of soil and water can be very heavy. Wind factor and drainage must also be taken into consideration. Small containers can easily be blown away, and soft-leaved herbs soon spoil with strong winds.

Potting up

All containers need drainage holes and all, except for hanging baskets, need a layer of gravel, perlite or broken pottery in the bottom to prevent waterlogging (for choice of containers and different pot sizes see opposite). Fill containers with a good potting mixture. This can be either peat based or soil based. Peat-based mixtures tend to be very light when allowed to dry out. (If this happens, submerge the pot in water to just below rim level and soak for several hours.) A soil-based mixture is more suitable for large plants.

A traditional potting compound can be made using seven parts loam, three parts peat and two parts grit or sharp sand, with some well-rotted compost or comfrey leaves (mixed with the peat the previous season so they have had time to decompose and have their nutrients absorbed). Sun-loving Mediterranean herbs benefit from a larger proportion of grit or horticultural sand in the mixture, say six parts loam and three parts sand. Do not use builder's sand, as it has a rounded surface and makes drainage worse.

Most gardening books recommend the use of sterilized loam in potting mixtures. However, the sterilizing process is time-consuming. I use organically enriched garden loam unsterilized in my potting compound, and although it gives me weed seedlings to contend with, in 10 years I have never experienced any soil-borne diseases. This may be because I keep any mixture loose and open, not stored in plastic, which would assist fungal spores to develop, and because herbs contribute to a healthy soil (see p. 267).

To provide the alkalinity herbs prefer, mix agricultural lime with the potting compost each year – a teaspoon of lime is enough for a $4\frac{1}{2}$ inch pot. A layer of charcoal granules near the bottom of the soil — about a tablespoon to a $4\frac{1}{2}$ inch pot — helps to keep the soil sweet by absorbing any waste products.

General care

Pots can be moved outdoors or plunged into soil in spring or early summer. Introduce plants to sunlight gradually. Clip or pick leaves often to encourage bushy new growth. In cold climates bring plants indoors, as described on p. 255, as soon as there is any danger of frost. For information on watering and feeding, see p. 266–7.

Repotting

When the roots of a herb are protruding through the base of a pot, it is time to repot it into a bigger pot. Usually the next size up is appropriate. Use the same soil mix.

The best time for repotting is in the spring. Avoid transferring at the end of the growing season, or when the plant is dormant, as no new roots will grow to anchor the plant into the new soil.

Carefully remove the plant from the original pot; then clear any weeds or moss from the soil's surface and line the new pot with drainage material and

a large spoonful of granulated charcoal. Add a little of the soil and check to see the plant will sit at the same level. Then loosen the roots, put in the herb, fill with soil, firm gently and water well.

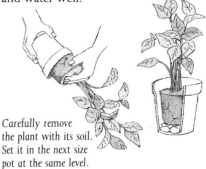

Carefully remove the plant with its soil. Set it in the next size pot at the same level.

Eventually, when the maximum pot size has been reached, remove the top layer of soil each spring and replace with a fresh mixture spiced with a slow-release fertilizer (see p. 267).

Newly potted herbs will not require fertilizing for at least a month or six weeks because of the nutrients already present in the fresh soil.

Perennial herbs should be repotted in stages until they are in $4\frac{1}{2}$–6 inch pots for good bushy specimens of smaller varieties and 8–10 inch pots for larger herbs. In general, the larger the pot, the better the crop. All the smaller herbs can be grown in pots (see p. 252 for instructions on growing seed indoors), but annuals grown for their seed may bolt because of the confined root space.

Taprooted herbs such as borage, parsley and dill do better in deep pots. For lovage and fennel, it is best to put three seedlings in a 6 inch pot and to use the leaves when the plants are young. After one restricted season they often make a desperate attempt to set seed and neglect to produce further succulent leaves. Alternatively, put three seedlings into a 12 inch pot for two years of growth.

CHOOSING CONTAINERS

Containers come in all shapes and sizes and in a wide range of materials. For individual herbs, pots are probably the most practical and useful. Plastic pots are reasonably priced, easy to clean and store, and lightweight. This last property makes it possible to judge the moisture content of the soil just by lifting the pot. If your plans include pots spending any time outdoors, ensure that the plastic will not crack in cold spells.

Clay pots

Unglazed clay pots have greater aesthetic appeal and allow excess water to evaporate through their fabric. Check the moisture content of the soil by sharply rapping the pot with your knuckles: a dull thud means the soil is too wet, a hollow ring means it is too dry. Soil in clay pots dries out more quickly than in plastic pots, so you will have to water more often. New clay pots should be soaked in water for 24 hours before use.

Understanding pot sizes

Traditional round pots are listed by a number, which is their diameter and roughly their height. So the 3 inch pot in which many herbs are sold is 3 inches across the rim and $3\frac{1}{2}$ inches from the top of the rim to

the base. Vigorous herbs quickly outgrow this size, so check when you buy a herb in such a pot, as it may already need repotting. If roots appear through the bottom, or the herb seems overcrowded, move it to the next size up. Suprisingly, a 4 inch pot holds double the soil volume of a 3 inch pot, and a $4\frac{1}{2}$ inch pot holds three times the amount of soil of a 3 inch pot.

New square pots are stamped as 6 k, 8 k, 10 k, etc. and although this is said to refer to the volume of the pot, the number is the same as the width across the top in centimetres.

PLANTING UP A LARGE CONTAINER

Always set a large container in position before filling it with soil and planting. Once filled, you will not be able to move it. Alternatively, keep it on a base with castors, so you can reposition it with ease. Fill some of the centre depth with lightweight rubble or perlite to save compost and weight, and fill with a soil-based potting mixture to within 1 in (2.5 cm) of the rim. Plant up with herbs which enjoy the same growing conditions, say parsley, chives and buckler leaf sorrel for a culinary collection set near the kitchen door.

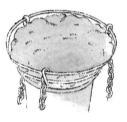

Insert long, open-ended tubes to help water reach the lower depths of tall containers.

Contained planting schemes

Grow more of the plants you use most often. Use a 12 in (30 cm) pot for sun-loving seedlings of sweet basil, lemon basil and sweet marjoram. Chervil, coriander and parsley could share a pot as they all prefer a bright position without constant direct sun, and like the environment to be a little cooler and wetter than the first group.

Several varieties of mint can be grown in one pot as they enjoy moderately wet soil and all tend to spread their roots. Angelica does not take kindly to being in a small pot, but planted in a cool location in a large container, a splendid tropical-looking specimen can be grown. Angelica and mint make excellent bed-fellows. When the angelica has reached the conclusion of its three-year life cycle, it would also be time to replant the mint.

Bay, rosemary, santolina, sweet myrtle, box, lemon verbena, sage and lavender make fine single specimens in $9\frac{1}{2}$–12 in (24–30 cm) pots, and the first five also lend themselves to topiary. These herbs might benefit from a carpet of aromatic herbs to keep the soil shaded and restrict evaporation – scented thymes in sunny spots; perennial apple-scented chamomile in dappled light or the tiny peppermint, *Mentha requienii*, in a cool location.

Unusual containers

An old rectangular sink at least 5 in (13 cm) deep and set on bricks to allow for drainage makes a convenient and attractive miniature herb bed. Large strawberry pots, troughs and wooden boxes and half barrels also make good containers.

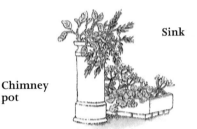

Chimney pot   **Sink**

HANGING BASKETS

A hanging basket is an ideal way to bring height into a patio or balcony, though it also demands some careful attention: herbs are vigorous plants to grow in a confined space. If they are too cramped or watered irregularly, they will soon drop their lower leaves and give a sad, spiky appearance.

Hang the basket on a well-secured, strong bracket. Ensure that it is set clear of the wall and that there is no danger of it falling. A planted-up basket can be heavy. Take care not to position hanging baskets between tall buildings where powerful wind tunnels often exist, causing damage to delicate herbs.

Baskets may need watering two or three times a day in high summer so you need to consider ways of watering conveniently. Small long-necked watering cans are ideal, or use a hose pipe to avoid lifting a heavy can.

HERBS FOR A HANGING BASKET

Select plants sympathetic to the shape of the container: plants whose leaves appear to grow in layers or horizontal mounds, or herbs with graceful arching or trailing branches. Avoid upright plants unless they are surrounded by others to soften the outline. The following are all attractive.

In a sunny location: different creeping thymes such as lemon-scented, caraway-scented thyme, pine-scented creeping thyme.
catmint (*Nepeta mussinii*)
ivies
prostrate winter savory
prostrate rosemary
prostrate sage
lady's mantle

For the shady side of a hanging basket: pennyroyal, variegated mints with ginger mint, periwinkle.

With so many trailing and horizontal herbs to choose from, it's easy to tuck in a parsley out of direct sunlight, or a clump of chives to provide a complete mini herb garden in a basket.

MAKING A HANGING BASKET

Follow the procedure below to plant up a hanging basket. Make a rough plan of the arrangement you want and check that you have enough room for all the plants.

3 *Place trailing herbs around the outer rim and plant two or three in the outside of the basket through the moss and the holes in the plastic lining. Put taller herbs in the centre.*

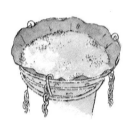

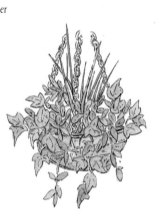

1 *To plant up a hanging basket, balance it on a bucket. If it is a wire basket, line with sphagnum moss, then black plastic punctured with drainage holes.*

2 *Half fill with a moisture-retentive compost. Loosen the soil of any pot-grown plants you wish to add and blend it into the new compost mixture.*

4 *Top up with compost and water well. Drain before hanging in position.*

WINDOW BOXES

Given a sunny aspect and proper attention to watering and pruning, a useful selection of herbs can be grown in a window box. Particularly appropriate for such a location are many of the culinary and aromatic herbs, arranged for convenience and so that their fragrance will waft indoors.

Before you plant a window box, check local bylaws and tenancy contracts, in case window boxes are prohibited, and make sure the window sill is sound and strong enough to take the weight. Whatever fixing you use, it must remain secure, as a falling window box could prove fatal to a pedestrian below. For extra security and peace of mind, attach the box to the wall with a chain or strap. When positioning the window box, consider where water will drain: use a removable drip tray if possible.

Choosing a window box

Plastic troughs are light and easy to maintain but wood is visually more pleasing. For timber, choose treated hardwood such as oak or elm, or marine plywood. Raise the base slightly on wedges to allow the bottom to dry out occasionally and give space for a drip tray. Clay window boxes are available at many garden centers and complement the foliage of many herbs. They are often supplied with raised supports. However, they may crack or flake in a cold winter.

FILLING A WINDOW BOX

Position the box and cover the first 1 inch with broken pottery or some other drainage material. Some growers recommend adding a sheet of heavy plastic punctured with drainage slits to help retain moisture and stop the soil being washed away. In a wooden box, if the plastic comes up the sides as well, it will extend the life of the timber.

In colder climates where the herbs are to be left outside during frosts, a layer of polystyrene will give the roots some protection from rapid freezing and thawing. Another solution is to keep perennial herbs in individual clay pots, which allow moisture to permeate through, and then plant these in a trough of moist peat compost, for extra insulation. Plant any annuals in the peat.

When filling a plastic box, add a thin layer of charcoal granules to keep the soil sweet. Then add a soil- or peat-based compost.

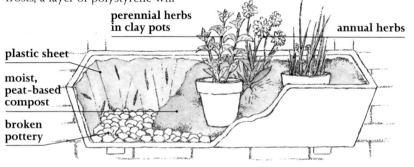

perennial herbs in clay pots

annual herbs

plastic sheet

moist, peat-based compost

broken pottery

HERBS FOR A WINDOW BOX

With a small space you will want to make every herb count. For culinary usefulness, grow parsley, chives, a small rosemary and a golden creeping lemon thyme, and basil if the position is sheltered. A calendula adds cheerful color and flower petals for salads and rice dishes. A nasturtium provides trailing leaves and colorful flowers which you can add to salads. If your position is hot and dry, try the saffron crocus (Crocus sativus) for its valuable crop.

Growing herbs indoors

Sun-loving herbs need at least six hours of sun a day to thrive, which is why many do not do well indoors. With inadequate light, plants become thin and elongated, producing smaller leaves and a poorer aroma. When selecting a location for herbs indoors, keep in mind that the reflective properties of glass can reduce light by 30 to 50 percent. Consider also the outside environment; a large white wall or glass surface facing a window can act as a mirror reflecting back much of the light; conversely an apparently sunny window can have its light reduced because of deep eaves or a wall. An interior white wall and glossy surfaces also make more light available. Turn herbs a little each day so all parts receive the same amount of sun, or consider artificial lighting as a supplementary source.

Basil requires the sunniest position and tolerates dry air. Thyme, sage, marjoram, pelargoniums and dwarf lavender also enjoy direct sun. Dill, savory and chives like full sun but a cooler temperature. Rosemary likes a bright situation (this can be reflected light) but prefers a cooler atmosphere of about 60 °F to produce its flowers. Coriander, salad burnet and parsley also prefer this combination.

Tarragon and lemon balm take full sun but tolerate light shade. Mint and chervil enjoy some sun but not the hot midday sun, and both like a moist, cool soil. Lemon verbena and bay prefer filtered sun with rich soil in a cool spot.

TEMPERATURE

Most herbs prefer a pleasantly warm temperature of between 60–70 °F with a 10 °F drop at night. Herbs will tolerate from 45–75 °F but do not thrive at the lower temperatures.

Draughts affect growth and survival. A door opened in cold weather causes a sharp drop in temperature, an open fire draws in a large amount of the air from any cracks or openings, creating draughts in a straight line to the fire, and single-glazed windows allow enormous temperature drops in the sill area during the night. Every sharp temperature drop is a stressful shock to a herb and weakens its constitution, so attempt to position herbs where there will be a minimum of shocks.

Although herbs do not like draughts, they do like some fresh air each day. This removes stale air, hinders airborne diseases and helps to disperse possible oil or gas fumes from heating systems.

WATERING

Potted herbs indoors and out are more vulnerable than plants in the open ground and more dependent on your care. Pots outside dry out very quickly, not just from the top but from every direction. During hot weather check the soil each day. In autumn water only when the soil is dry, particularly the aromatic herbs such as thyme and rosemary. Seedlings usually need daily watering. Herbs with large, soft leaves, in hot sun, in active growth or in small pots also need frequent watering.

Plants prefer a substantial watering when dry to a little water more frequently, as sometimes the bottom area of soil does not receive moisture. It is best to use tepid water and apply it in the morning, so excess moisture evaporates during the day. If uncertain about the need to water, wait another day, then water. For accurate guidance with indoor plants, small stick gauges are available which change color as the moisture level changes. Simply push them into the soil.

Do not overwater. Air is an important requirement for root hairs, and if vital air pockets in the soil are eliminated by waterlogging, a perfect environment is created for root-rot fungus to thrive.

If a pot with a peat-based mixture has dried out and become very light, this will create a gap between the pot and soil. Plunge the pot in water for 15 minutes or more to just below the rim of the pot. This allows the water to permeate the peat. If poured in, it will run down between the pot and the soil. Peat particles have a natural waterproof coating which helps retain moisture when it is wet but actually prevents water being absorbed if it has dried out. Many modern mixtures have a wetting agent added to counteract this.

Moisture in the atmosphere is also important to most herbs. Grouping plants together helps create a humid environment, as does a layer of sphagnum moss on the soil's surface; you can also place the pots on trays of moist pebbles, vermiculite or perlite. A quick spray of tepid water with a mist atomizer all around the plants is useful in hot weather, especially for herbs with soft leaves such as basil.

Ensure that all containers are adequately drained. Indoors they require a drip tray or outer container where excess water can collect. A large tray containing clean gravel is best as this holds the herbs above excess water, and can double as a humidifier.

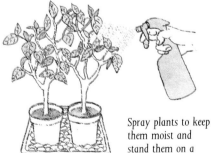

Spray plants to keep them moist and stand them on a gravel tray to drain.

FEEDING
Herbs that are regularly harvested need feeding with a weak liquid fertilizer every two weeks in spring and summer, reduced to a monthly feed as the growth rate slows. Do not feed plants during the winter, and never use more fertilizer than the manufacturer's instructions recommend.

Leaf blemishes
Pale yellow leaves or yellow spotting, as frequently seen on the outside leaves of parsley, fennel and overcrowded seedlings, are an indication that

fertilizer is needed. Other signs are lower leaves dropping early and weak growth with susceptibility to disease.

Signs of over-fertilization are brown patches or scorched edges to leaves and possibly malformed leaves. A blanket of green moss, liverworts or slime means an excess of nitrogen. This usually occurs in winter when plants are dormant, and it is less likely to develop in dry interiors.

Types of fertilizer
Liquid fertilizers, properly dissolved in water, are reliable and can be applied from above or below. Slow-release fertilizer tablets and sticks are available to push into the soil, but they can create spots of concentrated fertilizer. For indoor use, there are also mats impregnated with nutrients, which feed the plant through base watering.

If you buy larger evergreen herbs in pots, you may notice little white globules, smaller than peas, mixed with the soil. These are slow-release fertilizer pellets, which provide feed for a whole growing season.

Herbal fertilizers
You can grow and make your own herbal fertilizers from a surprising number of herbs. One comfrey plant in a small barrel or a 12 in (30 cm) pot will provide four crops a year. Comfrey fertilizer (see recipe on p. 131) supplies the three primary fertilizing ingredients: nitrogen, phosphorus and abundant potash, as well as several trace elements and minerals.

To make up a standard fertilizer, follow this basic recipe: pour 4 cups of boiling water over a good handful of fresh herb or 2 tablespoons dried herb, cover and allow to infuse for at least 10 minutes. Strain the infusion through cheesecloth before using.
Select from the following:
Coltsfoot (*Tussilago farfara*) for sulfur and potassium.
Couch grass (*Agropyron repens*), although a weed, is rich in minerals, potassium and silica.
Dandelion (*Taraxacum officinale*) supplies copper.
Dill (*Anethum graveolens*) is rich in minerals, potassium, sulfur and sodium.
Fat hen (*Chenopodium album*) contains iron and other minerals.
Fenugreek (*Trigonella foenum-graecum*) The sprouted seed heads are rich in nitrates and calcium.
Horsetail (*Equisetum hyemale*) is high in silica.
Nettle (*Urtica dioica*) is a treasure house of iron, nitrogen and several minerals and trace elements. Make a fermented brew following the comfrey recipe on p. 131, steeping the nettles for 3 weeks.
Sunflower (*Helianthus annuus*) The ash of sunflower stalks is high in potash.

Tansy (*Tanacetum vulgare*) is rich in potassium and other minerals.
Tea leaves contain nitrogen, phosphoric acid, manganese and potash. These are locked in the tannin but released by brewing.
Yarrow (*Achillea millefolium*) provides copper and is a good general fertilizer.

ARTIFICIAL LIGHTING
Special fluorescent lights are available that supply the radiation required by plants for photosynthesis. These will improve the growth of herbs indoors, particularly where there is little natural light. Alternatively, you can combine two domestic fluorescent lights, one "cool white" and one "warm white," for a similar effect.

Use available daylight first and top up with fluorescent lights in the evening to achieve the optimum 15 hours a day for good seed germination and maximum plant growth. These lights should be sited 6–9 inches above small herbs and 12–16 inches above larger herbs. If the lights are too close to the herbs, the leaves will become scorched; if too far away, the plants will grow tall and spindly.

CARE AND CLEANING
If your water has a high lime content, which manifests itself as a white deposit on the soil's surface, scrape it off periodically and top up with fresh compost. To remove lime from the surface of bay leaves, wipe gently with a clean damp cloth. You could use a water-filter jug for lime-free water.

A mist spray of water on the leaves of all indoor herbs helps to keep any dust from clogging their pores. An occasional wipe is necessary if you have any larger-leaved plants in the kitchen, where a fine film of grease builds up and acts as a magnet for dust. As a rule, the kitchen is not a good place to grow herbs because of the temperature variations and cooking fumes. Use a pipe cleaner or brush to dust woolly-leaved herbs, as shown below.

Remove any dead or damaged leaves and faded flowers rather than have them rot on the parent plant.

Use a small, soft paintbrush to clean woolly-leaved plants such as clary sage.

Keeping herbs healthy

Routine plant care, common sense and observation are the main requirements for maintaining healthy plants. Herbs are mainly disease-free, but over-crowding in pots or too much water can weaken plants and make them more vulnerable, so look first for physical conditions that may require attention.

PESTS: PREVENTION AND CURE

Whenever you buy or are given a new plant, check to make sure it has no small creatures lurking under leaves or in the leaf axils. A good prevention is to plunge each plant into a bucket of mild dishwashing-detergent solution. Hold your hand over the soil area, or cover with plastic or card, invert the plant and swish it around gently as shown below.

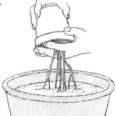

Dip new plants in a mild solution of dishwashing liquid to remove insects.

Organic insecticides

If you do have problems with insects, try to combat them with an organic or herbal insecticide. Unlike ordinary garden chemicals, these are non-persistent, generally remaining active for no more than a day. Rotenone is a vegetable insecticide taken from the roots of *Derris elliptica*, a tropical legume. It is available ready to mix from organic suppliers and comes with full instructions. Use against biting and sucking insects: red spider mites, wasps, cabbage caterpillars, raspberry and flea beetles, sawfly larvae and aphids. It is not selective and is harmful to cold-blooded creatures like toads, tortoises and fish, so keep it away from ponds. It breaks down quickly once exposed to air and sunlight and is harmless to humans, dogs, cats and birds. Spray on a windless day, and preferably in the late evening, to avoid harming helpful insects such as bees and butterflies.

Several herbs have insecticide properties and can be sprayed on troubled leaves. Use the formula for chamomile in the box below, unless indicated otherwise, adding a teaspoon of dishwashing detergent or soft soapflakes to help the mixture stick to the leaves.

Elder leaves for aphids: take 8 ounces of leaves, simmer in 4 cups of water for 30 minutes, stir well, strain and cool. Separately, dissolve a teaspoon of soapflakes or dishwashing detergent in $2\frac{1}{2}$ cups of cold water. Mix with the elder water.

Rhubarb leaves for aphids. Follow the above recipe, using roughly cut rhubarb leaves.

Basil leaves for aphids.

Garlic cloves for aphids: use two crushed cloves of garlic for each $2\frac{1}{2}$ cups of water.

Costmary leaves as a general insecticide.

Great fleabane (*Inula conyza*) **leaves and roots** make a strong insecticide.

Wormwood leaves protect against larger pests such as caterpillars, moths and flea beetles, as well as aphids. Make this decoction at half strength and use only on mature plants because of its toxic properties.

Pyrethrum, dried and powdered flowerheads This well-known natural insecticide has a rapid paralyzing effect on insects. It decomposes rapidly, especially in bright sunlight. It is sometimes found in commercial products mixed with other insecticides, or you can make up your own insecticide following the recipe on p. 67. Use against all common sucking insect pests; it is also effective against bed-bugs, mosquitoes, cockroaches and the domestic fly. Wear gloves when processing the flowerheads, as prolonged contact can cause allergic conditions in some people.

For scale insects on sweet bay or citrus plants, scrub the leaves with a strong dishwashing-detergent solution and a soft nail brush, or wipe with denatured alcohol, dislodging persistent scales with your fingernail.

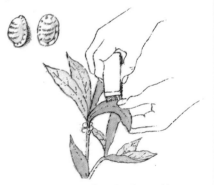

Remove scale insects from bay by scrubbing the leaves with a strong detergent solution, as described above.

DISEASES: PREVENTION AND CURE

Avoid using harmful chemicals on edible herbs. To help fight ailments, spray plants with one of these brews.

Chamomile flowers help prevent damping-off mold in seedlings. Pour 4 cups of boiling water over a handful of fresh or 2 tablespoons of dried herbs. Cover with a lid and steep for 10 minutes, then strain, cool and use at once.

Couch grass rhizome tea sprayed on leaves helps to prevent mildew and fungus diseases. Prepare and use as for chamomile flowers.

Horsetail (*Equisetum hyemale*) is useful against mildew, rust and other fungus diseases. Use only half a handful of fresh horsetail or half a tablespoon of dried to 4 cups of water. Boil for 20 minutes, covered, and stand for 24 hours before straining and using.

COMPANION PLANTING

Many gardeners have observed how certain herbs benefit the growth of nearby plants: garlic and chives under roses deter greenfly, nasturtium repels woolly aphids from apple trees and a nearby chamomile can act as a tonic to an ailing plant.

Science is beginning to discover how some plants communicate and assist others through their root secretions. Some tagetes secrete chemicals that kill ground elder and bindweed, reduce couch grass and stop eelworm from recognizing their host plant. Many aromatic leaves such as wormwood, hyssop and savory repel or mislead insects pests. Others, such as tagetes, calendula, nasturtiums, poppies and fat hen attract hoverflies, whose larvae feed on aphids. Refer to entries in the Herbal Index for further information.

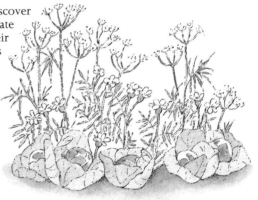

Plant dill and tagetes among cabbages to divert pests.

Harvesting herbs

Fresh leaves can be picked for immediate use at any time during the growing season (see below). Evergreen herbs such as thyme can be picked throughout the year, although new growth should be given the chance to harden before winter sets in. For all herbs there is an optimum time when their leaves, flowers, seeds or roots should be harvested for storage, as described below. See the Herbal Index for details on individual plants.

Place cut plants, leaves and flowers gently in a flat-bottomed basket, trug or wooden box. Do not put them in a sack or bag or they'll be crushed and bruised and start to sweat. In this condition, they are not worth preserving.

If collecting from the wild, be certain of identification: it is easy to confuse plants, and some are highly poisonous. Also check the legality, as most countries have some protected species, and do not collect too much from any one plant. Do not pick any parts that grow where car fumes or chemical sprays may have affected the plant. Ensure that herbs in your own garden have not been sprayed with chemical pesticides or herbicides.

Ideally, harvest only one species at a time. Sort and clean these before gathering parts from other plants.

Leaves

Collect in the morning, after the dew has evaporated. As the day warms up and photosynthesis gets under way, various organic components start moving around the plant system. Essential oils are concentrated in the leaves, ready to give off their protective cooling and antiseptic essence in the midday heat. To obtain the maximum potency and flavor, the leaves must be picked after some warmth has drawn up the oils but before any has escaped in the heat.

Leaves are most tender and sweet when the plant is young, up to flowering time. From this point the plant's priorities change and its energy goes into reproduction.

Pick the succulent leaves of sorrel, bistort, good King Henry, angelica, and all the salad herbs when young. This type of leaf is not generally suited to drying and should either be frozen in a cooked dish or preserved in oil or vinegar (see p. 188).

Treat all leaves gently, taking care not to bruise or crush them. Pick only healthy whole leaves without blemish, yellowing or insect damage.

Leaves of aromatic evergreens (rosemary, sage, thyme, savory) can be picked throughout the year, but for maximum flavor collect them just before flowering. Leaves of basil, mint, marjorams and lovage hold their pungent flavors well throughout the summer but they will be sweeter if picked before flowering. Later in the season, if mints have depleted the soil of plant food, the leaves begin to acquire a hint of turpentine.

With tall plants like marsh mallow, collect only the top growth.

Use pruning shears to collect whole stems of mints and small-leaved herbs such as thyme and marjoram, as this makes drying a more convenient process.

Whole plant

The best time to harvest a whole plant is just before the flowers open. If you want the green parts only, cut back annuals 3 inches above the ground but take no more than a third from perennials.

Flowers

Flowers are best collected at midday in dry weather. Pick them just as they open fully, their moment of greatest beauty. Snip lavender flower stalks whole and pick other flowers by hand, if possible without touching the petals. Treat all flowers with great care. Avoid damaged or wilted flowers, particularly if you wish to crystallize them. Once picked, keep flowers loose in open containers, as they bruise easily and soon begin to sweat.

Seeds and fruit

Pick seed on a warm dry day when it is fully ripe but before it has been dispersed. It should be buff, brown or black, with no green remaining, and it should be hard, with paper-dry pods. Shake small seed into a paper bag or cut the flower head on its stalk and hang it over a tray to catch the seed. Keep all seeds separate; label and date.

Remember to collect the seed of annuals and any others required for propagation, as well as culinary seeds such as fennel, dill, coriander, lovage and caraway.

Pick fruit when ripe but before it becomes soft. Berries and hops can be collected on their stalks and forked off when they are half dried.

Roots and rhizomes

Harvest roots in the fall when plant parts above ground are beginning to wither and die. This is also the time when the greatest concentration of therapeutic compounds is stored in the roots. Dig up annuals when their growing cycle has been completed at the end of the year. Gather perennial roots in their second or third year of growth, when the active components should have developed. Ginseng is believed to require seven years for maturity, though researchers are trying to find cultivars that develop faster.

Carefully dig up the whole root, taking care not to bruise or cut the sections. Separate the amount required and replant the remainder.

Most roots such as horseradish and comfrey can be scrubbed clean and have their fibrous hairs removed, but others, such as valerian, should not be scrubbed, as their precious constituents are contained in the epidermal (surface) cells.

In Britain it is illegal to dig up roots from any land other than one's own without the owner's permission.

Bark

Bark peels off readily in damp weather and should be collected from young branches or trunks, preferably on trees already cut down. Trees can be killed if too much bark is taken, especially in a circle around the trunk.

Preserving and storing herbs

Most herbs wilt soon after cutting. Putting them in a jar of water out of the sun helps for an hour or so, but to keep picked herbs such as parsley fresh for a few days, or to revive wilted cut herbs, place them in a plastic bag filled with air and tightly secured. Store in the refrigerator and they should remain in good condition for several days.

Many herbs keep their flavor well when dried, and some even seem to improve with drying. However, suc- cessful preserving requires care and specific conditions. For information, refer to entries in the Herbal Index.

DRYING HERBS

As soon as a leaf or flower is separated from the plant, metabolic changes begin. Individual cells start to die as their supply of moisture and nutrients ceases. Enzymes which previously helped to create active constituents now begin to break down these substances. With this decomposition, the medicinal values and flavor are reduced on a sliding scale. The sooner drying begins, and the quicker the system, the better the quality and color of the dried herb will be. The speed is limited, however, as moisture must be removed gradually from a plant. Drying leaves in the oven is not satisfactory, as the water evaporates too quickly and essential oils are lost. Microwave ovens speed up the process considerably without affecting the flavor of herbs, but they may destroy some of the therapeutic properties in the process.

Keep herbs quite separate when drying to avoid any confusion or tainting, especially if they are to be used medicinally. Do not introduce fresh plant parts into an area where drying is in process.

Drying leaves

Wipe off any soil or grit and avoid washing leaves unless absolutely necessary. Keep the leaves out of sunlight, as this extracts and evaporates essential oils.

Choose a warm, dry, dark situation with adequate ventilation – a linen closet, warm loft or garden shed for example. A drying temperature of 90 °F is ideal for the first 24 hours, with a reduced temperature of 75–80 °F thereafter. Leaves that are not unduly thick will take about four days at these temperatures. Allow one to two weeks in cooler temperatures.

Hang stems of leaves such as sage, rosemary, savory and thyme in small bunches, tied with string. Do not pack stems too tightly together, as air needs to circulate through and around the bunch. About 10 stems at a time should be the maximum. Hang bunches stem upward. If you're hanging them anywhere dusty, place loose paper bags over them with the bottom end open.

When drying small quantities, spread the leaves thinly on muslin, cheesecloth or brown paper punctured with fine holes. Stretch the material over a frame or wire cooling rack so air can circulate freely.

When drying is completed, the leaves should be paper-dry and fragile, but not so dry that they powder on contact. Avoid drying strongly flavored herbs such as lovage close to others, as their flavor may spread.

Storing dried leaves

Once dried, remove leaves from stems. Keep them whole so they retain their scent and goodness for as long as possible; break them up only if you have to fit them into jars. Crush them just before using.

Leaves should be stored in airtight dark glass bottles away from sunlight, moisture and dust. Plastic and metal containers are not suitable, as they may affect the chemistry of a herb.

Label bottles with the name and the date. If you notice any condensation on the glass, the leaves were not dried enough before storage. Remove them immediately and dry them further.

Some herbs are hygroscopic when dried – they absorb moisture from the air. This can reactivate their enzymes enough to cause chemical deterioration, so they should not be stored for too

long. Marsh mallow and lady's mantle leaves behave this way.

Check dried leaves periodically for moisture, molds and insects and discard them promptly if you discover anything. Most herbs deteriorate after a year, by which time you can replace them with a new harvest. Put excess sweet-smelling dried leaves into potpourri, herb bags or on an open fire. Use the pungent herbs to sprinkle over seed trays to discourage mice, or put them on the compost heap.

Drying flowers

Dry flowers in the same way as leaves. When dried correctly they should retain their color. Delicate flowers such as borage and sweet violets must be spread out carefully so they maintain their shape. Allow one to three weeks drying time, depending on the thickness of the petals. Store flat if possible. For calendula, remove the dried petals to store. Keep chamomile, lavender and smaller-headed flowers intact.

Drying seed and fruit

After removing the seed heads of annual and culinary herbs such as fennel and dill, hang them to dry over a box or sheet of paper, or with a paper bag or piece of fine muslin tied lightly over the head to collect seeds as they fall. Dry sunflower heads whole and separate the seeds for storage when they become loose.

Seeds dry very quickly in an airy, dry, warm environment, usually within two weeks, and should be labeled and stored in dark, airtight jars. Seed required for sowing should be kept in a cool, dark place, free of frost.

Berries and fruits such as rosehips take longer to dry and can be placed in a drying cupboard to speed up the process. Fleshy fruits need frequent turning until they are dry.

Drying roots

All roots should be clean, with fibrous parts removed before drying. Cut large thick roots in half lengthways and then into small pieces to facilitate drying. Roots require higher temperatures – 120 °F, even up to 140 °F. You can dry them in the oven, turning them regularly, until they are fragile and break easily. Peel the roots of marsh mallow and the rhizomes of licorice before drying.

Once dried, store roots in dark, airtight containers. Roots of parsley and angelica reabsorb moisture from the air. Discard if they become soft.

Drying bark

Bark may need washing to remove insects and moss; then dry it out in a dry, warm, airy, dark place as flat as possible. Store in airtight jars.

FREEZING HERBS

Freezing retains color and flavor, as well as most of the nutritive value of fresh young leaves. This is now the most popular way to preserve culinary herbs because it is convenient and fast (though it is reported that it is not suitable for those herbs required for therapeutic use). It is also a far more satisfactory method of preserving the more delicate culinary herb leaves such as fennel, salad burnet, chervil, parsley, basil, tarragon, sweet cicely and chives.

Some people recommend blanching first, which may be necessary for long-term storage and for large leaves. Rinse when necessary and shake dry beforehand.

The easiest way to freeze herbs is simply to pack them into plastic bags and label, either singly or in mixtures such as bouquet garni. Store small packets in larger, rigid containers in the freezer, to avoid the possibility of their being lost or damaged. Alternatively, put finely chopped leaves into ice-cube trays and top up with water. One average cube holds one tablespoon of chopped herb and one tablespoon of water – a convenient quantity for cooking. If the water is not required in a recipe, the ice cube can be placed in a sieve over a bowl and allowed to thaw.

Flowers and leaves such as borage or mint are particularly attractive frozen individually in ice cubes for drinks.

OTHER METHODS OF PRESERVING

The flavor of herbs can be preserved in herb vinegars and oils, as described on p. 188. This is an excellent method for well-flavored culinary herbs, and the resulting liquid makes an interesting addition to dressings, pickles and marinades. Use the same technique to make aromatic herbal or floral vinegars and oils for perfume, medicinal and cosmetic purposes.

There are numerous alternative techniques for preserving culinary herbs: in pickles, jellies, sugar and alcohol, as described on pp. 188–193.

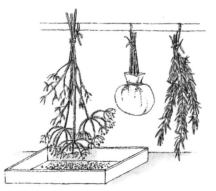

A selection of herbs being dried for their seeds and leaves.

A catalogue of herbs

In every country there are herbs employed by local people for seasoning, medicine or household uses which may be unknown to others. As these practices come to notice, some are investigated and brought to wider attention. This gives the subject of herbs frequent new surprises and is part of its continuing appeal.

One such example is the oil found in the jojoba plant, which has the same properties as the oil of the sperm whale and should mean a reduction in the killing of these huge creatures. Jojoba grows on semiarid land and could be cultivated as a cash crop on the desert margins.

This catalogue includes a selection of useful herbs, including trees and shrubs, and some lesser-known herbs which were popular in the past. It also includes spices, that unique group of plants which compelled explorers to discover new lands. *Do not try remedies without seeking medical advice, particularly if you are pregnant or undergoing any medical treatment.*

Spices

Capsicum annuum
Sweet pepper/Chili pepper
Solanaceae

Description Annual or biennial grown commercially in the tropics and subtropics. Grows from 1–3 feet high with pointed oval leaves and white flowers in summer. Fleshy, edible fruit with furrowed sides varies in color (yellow, brown, purple, bright red) when mature. When unripe it is green but still edible.

Cultivation Grow in a sunny position in rich soil. Avoid extremes in temperature. Sow in spring.

Uses Eat fruit in salads, as a vegetable or add to casseroles and stews. Fresh or dried fruit is used as a stimulant and digestive. Sprinkle $\frac{1}{2}$ teaspoon, finely chopped, in $\frac{1}{2}$ cup of boiling water or hot milk at the first sign of a chill. The dried fruit of a variety of C. annuum is crushed as paprika pepper. It has a sweet, mild flavor, which is free of the hot pungency of chili. It should be brilliant red; if brown it is probably stale. Paprika is high in vitamin C and should be used generously in stews and meat dishes.

Capsicum frutescens
Tabasco pepper/Cayenne
Solanaceae

Description Perennial shrub in the tropics and subtropics; annual elsewhere. Grows 2–6 feet tall. Woody stem, elliptical leaves and starlike white flowers with yellow centers, appearing in summer. Small, leathery, oblong pods, containing numerous pungent seeds, develop in various shades of red and yellow.

Cultivation Grow under glass in a sunny position. Sow in spring.

Uses Pulverize seed and use the hot spice discreetly. Pods contain vitamin C and magnesium. They stimulate blood circulation and the digestive system and help to ward off colds. Use to relieve colic, flatulence, stomach pains and cramp. Infuse weakly as a gargle for a sore throat.

Cinnamomum zeylanicum
Cinnamon
Lauraceae

Description Tropical evergreen tree. Reaches 20–30 feet tall with thick, smooth, pale bark, leathery, oval, green leaves with paler undersides and small, white flowers. Bark, leaves and oval, bluish fruit are fragrant.

Cultivation Grows best in pure sand in a sheltered place with constant rain, heat and even temperature. Propagate by seed, cuttings or division of roots.

Uses Dried inner bark of the branches employed as a spice in teas, cooked fruit, pickling liquids, honey, punches and mulled red wine. Ground spice added to sweet baked puddings, cooked fruit and some meat and fish dishes. Coarsely ground seed used in potpourri and seed oil in perfumery. Bark used medicinally as an antiseptic, astringent and stimulant; will relieve nausea, flatulence and diarrhea.

Crocus sativus
Saffron
Iridaceae

Description Bulbous perennial. Reaches 12–18 inches high. Numerous, narrow, grasslike, gray-green leaves; funnel-shaped, rich purple flowers appear in autumn. Each flower has three stigmas which protrude out of the flower, a feature which distinguishes it from the poisonous *Colchicum autumnale*.

Cultivation Grows in any rich, well-drained soil in a sunny, sheltered site. It requires a long hot summer to produce flowers. Break off outer corms and replant in late summer.

Uses Most delicately flavored spice; use stigmas to flavor and color rice, meat and fish dishes, soups, breads, cakes and biscuits. In herb liqueurs, it flavors and stimulates the appetite. Saffron's strong yellow dye is water-soluble. Use to tint hair and to scent perfumes. Stigmas aid digestion, reduce fevers and cramp. Formerly considered an aphrodisiac.

Cuminum cyminum
Cumin
Umbelliferae

Description Tender annual. Grows 6–12 inches tall. Leaves are slightly fragrant and threadlike; white or pinkish flowers appear in summer and are followed by aromatic seeds. These are similar in appearance to caraway seeds, except they are bristly.

Cultivation Grows in light, well-drained soil in sheltered, sunny site. Sow in late spring in warm situation.

Uses Powerfully flavored seeds, whole or ground, are added to many Middle Eastern and Indian dishes, especially to lamb, curries and yogurt. Also used for pickling and flavoring liqueurs and cordials. The seed oil is employed in perfumery and in veterinary medicine. Thought to relieve flatulence, colic, indigestion and diarrhea.

Curcuma longa
Turmeric
Zingiberaceae

Description Tender perennial. Grows to 2 feet high. Large, fragrant, ovoid roots, with deep orange flesh, send up large lance-shaped leaves in tufts. Clusters of pale yellow flowers in dense spikes appear from late spring to midsummer.

Cultivation Grows in rich loamy soil in humid conditions. Take root cuttings in autumn.

Uses Dried root has bitter, gingery flavor when soaked in water or alcohol. It also provides a culinary and medicinal coloring agent and will dye cloth a rich yellow. Soak unglazed white paper in a tincture and then dry for a yellow paper. Root may relieve catarrh and some blood problems and, used externally, heal bruising.

Elettaria cardamomum
Cardamom
Zingiberaceae

Description Tender perennial from the tropics. Reaches from 6–10 feet high. Leaves are lance-shaped and dark green, with paler, silky undersides; creeping roots are large and fleshy. Small yellow flowers spread along the ground during mid- to late spring, followed by green, three-celled pods containing dark red-brown seeds.
Cultivation Grows in rich, moist soil in shade. Sow seed or divide rhizomes.
Uses Whole seeds used to flavor marinades, liqueurs, punches, mulled wines and pickling liquids. Add ground seeds as a spice to fruit salads, curries, cakes, breads, biscuits and coffee. Chew seeds to freshen breath. Use in potpourri and in perfumes. Helpful for flatulence, indigestion and headaches.

Illicium verum
Star anise
Magnoliaceae

Description Tender evergreen tree. Grows from 15–30 feet high with aromatic, white bark, aromatic, glossy, elliptical leaves and whitish, yellow or purple flowers surrounded by many narrow petals. These are followed by star-shaped gray-brown fruits.
Cultivation Grows in well-drained soil in sunny, sheltered sites. Propagate by seed or stem cuttings.
Uses Seed oil provides important substitute for aniseed as a flavoring agent. Seed employed as a spice. Add to drinks. Seed promotes digestion and appetite, and relieves flatulence, coughs, bronchitis and rheumatism.

Myristica fragrans
Nutmeg and Mace
Myristicaceae

Description Bushy, tender, evergreen tree. Reaches up to 25 feet tall with smooth, gray-brown bark and aromatic, leathery, elliptical, glossy, dark green leaves. Yellow flowers are followed by globular red or yellow fruits, containing an aromatic, ovoid, brown kernel (nutmeg) surrounded by a red aril (mace).
Cultivation Grows in humus-rich loam in a heated greenhouse with high humidity and ambient temperature. Take hardwood cuttings in autumn.
Uses Dried kernel provides very strong, bitter flavor; add freshly grated to sweet and savory dishes, especially to milk and cheese dishes. Used to flavor mead, milk drinks, liqueurs and cordials. Add to potpourri. In very small quantities, nutmeg will improve appetites and digestion. It can be mildly hallucinogenic.

Note: *Use nutmeg very sparingly.*

Pimenta dioica
Allspice
Myrtaceae

Description Aromatic tender evergreen tree. Grows up to 40 feet tall. Leaves are leathery, glossy and oblong, in pairs along stem; small white clusters appear from summer to early autumn, followed by fleshy, purplish-black sweet fruits.
Cultivation In temperate climates, allspice is grown as a nonflowering ornamental in the greenhouse. Take cuttings or layer the stem.
Uses Dried, unripe fruit employed mainly as a spice and as a condiment; add to curries, rice, puddings, pickling liquids and mulled wines. Use to perfume soaps and notepaper. Grind seed and sprinkle over potpourri. Oil from fruit relieves colic and flatulence. Boil crushed fruit and apply on cloth to treat rheumatism and neuralgia.

Piper nigrum
Black pepper
Piperaceae

Description Tender perennial climbing shrub from the tropics. Grows to 20 feet or more. Strong, woody, twining stems bear broad, oval, glossy dark green leaves with prominent veins. White flower clusters appear in summer, followed by aromatic, globular, wrinkled red fruits.
Cultivation Grows in high humidity in shade. Needs supporting. Propagate by softwood cuttings.
Uses Dried unripe fruit used as a spice and a condiment; add freshly ground to all savory foods. It kills bacteria, so employ as a food preservative. Use as a diuretic, stimulant, digestive and anti-flatulence remedy. Good for constipation, nausea, vertigo and arthritis.

Syzygium aromaticum (Eugenia aromatica)
Clove
Myrtaceae

Description Tender evergreen tree from the tropics. Reaches 30 feet or higher, with large leathery, oval, glossy leaves in pairs. Bell-shaped red flowers appear for two separate periods during growing season. Pink flower buds turn reddish-brown after drying.
Cultivation Well-drained, acidic soil in shade. Protect from wind.
Uses For a spicy flavor, add whole, dried, unopened flower buds, known as cloves, to curries, stewed fruit, marinades, pickling liquids, mulled wine; grind cloves for breads, biscuits, cakes. Use in pomanders and potpourri. Chew as a breath freshener. Infuse as a tea to relieve nausea. Drop clove oil into a tooth cavity to stop toothache. Apply externally to ease neuralgia and rheumatism.

Vanilla planifolia
Vanilla
Orchidaceae

Description Tender epiphytic tropical orchid. Grows 30–50 feet tall. Long, leathery, fleshy, oval leaves grow on stout stems. Yellow or orange flowers appear after third year of planting and are followed by long aromatic pods.
Cultivation Grows in high humidity under shade, on poles or tree trunks. Propagate by stem cuttings.
Uses Dried, cured fruit pods, known as vanilla beans, principally used as culinary and commercial flavorings and as a pharmaceutical coloring agent. It was used by the Mexican Aztecs to flavor chocolate. Also used in cosmetics, especially perfumes. Add to potpourri. Sprinkle powdered beans over notepaper for an attractive scent.

Zingiber officinale
Ginger
Zingiberaceae

Description Tender creeping perennial from the tropics. Grows 3–4 feet high. Thick, aromatic, fibrous, knotty, buff-colored tuberous roots produce erect, annual stems bearing long, narrow, lance-shaped leaves. Sterile, fragrant, white flowers with purple streaks appear rarely.
Cultivation Grows in rich, well-drained loam in light shade. Propagate by root cuttings.
Uses Fresh ginger root peeled and sliced, or grated, can be added to stews, sauces and oriental dishes. Use ground root in gingerbread, cakes, biscuits, mulled wine, liqueurs and cordials. Preserve young green roots in syrup. Apply fresh root externally as a "rouge," as it stimulates circulation. Infuse root as a tea to cleanse the body's systems, ease a cold and to bring warmth on cold days. Chew root to soothe a sore throat. Recent research confirms that an infusion is excellent to settle the stomach and prevent nausea when traveling.

Trees and shrubs

Buxus sempervirens
Box
Buxaceae

Description Slow-growing, fairly hardy evergreen tree. Grows from 15–20 feet high. The rugged gray bark surrounds hard yellow timber. Dense branches bear leathery, glossy, oval, dark green leaves with paler undersides. Small pale yellow flowers appear from midspring. B.s. 'Suffruticosa' is a dwarf form for edging.
Cultivation Prefers alkaline soil. Take stem cuttings in spring.
Uses Whole plant, when close clipped, makes an excellent edging to a formal herb garden. The timber is very durable.

Camellia sinensis
Tea
Theaceae

Description Tender evergreen shrub. Grows from 7–8 feet high under cultivation; up to 30 feet high in the wild. Rough gray branches bear toothed, elliptical, dark green leaves; white flowers appear in spring and are followed by flat rounded fruits.
Cultivation Requires deep acid soil in equable temperature and high humidity. Propagate by seed.
Uses Dried green leaves yield "green tea," which is the primary drink in China and has medicinal virtues listed 5,000 years ago. It aids digestion of oily foods and is thought to normalize metabolism. To make black tea, the leaves are fermented, which increases the tannin, caffeine and stimulant properties. Drink in moderation.

Citrus limon
Lemon
Rutaceae

Description Tender, subtropical, evergreen tree. Grows 10–20 feet high with gray bark, elliptical leaves; clusters of white flowers, with pink outsides, appear at all seasons and are followed by sour-tasting, bright yellow fruits, indented with oil glands.
Cultivation Prefers a light, well-drained fertile soil in a site protected from wind. Propagate by seed.
Uses Fruit, juice and peel, which are rich in vitamins and minerals, are widely used in cooking, sweets and drinks, and as an antioxidant. Add to potpourri, herb pillows, soaps and perfumes. Has many household uses: cleans brass, silver, marble and rust stains. Use as an astringent and skin tonic. Bleaching properties may remove nicotine stains from nails and teeth, fade freckles and condition blond hair. Juice soothes colds, coughs, sore throats, headaches, rheumatism and fevers. Use as an antiseptic to neutralize bacteria.

Eucalyptus globulus
Eucalyptus
Myrtaceae

Description Evergreen tree whose young leaves are susceptible to frosts. Grows to 300 feet or more. Bark is peeling and papery; leaves when mature, are leathery, lance-shaped, bluish-green and covered with oil-bearing glands. Small, petal-less, white flowers appear in summer.
Cultivation Grows in a wide variety of soils and conditions. Sow in spring.
Uses Leaves provide an effective flea repellent. Timber is used as an exterior building material. Leaves are included in dry potpourris. Volatile greenish-yellow oil from mature leaves useful for catarrh, sore throats, bronchitis, indigestion, fevers and as an inhalant, antiseptic, deodorant and stimulant. Apply, diluted, externally for burns, wounds and ulcers.

Note: *In large doses, eucalyptus is toxic.*

Gaultheria procumbens
Wintergreen
Ericaceae

Description Hardy evergreen shrub. Grows up to 5–6 inches high. Its creeping stems produce stiff branches. Leaves are strongly aromatic, leathery, glossy and oval; drooping, bell-shaped white flowers, which appear in mid- to late summer, are followed by fleshy bright red berries.
Cultivation Grows in acidic soils in light shade. Sow seed, take stem cuttings or layer in spring or autumn.
Uses Leaves contain magnesium and potassium and painkilling ingredients in an oil readily absorbed by the skin. Diluted oil can be applied externally for rheumatism, inflammation and skin diseases. Infuse leaves as a tea and as a gargle for headaches and sore throats.

Ginkgo biloba
Maidenhair tree
Ginkgoaceae

Description Very slow-growing hardy tree that has a fossil record dating back some 200 million years. Grows 30–50 feet tall. The trunk is light brown with corky fissures. The leaves are fan-shaped and bright green, turning yellow in autumn. Flowers are rare and on separate trees: male flowers small, green catkins; female ones small, globular and green, followed by small, plum-shaped, foul-smelling fruits.
Cultivation Grows in any fertile, well-drained soil in sun or light shade. Propagate by stem cuttings in spring.
Uses Inner bark yields a pale brown dye. Roasted or pan-fried seeds are pleasant to eat and relieve hangovers. In China, the seeds and leaves are used for coughs and asthma.

Hamamelis virginiana
Witch hazel
Hamamelidaceae

Description Hardy tree. Grows 8–10 feet high with brown bark and toothed, elliptical leaves with hairy undersides. Scented, yellow flowers, with straplike petals, appear late autumn.
Cultivation Grows in moist, lime-free soil in sun or light shade. Propagate by layering in autumn.
Uses Forked branches formerly used as water divining rods. Apply distilled extract from young flower-bearing twigs (available commercially as witch hazel) externally for bruises, sprains, varicose veins, hemorrhoids, insect bites and to stop bleeding. Used as an astringent cosmetic.

Note: *A tincture from the bark or leaves may disfigure skin.*

Ilex aquifolium
English holly
Aquifoliaceae

Description Hardy evergreen tree. Reaches up to 30 feet in height. Green branches bear leathery, glossy, wavy edged, prickly, oval dark green leaves. Small, fragrant white flowers appear in clusters in early and midsummer and are followed by globular red or yellow fruits. Some trees are hermaphrodite; others require a male tree nearby for successful pollination.
Cultivation Prefers growing in humus-rich, moist, well-drained soils in light shade. Sow seed in spring.
Uses Whole plant makes a decorative garden plant and is excellent for hedging. Timber used for engraving and for walking sticks. Burn green branches as firewood. Infuse leaves as a tea for coughs, colds, catarrh, influenza, fevers and rheumatism.

Morus nigra
Black mulberry
Moraceae

Description Hardy tree. Grows to 30 feet. Bushy, with thick, toothed, heart-shaped leaves and unisexual green catkins in clusters, which appear in late spring and early summer. They are followed by oblong purplish-red fruits.
Cultivation Grows on well-drained, loamy soil in a warm position; protect from cold winds and frosts. Sow in spring. Take stem cuttings in early spring. Layer in autumn.
Uses Fruit is rich in vitamin C and sugar; eat raw or cooked and make into wines and jams. Leaves were used for silkworm rearing (until replaced by white mulberry) and diabetes. Fruit provides a laxative, a convalescent syrup, and coloring and flavoring for other medications. White mulberry (M. *alba*) has similar properties.

Myrica gale
Sweet gale/Bog myrtle
Myricaceae
Description Bushy deciduous shrub, up to 4–5 feet tall, with fragrant wood and leaves when bruised. Toothed, glossy, lance-shaped leaves have slightly hairy, paler undersides and a few shining oil glands. Catkins of brown or yellow-green unisexual flowers appear in late spring and early summer, followed by small, flattened fruit catkins, which contain wax.
Cultivation Grows in damp, acidic soil in shade. Take stem cuttings, divide root or transplant suckers in spring or early autumn.
Uses Dried leaves and fruits used as a spice in soups and stews. Leaves provide a flavoring for beer and, when dried, will perfume linen. Roots and bark yield a yellow woolen dye. Fruits used to make an insecticide and aromatic candles. Infuse leaves as a tea for stomach disorders.

Phyllostachys nigra
Bamboo
Gramineae
Description Temperate evergreen perennial. Grows 26 feet high in clumps. Stems, which are dense, woody and resilient, change from green to brown-black at maturity. Leaves are long, narrow and pointed. Bamboo seldom flowers.
Cultivation Grows on moist soil in sun or light shade, protected from cold winds. Propagate by plant or rhizome division in late winter or early spring.
Uses Young shoots are edible in spring. Stem provides materials for garden stakes, building, basketwork and musical instruments. Detoxifies the body and is diuretic. Roots soothe high fevers and fretfulness in infants.

Populus balsamifera
Balsam poplar
Salicaceae
Description Hardy aromatic tree. Grows 100 feet high. Highly aromatic, sticky, resinous leaf buds during winter develop into toothed, heart-shaped, dark green leaves with hairy white undersides. Drooping yellow catkins appear in spring.
Cultivation Grows in any conditions and soil. Propagate from suckers or 12 inch cuttings in autumn.
Uses Add buds to potpourri. Oil in leaf buds is used to give a resinous balsamic fragrance to many articles. In a tincture, leaf buds relieve coughs, laryngitis, bronchitis, stomach and kidney complaints, and rheumatism. Use also as an antiseptic, stimulant, tonic and diuretic. Apply as ointment for cuts, bruises and general pain relief.

Prunus dulcis
Almond
Rosaceae
Description A somewhat frost-sensitive tree. Grows 30 feet tall with finely toothed pointed oval leaves. Pink or white flowers in late spring precede ovoid light green fruits containing two nuts.
Cultivation Grow in well-drained soil in full sun, protected from cold winds. To propagate, bud onto stock in spring.
Uses Nuts used in cakes, sweets, savory dishes, confectionery and liqueurs. Use ground nuts to make marzipan. Hard pale red timber provides tool handles, veneers and ornaments. Oil is valued for perfumes, skin creams, facial masks and is the most popular carrier oil in aromatherapy massage. It is a soothing oil for sunburn, cough medicine and a laxative.

Quercus robur
Oak
Fagaceae
Description Hardy tree, grows to 110 feet with lobed oval leaves, long male catkins and small green-yellow flowers in spring. Autumn brings oblong cupped fruits (acorns) and sometimes oak galls – ball-like growths that result from gall wasp larvae.
Cultivation Grows in any soil in any situation. Sow seed or graft in autumn.
Uses Roast acorns for a coffee substitute. Strong durable timber is used to build ships, buildings, furniture and weapons, as fuel and to smoke ham. Bark yields tannin for leather, twine and various dyes. Galls yield black ink (see p. 202). A decoction of unblemished bark collected in late spring is an effective astringent to take internally for diarrhea, hemorrhoids, varicose veins, a gargle for sore throats or applied directly to bleeding gums or piles. Use in a lotion for cuts, burns and hemorrhoids.

Rubus laciniatus
Bramble
Rosaceae
Description Biennial shrub. Reaches up to 10 feet tall with thorny biennial stems and toothed leaves. Pink or white flowers appear from summer and are followed by blackberries.
Cultivation Grows in most situations. Tip layer in summer, sow in autumn.
Uses Fruits are high in vitamin C; eat raw or cooked in puddings, jams, jellies, wine and vinegar. Organic acids in fruit are useful in face masks. Roots provide orange dye. Infuse leaves and shoots in bath water to revive skin. Decoct leaves as a tonic, gargle, or poultice for skin ulcers.

Simmondsia chinensis
Jojoba
Buxaceae
Description Tender woody evergreen shrub. Grows from 2–8 feet high with hairy young stems and lance-shaped gray-green leaves. In spring there are clusters of cup-shaped, greenish male flowers or single bell-shaped female flowers which develop ovoid, single-seeded capsules. Seeds contain a scentless, clear, waxy oil.
Cultivation Grow in well-drained dry soil in full sun. Propagate by seed.
Uses The seed oil is the only known plant equivalent to sperm whale oil. Used as a diet oil, as it passes largely unutilized through the digestive tract. Use in soaps, shampoos, hair tonics and skin creams. Add to furniture polish or car wax, or use as a lubricant for high-speed machinery. Seed makes excellent basic fodder for cattle.

Taxus baccata
Yew
Taxaceae
Description Evergreen tree. Grows to 50 feet high. Flaking reddish-brown bark and long, narrow, glossy, dark green needles with paler undersides. Yellow male flowers appear in spring, as do female ones, which are small and green. These develop into bell-shaped red or yellow fruits.
Cultivation Grows best on alkaline soil; tolerates shade. Sow seed or take heeled cuttings in early autumn.
Uses Orange-brown timber is water-resistant and hard; use for furniture, archery bows and as firewood. A homeopathic tincture made from leaves and berries is used medicinally.

Note: *All parts of yew are poisonous, including the seed.*

Vitex agnus-castus
Chaste tree/Monk's pepper
Verbenaceae
Description Fairly hardy tree or shrub. Reaches up to 20 feet. Leaflets are aromatic, long, oval and dark green; clusters of fragrant, lilac-blue flowers, in long, erect spikes, appear in autumn and are followed by small, spherical fruits containing aromatic seeds.
Cultivation Grows in full sun on light, well-drained, acidic soil, protected by a wall. Sow seed in spring. Layer in spring or summer. Take cuttings in early autumn.
Uses Ground seed used as a peppery condiment. Stems are woven in basketwork. Dried fruits contain hormonal constituents which normalize pituitary gland functions and relieve menopausal changes. They have a reputation as an anaphrodisiac for men; hence the name Monk's pepper.

Other herbs

Acorus calamus
Sweet flag
Araceae

Description A perennial marsh plant from temperate regions with a knobbly aromatic rhizome. The irislike leaves reach 3 feet with tiny green flowers appearing in midsummer on a curved, protruding spike halfway up the stalk.
Cultivation Grow in a sunny position in shallow water or rich, marshy soil. Plant pieces of rhizome with small roots attached in spring or autumn.
Uses The whole plant has a rich cinnamon-spicy fragrance. Dry leaves and two-year-old rhizome for pot-pourri and sweet bags. It was formerly a strewing herb and used to flavor meat dishes. May be carcinogenic.

Agastache foeniculum (A. anethiodora)
Anise hyssop
Labiatae

Description Hardy perennial. Grows 2–3 feet high. Oval, pointed leaves, with whitish undersides, have an aniseed scent. Long spikes of purple-blue flowers appear in late summer.
Cultivation Grows in rich, moist soil in a sunny site. Propagate in spring by seed or divide creeping root.
Uses Use dried leaves as a seasoning or infuse as a tea. An excellent bee herb.

Anchusa officinalis
Alkanet/Bugloss
Boraginaceae

Description Biennial or perennial. Grows to 12 inches high. Similar to borage, with rough leaves, thick tap root and small bright blue flowers in early summer.
Cultivation Tolerates any soil. Sow in spring; divide in autumn.
Uses Add flowers and young leaves to salads. Decoct root for blood cleanser and expectorant for coughs. Root gives a strong red dye in alcohol or oil. Once used as face rouge. Valuable bee plant.

Arnica montana
Arnica
Compositae

Description Hardy perennial, growing 1–2 feet tall. Oval, hairy leaves form rosettes and large, scented yellow flowers appear all summer.
Cultivation Plant in sandy, acidic soil, rich in humus, in a sunny position. Divide creeping rhizomes in spring. Sow in spring; slow to germinate.
Uses A good bee plant. Leaves and roots smoked in herbal tobaccos. Use a tincture of flowers for sprains, wounds and bruises, relief from rheumatic pain and on chilblains when skin not broken. Add to a relaxing footbath.

Note: *Potentially toxic if taken internally.*

Bellis perennis
Lawn daisy
Compositae

Description Hardy perennial. Grows from 3–6 inches tall with flat rosettes of finely hairy, serrated leaves. Single or double white or pink flowers with golden centers bloom from spring through to autumn.
Cultivation Easy to grow on fertile soil in sun or part shade. Divide in spring or sow in spring or late summer.
Uses Add young leaves and petals to salads; add flowers to potpourri. Good nectar plant for bees and butterflies. Infuse flowers for a spring tonic bath to revive dull skin or drink for enteritis, diarrhea or as an expectorant for coughs and colds. Crushed fresh leaves or a decoction helps to heal wounds and bruises.

Calamintha grandiflora
Calamint
Labiatae

Description Perennial herb. Reaches a height of 12 inches. Its square, hairy, woody stems rise from creeping rootstalk. Dense whorls of bluish flowers, appearing from midsummer until early autumn, are borne beside each pair of mint-scented toothed, oval leaves.
Cultivation Prefers chalky soil in dry woodlands and wasteground. Sow in spring. Take stem cuttings in spring. Divide root in late spring or autumn.
Uses Calamint contains camphorlike essential oils. Infuse dried leaves as a tea for flatulent colic and as an invigorating tonic. Leaves also produce peppermint-flavored tisane. Use fresh in a poultice for bruises. Take as a syrup or decoction for coughs.

Carthamus tinctorius
Safflower
Compositae

Description An annual that is not related to saffron, although the flowers are used similarly; grows up to 2–3 feet tall. Prickly oval leaves grow along its stiff whitish stem, which branches near the top and terminates with an orange-yellow flower in summer. It has shiny, white fruits.
Cultivation Sow in spring.
Uses Seed is rich in linoleic acid, an essential fatty acid, and thus excellent for culinary purposes, to lower blood cholesterol and help prevent heart disease. Flowers yield yellow and red dyes, which when mixed with powdered talc form "rouge." Add flowers to potpourri. Infuse flowers as a laxative, diuretic, and perspiration inducer, and to alleviate skin diseases.

Note: *Do not take large amounts during pregnancy.*

Cymbopogon citratus
Lemon grass
Gramineae

Description Tender perennial grass from the tropics. Grows up to 6 feet tall. Densely tufted with fragrant, very long, thin, pointed leaves with prominent mid-veins. Greenish flowers, with reddish tinge, appear in nodding clusters in summer.
Cultivation Grow in moist soil in full sun in the greenhouse, with a minimum temperature of 55 °F. Propagate by division.
Uses Chop tender stalks into salads. Infuse leaves as a herbal tea. Use oil to clean oily skin and as a relaxant in bathwater. Add to perfumes and soaps.

Dictamnus albus
White dittany/Burning bush
Rutaceae

Description This hardy perennial with a penetrating orangelike scent exudes so much inflammable vapor in heat or dry, cloudy weather that it can sometimes be ignited. Grows 2 feet high with round, hairy stems and fragrant, toothed, oval leaflets; all parts are covered with glandular dots. Long spikes of large, red, white, blue or striped flowers appear in summer.
Cultivation Grows in well-drained, alkaline soil in sunny gardens and warm places such as sheltered woodlands. Sow in late summer in situ.
Uses Dry leaves for potpourri. Infuse leaves as a herbal tea. Distilled water used as a cosmetic. Leaves and flowers produce tincture for rheumatic pains. In the past leaves were infused for nervous complaints. Decoction of rootstalk was used for fever and stomach cramps, and, combined with seeds, for kidney and bladder stones. One constituent, dictamine, is toxic in strong doses. Avoid during pregnancy.

Echium vulgare
Viper's bugloss
Boraginaceae

Description Biennial, closely related to borage. Grows up to 2–3 feet tall with oblong prickly leaves and stem, often spotted with red. Pink buds open into blue-violet flowers from early summer to early autumn.
Cultivation Easily grown in dry or stony, chalky or sandy soils, especially near the sea. Sow in late summer in situ. Self-seeds profusely.
Uses Add flowers to salads, make into a cordial and crystallize them. Infuse lower leaves to produce sweating in fevers; also to relieve headaches, colds, nervous complaints and inflammatory pain. Seeds used to be decocted and mixed in wine, to "comfort the heart and drive away melancholy."

Equisetum arvense
Horsetail/Bottlebrush
Equisetaceae
Description A resilient perennial, practically unchanged in form since prehistoric times. Grows up to 18 inches tall with whorls of small green branches around larger central stems. *E. hyemale* grows to 5 feet.
Cultivation Grows in dry, stony soil. Spreads easily by creeping rhizomes and airborne spores.
Uses Whole plant yields a yellow ocher dye. Stems have a high silica content and can be used to scour metal and polish pewter and fine woodwork. They contain vitamins and minerals and make a strength-giving tea which enriches the blood and hardens fingernails. A decoction is also astringent when applied externally. A poultice helps to heal wounds and ulcers.

Eryngium maritimum
Sea holly
Umbelliferae
Description Hardy perennial forming a semispherical bush, growing from 1–3 feet high. Leaves are very stiff, fleshy, prickly and blue-green edged with white. Tiny, thistlelike, metallic-blue flowers appear in mid- to late summer. The edible root is extremely long, brittle, fleshy and white.
Cultivation Well-drained sandy soil in full sun near the sea. Sow seed and divide roots in autumn.
Uses Crystallize roots as an aphrodisiac and nerve tonic. Boil young flowering shoots and serve like asparagus. Leaves are also edible. Use powdered root in a poultice to aid tissue regeneration. Drink root decoction as a tonic, diuretic and for cystitis, urethritis and inflamed prostate gland.

Euphrasia officinalis
Eyebright
Scrophulariaceae
Description Annual. Grows from 2–8 inches high with deeply cut, hairy, toothed, oval leaves and square, branched stems. Numerous small white flowers with purple and yellow spots or stripes appear from midsummer to late autumn.
Cultivation Difficult to grow, as it is semiparasitic on certain grass species. Sow in spring on chalky soil.
Uses Infuse whole plant or crush fresh stem, and use strained juice to relieve eye inflammations, eye strain and other eye ailments; also for hay fever, colds, coughs and sore throats. *E. rostkoviana* is the most useful species for eye treatments. Apply externally as an eye compress and in a poultice to aid wound healing.

Note: *Seek medical advice before treating eyes.*

Galega officinalis
Goat's rue
Leguminosae
Description Hardy perennial. Reaches 3 feet high. Bushy, with smooth, hollow, branched stem, lance-shaped, bright green leaflets and pealike purplish-blue or white flowers from midsummer to midautumn, followed by long, erect red-brown pods. The plant produces a disagreeable odor when bruised.
Cultivation Grows in deep, moist soil in a sunny position. Sow in spring. Divide roots in spring or autumn.
Uses Fresh juice clots milk and may be used in cheesemaking. Infuse dried flowering tops to stimulate the flow of milk in nursing mothers and animals. Pulverize the dried herb as a diuretic; also to reduce fevers. The seeds apparently lower blood sugar levels and may assist diabetics. Use only under strict medical supervision.

Galium verum
Lady's bedstraw
Rubiaceae
Description Hardy perennial; grows from 1–3 feet tall. Delicate whorls of thread-like leaves on square stems. Dense clusters of tiny, honey-scented yellow flowers appear all summer.
Cultivation Thrives in deeply dug, well-drained manured loam in sun or partial shade. Divide underground runners or sow seed in spring or autumn. Seed needs striation; graze between sandpaper.
Uses Strong decoctions of whole plant curdle milk when boiled for cheese-making, while flowers give cheese a golden color. Dried leaves contain coumarin and smell of new-mown hay. Add leaves and flowers to potpourri and herb pillows. Used in the past to stuff mattresses. Roots and lower stems yield red dye, flowers give yellow dye.

Genista tinctoria
Dyer's greenweed
Leguminosae
Description Hardy deciduous shrub. Grows from 1–3 feet tall. Leaves are small, oblong, glossy dark green; yellow pea-flowers appear in midsummer, followed by long, narrow seed pods in autumn.
Cultivation Grows on dryish, sandy soils. Sow in spring. Take cuttings in late summer.
Uses Flowers yield a yellowish-green dye. Formerly used as a diuretic but now considered poisonous.

Glycyrrhiza glabra
Licorice
Leguminosae
Description Herbaceous perennial. Grows from 2–5 feet tall with long, narrow, dark green leaflets. Its taproot has several long branches, which are wrinkled and brown, with yellow flesh. Yellow or purplish flowers appear in summer, followed by reddish-brown pods.
Cultivation Grows readily in deep, moist, rich, sandy loam. Divide roots in autumn or spring.
Uses Root flavors beers, confectionery, tobaccos and snuffs. Root pulp is incorporated in mushroom compost. Root contains glycyrrhizin, a substance many times sweeter than sugar, which may be taken by diabetics. Infuse as a refreshing tea and as a remedy for coughs and chest complaints. Strong decoction makes a laxative for children and may reduce fever.

Hydrastis canadensis
Goldenseal
Ranunculaceae
Description Hardy herbaceous perennial. Grows from 6–12 inches tall with hairy stems, toothed, lobed leaves and thick, knotted, yellow rootstalk. Greenish-white flowers (without petals) appear in late spring and early summer, followed by raspberrylike inedible fruits.
Cultivation Grows in well-drained, moist, rich soil in partially shaded sites. Divide rootstock in early autumn.
Uses Root yields a yellow-orange dye. Take a few drops of tincture to relieve constipation or add them to distilled water to make a lotion for skin ulcers. Use as a weak infusion for conjunctivitis and as an antiseptic mouthwash.

Hypericum perforatum
St John's wort
Hypericaceae
Description Fragrant, hardy, shrubby perennial. Grows from 1–3 feet tall. Leaves are pale green, oblong and covered with tiny perforations – the oil glands. Lemon-scented yellow flowers appear in summer and early autumn.
Cultivation Tolerates most soils in sun and light shade. Propagate from runners at base in autumn or seed.
Uses Leaves make an interesting salad herb. Flowers yield a yellow wool dye with alum, or violet-red silk dye with alcohol. Infused flower oil helps healing of bruises, wounds, varicose veins, ulcers and sunburn. Flowers have been infused as a pain-reducing sedative tea for anemia, rheumatism, headaches and nervous conditions. Now considered unsafe by some so use with caution. May cause photo-dermatitis.

Indigofera tinctoria
Indigo
Leguminosae
Description Perennial semitropical shrub. Pairs of oval leaves grow along its stems and clusters of small purplish flowers appear in summer.
Cultivation Must be grown in a greenhouse in temperate climates. Sow seed and take cuttings in spring.
Uses Famed for its rich blue dye since ancient times. Demand for it has not ceased since it was first introduced to the West three centuries ago, although its production as a colorfast blue dye agent involves surprisingly complex procedures, such as fermentation.

Iris x germanica var. florentina
Orris root
Iridaceae
Description Hardy perennial. Reaches up to 2–3 feet high. Its stout rhizomatous roots smell of violets and its leaves are sword-shaped. Large white flowers, tinged with pale lavender and with a yellow beard, appear in early to midsummer.
Cultivation Grows in deep, rich, well-drained soil in a sunny position. Divide roots in late spring or early autumn.
Uses Roots provide bitter flavoring for certain liqueurs. Powdered root imparts a refreshing scent to linen; also used as a base for dry shampoos, tooth powders and face packs as well as perfumery. Powdered root used as a fixative in potpourri. The root is a powerful purgative and now considered too strong to use medicinally. Dried root used to be used for coughs, hoarseness, bronchitis, colic and congestion in the liver. It also used to be chewed for disagreeable breath.

Lawsonia inermis
Henna
Lythraceae
Description Perennial tropical shrub. Can grow up to 10 feet high. Bushy, with narrow, gray-green leaves and small, sweet-scented pink or cream flowers, which give way to clusters of blue-black berries.
Cultivation Requires dry, well-drained soil and a tropical climate.
Uses Dried leaves produce a strong red dye and have been used for centuries in the East to color hair, skin and nails. Dried leaves also have astringent properties. Apply in a cold compress to soothe fevers, headaches, stings, aching joints and skin irritations.

Leonurus cardiaca
Motherwort
Labiatae
Description Hardy perennial with pungent odor and bitter taste. Reaches up to 3–5 feet tall. Thick, grooved, hairy, square stems bear hairy, lobed, toothed, dark green leaves with paler undersides. Whorls of pale pink to red-purple flowers appear from midsummer to midautumn.
Cultivation Grows on well-drained, light, limy soil in full sun. Sow in spring. Divide roots in late spring or midautumn. Self-seeds freely.
Uses Whole plant yields a dark green wool dye and is also slightly astringent. Infusion of dried plant may ease false labor pains. Also can be used as a heart tonic and to lower blood pressure. May cause contact dermatitis.

Linum usitatissimum
Flax
Linaceae
Description Hardy annual. Grows from 1–4 feet tall with narrow, hairy, sword-shaped leaves and red, white or blue flowers appearing in early to late summer. These are followed by spherical capsules with shiny, light brown seeds high in oils with linoleic acid.
Cultivation Grows in dryish, well-drained soil in an open sunny position. Sow in spring or early summer.
Uses These go back to the earliest times. Seed and unripe capsules provide food when roasted. Seed oil (linseed) is important in paint and varnish manufacture. Stems can be used to make paper and cloth. Seeds provide a setting lotion for hair and, when eaten whole, a laxative. A seed infusion may help pulmonary infections. Use as a poultice for boils and inflammations.

Note: *Contains toxins. Use with caution.*

Lupinus polyphyllus
Lupine
Leguminosae
Description Herbaceous perennial. Grows $2\frac{1}{2}$–4 feet high with whorls of long, narrow leaves and pea-shaped, deep blue, purple, pink, white or yellow flowers. These appear in late spring and early summer and are followed by flattened, spherical white seeds in long pods.
Cultivation Grows in light, sandy soil in sun or light shade. Sow in spring.
Uses Bruise seeds as a facial steam, or make into skin lotion, to cleanse oily skin. The plant may have a role in absorbing radiation.

Note: *The raw seed of some species is toxic when eaten.*

Onobrychis viciifolia
Sainfoin
Leguminosae
Description Attractive bushy perennial. Grows 4 inches–$2\frac{1}{2}$ feet high. Leaflets are narrow and in pairs, and cone-shaped spikes of pink flowers, streaked with red, appear from late spring to late summer. This is likely to be the Anglo-Saxon herb "Atterlothe," the last unidentified plant of the Nine Sacred Herbs listed in the eleventh-century herbal, the *Lacnunga*. The Archeological Unit of Bury St. Edmunds in England translated the word as "cock spur grass," and Culpeper's herbal of 1645 listed a "cock's head fitch" an *Onobrychis*.
Cultivation Grows in dry, well-drained soil. Scratch seeds, then sow in situ in spring or early autumn.
Uses Makes good honey, as its pollen is attractive to bees. Use as a fodder plant.

Panax quinquefolius
American ginseng
Araliaceae
Description Hardy perennial. Grows from 1–$1\frac{1}{2}$ feet tall with finely toothed, oval leaflets and aromatic, fleshy, spindle-shaped pale yellow to brown root. After 3–4 years, small yellow or pink flowers appear in late summer, followed by bright red berries.
Cultivation Grows in cool humus-rich soil in shade. Sow seed in early spring in shaded cold frames. Transplant outside. Harvest after 3–9 years.
Uses Infuse dried root as a tonic drink for increased mental and physical vigor, against depression caused by exhaustion, or external stress, as an appetite and digestive stimulant, and for relief from nausea. It is helpful for coughs and chest disorders. Oriental ginseng (*P. pseudoginseng*) has similar uses.

Polygonum bistorta
Bistort/Snakeweed
Polygonaceae
Description Hardy perennial. Reaches up to 3 feet high. Leaves are broad, oval and blue-green with heart-shaped base; knobbly, twisted blackish-brown rhizomes have red flesh. Pink flowers, in dense spikes, appear late spring.
Cultivation Grows in moist soil in sun or shade. Divide creeping rootstock in spring or early autumn; can be invasive.
Uses Young raw leaves are pleasant to eat. Rhizome be used to tan leather. Pulverize dried rhizome and use as a very astringent tea for both internal and external bleeding, diarrhea and as an enema. Decoct as a mouthwash for ulcers and as a remedy for coughs, sore throats and dysentery. Applied direct to a wound, the rhizome powder helps to stop bleeding.

Reseda luteola
Weld
Resedaceae

Description Biennial. Grows from 2–5 feet high with rosettes of long, wavy-edged leaves in its first season; graceful, curved spikes of small yellow-green flowers appear during summer of second season.
Cultivation Grows in fertile, well-drained alkaline soil in full sun. Sow seed in late summer. Seed stays fertile for many years.
Uses Whole flowering plant yields a strong, clear yellow dye for woolens and silks. Once mixed with woad to create "Saxon green."

Rubia tinctorum
Madder
Rubiaceae

Description A perennial climber with prickly, weak stems. Grows from 2–3 feet high with whorls of large, rough, prickly-edged, lance-shaped leaves; root is thick, fleshy and reddish-brown. Small yellow-green flowers appear from early summer to early autumn, followed by spherical black fruits.
Cultivation Grows in well-drained soil in full sun or light shade. Sow seed in spring or autumn in well-dug loam. Divide creeping root.
Uses Root and leaves of this traditional dye plant yield pink, red (alizarin crimson) and brown dyes, depending on the mordant used, for cloth and leather. Leaves can be used as metal scourers. Powdered root may heal urinary disorders and prevent kidney stone formation. Leafy stems, when infused, may relieve constipation.

Scutellaria lateriflora
Skullcap
Labiatae

Description Hardy perennial. Reaches from 1–3 feet tall. Branching stems bear oval, toothed leaves and small pretty blue flowers appear along the stem during summer. Roots are fibrous and yellow.
Cultivation Grows in ordinary well-drained soil in sun or light shade. Sow under gentle heat in late winter. Divide roots in early spring.
Uses Whole plant very effective as a soothing antispasmodic tonic and remedy for hysteria. Infuse powdered herb as a tea for premenstrual tension, rheumatism, neuralgia and severe hiccups.

Note: *Large doses may cause giddiness, confusion, twitching and stupor.*

Sesamum indicum
Sesame
Pedaliaceae

Description Strong-smelling tender annual, native to the tropics. Reaches up to 3 feet high with lance-shaped leaves; drooping purple to white flowers are followed by long capsules containing numerous flat white or yellowish seeds.
Cultivation Prefers sandy loam in a sunny position. Propagate by seed.
Uses Seeds provide excellent source of protein, niacin, phosphorus, sulfur and carbohydrates, and have a sweet, nutty flavor; sprinkle over breads, biscuits, vegetables and casseroles. Sesame seed paste (tahini) is mixed into spreads, sauces, casseroles and pâtés. Seeds will also relieve constipation, hemorrhoids and genito-urinary infections.

Stachys officinalis
Betony
Labiatae

Description Hardy perennial. Reaches up to 2 feet tall. Hairy, square stems bear aromatic, slightly hairy, round-lobed leaves; dense spikes of pink or purple flowers appear from mid- to late summer.
Cultivation Grows in ordinary soil in sun or shade; prefers some humus. Sow seed in spring. Divide roots in spring or autumn.
Uses Try dried leaves as a tea substitute. Fresh plant yields yellow dye and hair rinse to highlight golden tones in gray hair. Leaves now chiefly employed in herbal smoking mixtures and snuffs; in poultices, and also in homeopathic tinctures for diarrhea. Whole plant has aromatic, astringent and blood-purifying properties. Infuse as a sedative and antispasmodic for migraines and indigestion.

Stellaria media
Chickweed
Caryophyllaceae

Description Vigorous creeping annual, from 4–12 inches long. Succulent, oval leaves grow on very straggly, brittle, much branched stems that are hairy on only one side. Small, star-like, white flowers appear from early spring until autumn.
Cultivation Easy to grow in any soil in any position, but prefers moist places. Sow in spring. Self-seeds readily.
Uses Leaves contain vitamin C and phosphorus and are delicious eaten raw in salads or boiled as a vegetable. Fresh leaves in a poultice relieve inflammation and ulcers. Decoct whole plant to treat constipation, piles and sores. Apply in an ointment to heal eczema, psoriasis and other irritating skin diseases.

Taraxacum officinale
Dandelion
Compositae

Description Very common hardy perennial weed. Grows from 2–12 inches high. Long, milky taproot and stem bear oblong, toothed leaves in flat rosettes. Golden flowers appear from spring to midautumn and are followed by globular clusters of tufted seeds.
Cultivation Grows in most soils in open sunny positions. Sow in spring to early autumn. Self-seeds profusely.
Uses Leaves — which are high in vitamins A and C, niacin and various minerals — and roots can be eaten raw in salads. Grind dried and roasted root as a coffee substitute. Root yields a magenta wool dye. Latex in the leaves is a rich emollient for facial steams, cleansing milks and moisturizers for all skins. Add to bathwater as a tonic. Decoct flowers as a cosmetic wash. Root increases bile production and is an effective diuretic; also good for rheumatism, gout, eczema, constipation and insomnia.

Tussilago farfara
Coltsfoot
Compositae

Description Hardy perennial. Reaches from 3–12 inches high with small, white, spreading roots and toothed, dark green leaves with gray undersides; small yellow flowers appear in spring.
Cultivation Grows readily in most soils; can be invasive. Sow in spring. Take root cuttings in spring and autumn. Divide plant in autumn.
Uses Eat fresh leaves in a salad; dried leaves are included in herbal tobaccos. All parts of coltsfoot contain a mucilage, which is good for coughs and bronchitis. Decoct leaves for colds, flu and asthma.

Urtica dioica
Nettle
Urticaceae

Description Perennial with separate male and female plants. Grows up to 4 feet high. Leaves are toothed, pointed and oval; they sting when touched. Bristly, square stems also bear minute, greenish flowers from early summer to early autumn.
Cultivation Grows readily on any soil. Sow in spring. Divide roots in spring.
Uses Young shoots are rich in vitamins and minerals; eat in a salad, boil as a vegetable, or drink as a herbal tea. Use to make nettle beer. Whole plant yields a greenish-yellow wool dye. Nettle fibers spun into rope and made into cloth and paper. Astringent young leaves used in facial steams, bath mixtures and hair preparations. Infuse or decoct herb as a digestive, diuretic and astringent.

Glossary

acid A term applied to soil with a pH content of less than 6.5 and which contains no free lime.

alkaline A term applied to soil with a pH content of more than 7.3. Some herbs actively prefer an acid soil, but most will thrive in alkaline soil.

annual A plant that grows from seed, flowers, and then dies all in one growing season.

astringent A substance that contracts living tissue. An astringent cosmetic preparation tightens the skin.

axil The angle between the upper side of a leaf stalk and its stem.

biennial Taking two growing seasons to complete a life-cycle. A biennial plant produces stems and leaves during the first growing season and flowers and seeds during the second, after which time it dies.

bract A small, modified leaf at the base of a flower.

compress A piece of linen or cloth soaked in a herbal infusion or decoction and applied externally.

cordial A warming and reviving drink. The term is also applied to a medicine that stimulates the heart.

coumarin A compound present in certain plants which, if taken in large amounts, can cause hemorrhage. It gives the plant the smell of new-mown hay after it has been dried.

crown The base of a herbaceous perennial plant from which the roots and shoots grow.

cultivar A cultivated variety of plant, rather than one that occurs naturally in the wild.

cutting A leaf, bud or part of the stem or root removed from a plant to form the basis of a new plant.

deadhead To remove withered flowers, usually to prevent seeding.

deciduous A plant, especially a tree or shrub, that sheds its leaves at the end of the growing season.

decoction A herbal dose obtained by boiling or simmering a certain weight of herb in a certain quantity of liquid for a given length of time. A standard decoction is made with 1 ounce of herb to $2\frac{1}{2}$ cups of water. To make a mild decoction, halve the quantity of herb; for a strong decoction, double the quantity.

distillation The process of separating components of a liquid with different boiling points by heating the liquid until it becomes a vapor, then condensing the vapor and collecting the resulting liquid.

diuretic A substance that promotes the flow of urine.

effleurage A light sweeping stroke used in massage.

emetic A substance that causes vomiting.

emollient A softening substance.

enfleurage The extraction of perfumes from flowers by the use of fats.

evergreen A plant that bears living foliage year round.

expectorant A substance that encourages phlegm to be coughed up from the lungs.

genus A group of closely related plants belonging to the same family.

half hardy May not survive cold frosts. Some half-hardy plants can be grown outdoors only during the summer. Others, particularly some shrubs, will successfully overwinter outdoors in sheltered positions in regions where the climate is mild.

hardy Capable of surviving the winter outdoors without protection.

herbaceous Usually refers to perennial plants whose stems are not woody and which die down at the end of each growing season.

infusion A herbal dose obtained by pouring a certain quantity of boiling liquid over a certain weight of herb and leaving it to steep for a given length of time. For a standard infusion use 1 ounce dried herb to $2\frac{1}{2}$ cups of water. To make a mild infusion, use half the amount of herb; for a strong infusion, use double the amount.

maceration The extraction of a drug from a herb by steeping it in a solvent.

mucilage A gelatinous substance which occurs naturally in some herbs and is used to soothe and treat inflammation of the skin.

mulch A soil covering laid down to protect plant roots, to hold moisture or to control weeds.

narcotic A substance which in small doses deadens pain but in large doses can damage the nervous system and lead to unconsciousness and even death.

nervine A substance or remedy used to treat nervous disorders.

perennial Living from year to year. The stems and leaves of a perennial plant die down in the winter, and new shoots appear each spring. The term is usually applied to herbaceous plants.

pH scale A system devised for measuring the acid-alkaline content of soils. Numbers below 7 denote acidity; higher numbers show alkalinity.

poultice Crushed herb or plant extracts heated and applied to bruised or inflamed skin.

propagate To increase and reproduce plants.

prostrate Growing flat over the surface of the soil.

purgative A strong laxative taken to empty the bowels.

rhizome A horizontally creeping, swollen underground stem that stores food and from which roots and shoots are produced.

rootstock The crown and root system of herbaceous perennials and suckering shrubs. The term is also used to describe a vigorous plant onto which another plant is grafted.

runner A stem that spreads along the soil surface, rooting wherever it comes in contact with moist soil to form a new plant.

salve A soothing ointment.

self-seed A term applied to plants that drop their seed around them, from which new plants will grow, sometimes with poorer and more varied flowers.

shrub A perennial whose branched stems are woody, and which does not grow more than a few feet high.

species A classification applied to a plant or plants within a genus. Grown from seed, species remain consistently true to type.

stamen The male, pollen-bearing part of a flower.

subshrub A low-growing shrub whose base is woody but whose stems are soft.

sucker A shoot which grows up from below ground level.

tincture A solution of extracts of medicinal plants obtained by steeping the plants in alcohol or in a solution of alcohol and water.

topiary The clipping of evergreen trees and shrubs into geometric and fanciful shapes.

tuber A swollen root or underground stem in which food is stored.

umbels A flat-topped mass of small flowerheads on stalks that radiate out from a central point.

variegated A term used to describe leaves that have markings in a secondary color.

variety A term applied originally only to a naturally occurring variation of a species, but now often used also to describe a cultivar.

Useful addresses

When writing to any of the addresses listed below, we suggest you enclose a self-addressed stamped envelope to ensure a reply.

GENERAL SOCIETIES

American Herb Association
Box 353
Rescue, CA 95672
Provides members with current information on herbs. Publishes a newsletter and book service.

The Botanic Medicine Society
Box 103
Norval, Ontario
LOP 1KO
Provides information on herbalism.

Herb Research Foundation
Box 2602
Longmont, CO 80501
Promotes research into the medicinal properties of herbs. Publishes a journal for members.

The Herb Society of America
2 Independence Court
Concord, MA 01742
Provides information on herb suppliers. Membership is by invitation only.

The School of Herbal Medicine
Box 2446
San Rafael, CA 94912
American branch of the National Institute of Medical Herbalists in Great Britain. Offers correspondence courses.

HERB SUPPLIERS

The following selected addresses supply plants, seeds, products and accessories. To find out what they stock, ask for a catalogue. Note that you may have to pay for it. To find a supplier near you, consult the yellow pages under "Herbs."

Alloway Herb Farm
456 Mud College Road
Littlestown, PA 17340

Berkshire Garden Center
Routes 102 and 183
Stockbridge, MA 01262

Brooklyn Botanic Garden
1000 Washington Avenue
Brooklyn, NY 11225

Caprilands Herb Farm
534 Silver Street
Coventry, CT 06238

Casa de Luz Herbs
3568 S. Campbell Avenue
Tucson, AZ 85719

Casa Yerba Gardens
Box 21
Star Route 2
Days Creek, OR 97429

Catnip Acres Farm
67 Christian Street
Oxford, CT 06483

Companion Plants
7247 N. Coolville Ridge Road
Athens, OH 45701

Dionysos' Barn
Box 31
Bodines, PA 17722

Faith Mountain Herbs
Box 199, Main Street
Sperryville, VA 22740

Fox Hill Farm
Box 9, 444 W. Michigan Ave
Parma, MI 49269

Fox Ridge Herbs
4918 Red School Road
Central City, IA 52214

Fragrant Fields
Route 2, Box 199
Dongola, IL 62926

Goodwin Creek Gardens
Box 83
Williams, OR 97544

The Greig Herb Farm
Pitcher Lane
R.D. 3, Box 466
Red Hook, NY 12571

Hancock Shaker Village
P.O. Box 898
Pittsfield, MA 01202

Harmony Herbs, Inc.
527 E. Church Street
New Harmony, IN 47631

The Herb Cottage
Washington Cathedral
Mt. St. Alban
Washington, DC 20016

The Herb Garden
Haynes Road
Deerfield, NH 03037

The Herb Patch
20 Main Street
Concord, MA 01742

Hilltop Herb Farm Inc.
P.O. Box 1734
Cleveland, TX 77327

Meadowbrook Herb Garden
Route 138
Wyoming, RI 02898

Merry Gardens
P.O. Box 595
Camden, ME 04843

Otto Richter & Sons, Ltd.
Box 26
Goodwood, Ontario
Canada, LOC 1AO

Rutland of Kentucky
P.O. Box 182, Jail Street
Washington, KY 41096

Sandy Mush Herb Nursery
Route 2, Surrett Cove Road
Leicester, NC 28748

Shaker Herb Farm
11813 Oxford Road
Harrison, OH 45030

Sinking Springs Herb Farm
234 Blair Shore Road
Elkton, MD 21921

Tansy Farm
5888 Else Road
Agassiz, B. Columbia
Canada VOM 1AO

Taylor's Herb Garden, Inc.
1535 Lone Oak Road
Vista, CA 92083

Triple Oaks Nursery and Florist
Franklinville, NJ 08322

Village Arbors
1804 Saugahatchee Road
Auburn, AL 36830

Well-Sweep Herb Farm
317 Mt. Bethel Road
Port Murray, NJ 07865

Wyrttun Ward
Beach Street RFD,
Middleboro, MA 02346

PRODUCT SUPPLIERS

Aphrodisia Products, Inc.
282 Blecker Street
New York, NY 10014

Aroma Vera Co.
P.O. Box 3609
Culver City, CA 90231
For essential oils.

Caswell-Massey Co. Ltd.
Catalogue Division
111 Eighth Avenue
New York, NY 10011

Haussmann's Pharmacy
534 West Girard Avenue
Philadelphia, PA 19123

Indiana Botanic Gardens, Inc.
P.O. Box 5
Hammond, IN 46325

Nature's Herb Co.
281 Ellis Street
San Francisco, CA 94102

Northwest Handcraft House
110 West Esplanade
N. Vancouver, B. Columbia
Canada V7M 1AE
For dyestuffs.

Penn Herb Co.
603 North Second Street
Philadelphia, PA 19123

Straw into Gold
P.O. Box 2904
Oakland, CA 94618
For dyestuffs.

Weleda Inc.
841 S. Main St.
Spring Valley, NY 10977
For essential oils.

Bibliography

GENERAL

Clarkson, Rosetta E. *The Golden Age of Herbs and Herbals* Dover, New York, 1972
Clarkson, Rosetta E. *Herbs and Savory Seeds* Dover, New York, 1972
Culpeper's Complete Herbal Sterling, New York, 1959
Garland, Sarah *The Herb and Spice Book* Francis Lincoln, London, 1979
Grieve, Mrs. M. *A Modern Herbal* Dover, New York, 1971
Grigson, Geoffrey *The Englishman's Flora* Phoenix House, London, 1959
Grigson, Geoffrey *A Herbal Of All Sorts* Phoenix House, London, 1959
Hall, Dorothy *The Book of Herbs* Charles Scribner's, New York, 1974
Hortus Third: A Concise Dictionary of Plants Cultivated in USA and Canada Macmillan, New York, 1976
Kerik, Joan *Living with the Land: Use of Plants by the Native People of Alberta,* Provincial Museum of Alberta, Canada, 1978
Leyel, Mrs. C. F. *Herbal Delights* Faber & Faber, London, 1987
Lust, John *The Herb Book* Bantam, New York, 1974
Macleod, Dawn *A Book of Herbs* Duckworth, London, 1968
Quelch, Mary Thorne *Herbs and How to Know Them* Faber & Faber, London, 1946
Simmons, Adelma G. *Herb Gardens of Delight* Clinton Press, USA, 1974
Stodola, Jiri and Volak, Jan *The Illustrated Book of Herbs* Octopus, London, 1984
Stuart, Malcom *The Encyclopedia of Herbs and Herbalism* Grosset & Dunlap, New York, 1979
Weiner, Michael A. *Earth Medicine — Earth Foods* Collier Macmillan, New York, 1972

CULINARY

Apicius *The First Century AD Roman Cookery Book* British Book Center, New York, 1974
Boxer, Arabella & Back, Philippa *The Herb Book* Octopus, London, 1980
Clifton, Claire *Edible Flowers* McGraw, New York, 1984
Evelyn, John *Acetaria: A Discourse of Sallet* (1699) Prospect Books, London, 1982
Larkcom, Joy *The Salad Garden,* Viking, New York, 1984
Loewenfeld, Claire & Back, Philippa *The Complete Book of Herbs and Spices* Little, Brown & Co., New York, 1976
Mabey, Richard *Food For Free* Fontana, London, 1975
Rohde, Eleanour Sinclair *Rose Recipes from Olden Times* Dover, New York, 1973
Stobart, Tom *Herbs, Spices and Flavourings* Penguin, New York, 1977

COSMETIC AND HOUSEHOLD

Buchman, Dian Dincin *Feed Your Face* Duckworth, London, 1973
Duff, Gail *A Book of Pot-Pourri* Beaufort Books, New York, 1985
Heriteau, Jaqueline *Potpourris and Other Fragrant Delights* Simon and Schuster, New York, 1975
Little, Kitty *Kitty Little's Book of Herbal Beauty* Penguin, London, 1981
Mabey, Richard *Plants with a Purpose* Collins, London, 1977
Maxwell-Hudson, Clare *The Natural Beauty Book* Macdonald, London, 1983
Palmer, Catherine *Beauty for Free* Jonathan Cape, London, 1981

DYEING WITH HERBS

Dalby, Gill *Natural Dyes, Fast or Fugitive* Ashill Publications, England, 1985
Dye Plants and Dyeing, Brooklyn Botanic Garden, New York, 1964
Goodwin, J. *A Dyer's Manual* Pelham Books, London, 1982
Grae, Ida *Nature's Colors* Collier Books, New York, 1979
Robertson, S. *Dyes from Plants* Van Nostrand Reinhold, New York, 1977
Wickens, H. *Natural Dyes for Spinners & Weavers* Batsford, London, 1983

ESSENTIAL OILS AND AROMATHERAPY

Genders, Roy *Scented Flora of the World* St. Martin's, New York, 1977
Price, Shirley *Practical Aromatherapy* Thorsons, New York, 1983
Stead, Christine *The Power of Holistic Aromatherapy* Javelin, England, 1986
Tisserand, Maggie *Aromatherapy for Women* Thorsons, New York, 1984
Valnet, Dr Jean *The Practice of Aromatherapy* C. W. Daniel, Saffron Walden, 1982

GARDENING

Bacon, Francis *Collected Essays,* Rowman & Littlefield, New York, 1976
Beckett, Kenneth & Gillian *Planting Native Trees and Shrubs* Jarrold, London, 1979
Graham, Dorothy *Chinese Gardens* George Harrap, New York, 1938
Hills, Lawrence *Fertility without Fertilisers* Henry Doubleday Assoc., 1975
Huxley, Anthony *An Illustrated History of Gardening* Paddington Press, New York, 1978
Lamb, Kelley & Bowbrick *Nursery Stock Manual* Grower Books, London, 1975
Philbrick, Helen & Gregg, Richard *Companion Plants and How to Use Them* Stuart & Watkins, London, 1967
Rohde, Eleanour Sinclair *The Scented Garden* Gale, New York, 1974
Stevens, John *The National Trust Book of Wild Flower Gardening* Dorling Kindersley, London, 1987

MEDICINAL

Anderson, Dr Anne *Herbs of Long Ago — Canadian Indians* University of Alberta, Canada, 1982
Binding, G. J. *About Garlic: The Supreme Herbal Remedy* Thorsons, New York, 1976
Ceres *Herbs To Help You Sleep* Thorsons, New York, 1981
Chancellor, Philip *Handbook of the Bach Flower Remedies* Keats, New Canaan, Conn., 1980
Fu Weikang *Traditional Chinese Medicine and Pharmacology* Foreign Languages Press, Beijing, China, 1985
Gerard, John *Gerard's Herbal* (1636) Minerva, London, 1974
Gosling, Nalda *Herbs for Colds and 'Flu* Thorsons, New York, 1976
Griggs, Barbara *The Home Herbal* Jill Norman & Robert Hale, London, 1986
Hoffmann, David *The Holistic Herbal* The Findhorn Press, Scotland, 1986
Hunan Province, China Health Committee *A Barefoot Doctor's Manual* Cloudburst Press, Seattle, 1977
Inglis, Brian *Natural Medicine* Collins, London, 1979
Kaptchuk, Ted J. *The Web That Has No Weaver: Understanding Chinese Medicine* Congdon & Weed, New York, 1983
Marcin, Marietta Marshall *The Complete Book of Herbal Teas* Congdon & Weed, New York, 1983
Palaiseul, Jean *Grandmother's Secrets* G. P. Putnam's Sons, New York, 1974
Parvati, Jeannine *Hygieia: A Woman's Herbal* Freestone, New York, 1979
Sfikas, George *Medicinal Plants of Greece* Efstathiadis Group, Athens, 1981
Smith, William *Herbs to Ease Bronchitis* Thorsons, New York, 1973
Thomson, William *Herbs That Heal* A. & C. Black, London, 1976

OTHERS

de Bairacli Levy, Julietta *Herbal Handbook for Farm and Stable* Faber & Faber, London, 1975
Bohm, David *Wholeness and the Implicate Order* Methuen Inc., New York, 1980
Bremness, Lesley *The Herb Garden: Growing and Using Herbs* Netherfield Herbs, England, 1984
Dyer, T. F. Thiselton *The Folk-Lore of Plants* Appleton, New York, 1889
Graves, Robert *The White Goddess* Hippcrene Books, New York, 1972
Lovelock, J. E. *Gaia, A New Look at Life on Earth* Oxford University Press, 1979
Petulengro, Leon *Herbs and Astrology* Keats, New Canaan, Conn., 1977
Richardson, Maureen *Plant Papers* The Herb Society, London, 1981
Rohde, Eleanour Sinclair *Shakespeare's Wild Flowers, Fairy Lore, Gardens, Herbs, Gatherers of Simples & Bee Lore* Medici, London, 1935
Singleton, Esther *The Shakespeare Garden* Methuen, London, 1923
Tompkins, Peter and Bird, Christopher *The Secret Life of Plants* Avon Books, New York, 1974
Uyldert, Mellie *The Psychic Garden* Thorsons, New York, 1980
Zukav, Gary *The Dancing Wu Li Masters* Bantam Books, New York, 1980

Index

M

N

O

P

Acknowledgments

Author's acknowledgments
I would like to thank Jill Norman for introducing me to Dorling Kindersley, and Daphne Razazan for her committed vision of the book. I am especially indebted to my editor Carolyn Ryden for managing patiently and kindly to refocus my thoughts when I strayed too far from the central theme. My gratitude too to Tina Vaughan for her careful and imaginative art direction, and to Jill Dow for the dedicated accuracy of her garden drawings. Special thanks to photographer Dave King and his assistant Jonathan Buckley who made repeated good-humored trips to our nursery and country lanes to capture each herb at its best.

My thanks to two talented chefs for contributing original recipes: Jan Butcher of Beanfeast and Ruth Bolton of The Chalice Restaurant, Bury St Edmunds. Thanks also to Eileen Clarke for her inspiring recipes and ideas.

I am also grateful to Ann Mulley for her meticulous dye experiments and to Sonia Berrisford-Hobbs for creating such wonderful decorations. Thanks also to Vivienne Boulton for her herbal handicraft experiments, to Joy Larkcom for supplying unusual salad herbs, to Chao Hen of Hangzhou, my guide to gardens and herbs in China, to John Stephen of the Cotswold Perfumery Ltd. for information on perfume ingredients, and to Mary Chipper for her helpful advice on aromatherapy and for keeping Netherfield Herbs going while I was busy researching and writing.

Finally, special thanks to my family who were patient guinea pigs for numerous herbal experiments – eating herbs, drinking herbs and applying herbs in lotions and potions. Extra thanks to my eldest son, Toby Lowe, for literary criticism and keeping the gremlins at bay in my word processor, and most important to my husband J. Roger Lowe for his clarity and strength.

Dorling Kindersley would like to thank Lindy Newton, Clare Mitchison and Barbara Croxford for editorial work; Richard Bird for the index; Audrey Bamber for proofreading; Ann Warren-Davis MNIMH for her constructive comments on the chapter on herbal medicine; Val Baxter for use of her kitchen and garden; Margaret and Geoffrey Ellis and Joy Larkcom for permitting photography in their gardens; Phil Ladd for supplying herbs; Maureen Richardson for supplying herbal papers; Sue Brown; Linda Fraser; Steve Wilson; Henrietta Winthrop; SPAN for their speedy and accurate typesetting.

The following companies provided props for photography: Elizabeth David, 46 Bourne St, London SW1; Philip Poole 'His Nibs', 182 Drury Lane, London WC2; David Mellor, 4 Sloane St, London SW1 (and branches at 26 James St, London WC2; 66 King St, Manchester); Naturally British, 13 New Row, London WC2; Tables Laid, Novello St, London SW6; Josiah Wedgwood & Sons, 32 Wigmore St, London W1.

Illustrators
Jill Dow 19, 20–1, 22, 24, 27, 28, 30–1, 32, 33
Nick Hall 232–3, 234
Lorraine Harrison 17, 19, 20, 26, 31, 150, 163, 194, 212, 228, 238, 251, 252–68, 270

Photographic credits
All photography by Dave King except for:

A-Z Botanical Collection Ltd 141TR
Heather Angel (Biofotos) 18, 25TR
Clive Boursnell 2–3, 6–7, 14–15, 23BL
Lesley Bremness 13, 29, 105TR
Pat Brindley 47TR
Jonathan Buckley jacket flap
Linda Burgess (Botanical Pictures) Endpapers, 1, 10, 23TR, 36–7
Eric Crichton 34, 75TR, 76TR, 89TR, 90TR, 112TR, 119TR
Philip Dowell 46, 47, 118–9, 208–9
Julie Fisher 217, 221
Chao Hen 25B
Monique le Luhandre (Monstyle) 215, 223
Tania Midgley 11
The National Trust 6, 257
Peter Smith 169, 171, 175, 179, 181, 184, 187, 189, 192–3
Jessica Strang 23BR, 35
Michael Warren (Photos Horticultural) 9, 147TR

Key T = top, B = bottom, R = right, L = left